Anatomy and Physiology for Therapists

Jeanine Connor

Venetia Harwood-Pearce

Kathy Morgan

www.heinemann.co.uk
✓ Free online support
✓ Useful weblinks
✓ 24 hour online ordering

01865 888058

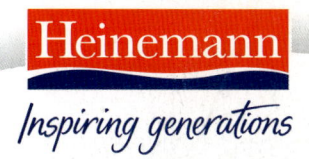

Heinemann
Inspiring generations

Heinemann is an imprint of Pearson Education Limited, a company incorporated in England and wales, having its registered office at Edinburgh Gate, Harlow, Essex, CM20 2JE. Registered company number: 872828

Heinemann is a registered trademark of Pearson Education Limited

Text © Jeanine Connor, Venetia Harwood-Pearce and Kathy Morgan, 2006

First published 2006

10
10 9 8 7 6 5

British Library Cataloguing in Publication Data is available from the British Library on request.

ISBN: 978 0 435449407

Copyright notice
All rights reserved. No part of this publication may be reproduced in any form or by any means (including photocopying or storing it in any medium by electronic means and whether or not transiently or incidentally to some other use of this publication) without the written permission of the copyright owner, except in accordance with the provisions of the Copyright, Designs and Patents Act 1988 or under the terms of a licence issued by the Copyright Licensing Agency, 90 Tottenham Court Road, London W1T 4LP. Applications for the copyright owner's written permission should be addressed to the publisher.

Edited by Caroline Low
Designed by Jackie Hill
Produced by Hardlines

Original illustrations © Harcourt Education Limited, 2006

Illustrated by Hardlines

Cover design by Tony Richardson, Wooden Ark Studios

Printed in China(EPC/05)

Cover photo: © Science Photo Library

Picture research by Chrissie Martin

Index by Indexing Specialists (UK) Ltd

Acknowledgements
I feel as if Anatomy and Physiology for Therapists has been a real team effort, and I would therefore like to acknowledge Venetia and Kathy for their co-authorship and sense of humour, which has made writing this book a most pleasurable experience. It seems we have worked with a larger than normal team of Editors (mostly trying to reduce our vastly over budget word count) who have done a fantastic job of refining and redesigning. I would also like to thank my friends and family for their interest and encouragement, especially Steve and Jo who both ran a very critical eye over my first chapter and offered honest, constructive feedback. And, as always, I would like to thank Pen for her invariable enthusiasm and confidence in my work. This is the book that she and I wanted to publish when we first met in a coffee shop at Paddington Station more than six years ago. As you can see, we got there in the end.

Jeanine Connor

I would like to acknowledge the effort and professionalism of the team who have produced this book; in particular Pen for getting this project off the ground and my co-authors Kathy and Jeanine, whose humour helped enormously in the developmental stages. Thanks also to friends and work colleagues for their support and my husband Harry for his help and encouragement.

Venetia Harwood-Pearce

I am so pleased that the dream of writing an anatomy and physiology book especially for therapists has become a reality at last. I would like to thank my co-authors for all their ideas and inspiration when we planned the project and during the writing. Also, thanks to Pen and her dedicated team at Heinemann. To my children, friends and colleagues who cheered me on and gave me ideas, a big thank you. Lastly thanks to my husband Roger, who helped with proof reading, checking details and providing endless encouragement throughout.

Kathy Morgan

The authors and publisher would like to thank the following individuals and organisations for permission to reproduce photographs:

Corbis p.2, 45; **Getty Images/Photodisc** p.45, 61; **Harcourt Education Ltd/Gareth Boden** p.29, 105, 107, 176; **iStockPhoto** p.5, 28, 57, 81, 121, 146, 181; **Photos.com** p.1, 47; **Science Photo Library** p.36, 44; **Trevor Clifford/Shanon Parker-Bennett** p.74

Every effort has been made to contact copyright holders of material reproduced in this book. Any omissions will be rectified in subsequent printings if notice is given to the publishers.

Tel: 01865 888058   www.heinemann.co.uk

Congratulations!

This is the book that we know therapists have been waiting for! You have just bought the only anatomy and physiology book you will ever need. We are therapists and lecturers who have notched up nearly 50 years experience between us, and students have told us how hard it is to find an anatomy and physiology book that meets their requirements. This is that book! Many of you may have found science a difficult and daunting subject at school; you may even be wondering why you have to learn anatomy and physiology at all. We will show you that the human body is a wonderful piece of equipment and, while we acknowledge that studying it may be difficult, it need not be daunting and it is certainly not boring. You may have a course textbook which includes anatomy and physiology; this book should be used in conjunction with other textbooks to provide an in-depth understanding. To help you with your learning we have supplied you with a selection of diagrams which you can download from www.heinemann.co.uk/anatomy

This book is divided into chapters based on all the systems of the body. In addition, there is an entire section which is called *All about Anatomy and Physiology*: this will help to explain difficult words and phrases.

The features of this book include:
Fascinating facts: these are nuggets of information, not necessarily related to your course, but you will find yourself saying to family and friends 'Did you know that...'
Links to practice: we have placed a great emphasis on linking theory to practice so that at every stage of your study you will know what you need to learn as well as why you need to learn it.
Proving the point: these are activities for you to try either in class or at home.
Links to learning: where relevant, we make connections to other areas of learning to reinforce your knowledge.
Case studies: these give you the opportunity to link theory to practice. The activities are differentiated in order to cater for different levels and qualifications.
Knowledge check: every chapter ends with 20 questions that relate directly to your course.
Illustrations: there are plenty of full-colour, clear illustrations.

Each chapter has sections on Disorders and diseases and The effects of ageing in relation to the system it covers.

Glossary terms are highlighted in colour and their definitions can be found in the back of the book.

We have found writing this book an exciting and rewarding experience – we hope you enjoy reading it and learning from it!

Jeanine Connor
Venetia Harwood-Pearce
Kathy Morgan

Contents

SECTION 1	All about Anatomy and Physiology	1
SECTION 2	Anatomy and Physiology for Therapists	
CHAPTER 1	Cells and Tissues	11
CHAPTER 2	The Skin, Hair and Nails	31
CHAPTER 3	The Skeletal System	47
CHAPTER 4	Muscles and the Muscular System	61
CHAPTER 5	The Blood Circulatory System	77
CHAPTER 6	The Lymphatic System	99
CHAPTER 7	The Respiratory System	111
CHAPTER 8	The Nervous System	121
CHAPTER 9	The Endocrine System	135
CHAPTER 10	The Digestive System	149
CHAPTER 11	The Excretory and Urinary System	167
CHAPTER 12	The Reproductive System	181
GLOSSARY		193
INDEX		198

All about Anatomy and Physiology

SECTION 1

The evolution of the human body

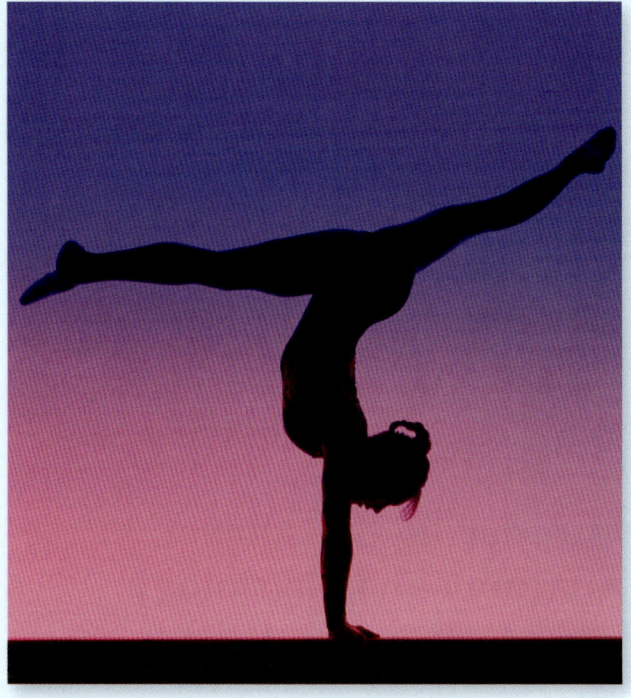

▲ The human body is an amazing machine.

The human body has evolved over millions of years to work effectively and efficiently in the modern world. Primarily, it functions without conscious effort and quite often, we only become aware of different parts of the body when they go wrong. Amazingly, almost every part of the body is continually renewing itself and is self-healing.

Before you begin learning about the science of this amazing machine, this section introduces you to some of the fascinating facts about the human body.

Millions of years ago, humans evolved from their animal ancestors and the human body began to change. Instead of walking on four legs, humans became upright and walked on two legs. This had a number of advantages:

- being upright enabled humans to see and hear things more clearly in their environment
- using the lower limbs only for walking left the upper limbs free to do other things, such as carry tools.

Fascinating fact

A person's eyes are the same size from birth until death.

Link to learning

You probably know a few fascinating facts about the human body already – share these with your peers and perhaps design a poster for the classroom.

You will learn

In this section you will learn about:
- the evolution of the human body
- similarities and individual differences in the human body
- definitions in anatomy and physiology
- common prefixes and suffixes
- levels of biological organisation
- the interdependence of the body's systems
- main biological functions
- anatomical terms and features
- assessing the client.

Similarities and individual differences in the human body

As well as developing differences from their animal ancestors, humans began to develop differences among themselves. For example, people that lived in very hot climates developed dark skins to protect them from the strong ultraviolet rays of the sun, while humans that lived in cooler climates developed paler skins as they required less protection from the sun.

There are many more similarities between humans than there are differences. Even though we are

PAGE 1

SECTION 1

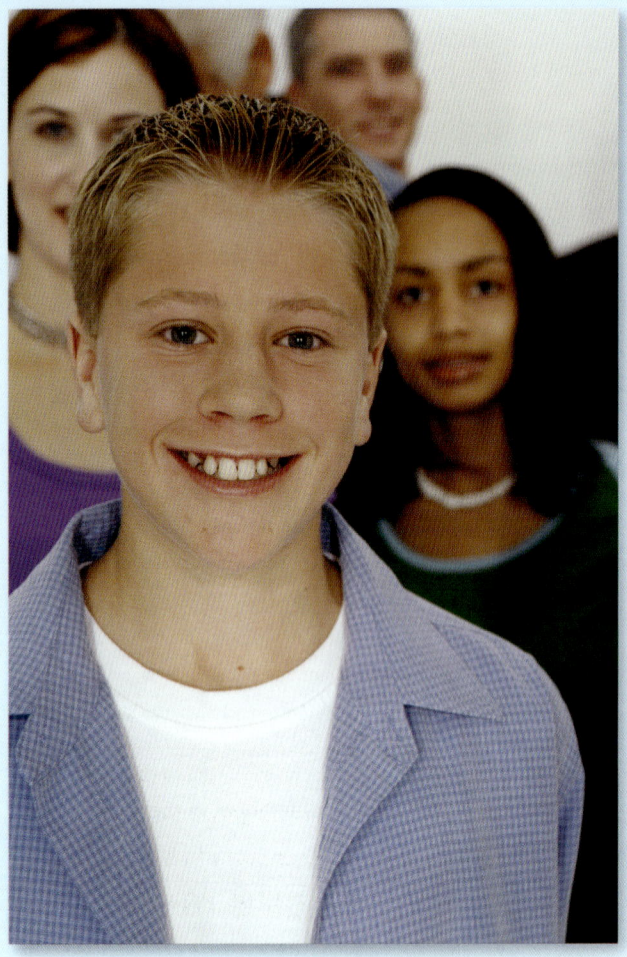

▲ The human body comes in a variety of shapes, sizes and colours.

Proving the point
- Stand with your arms outstretched and ask a partner to measure the distance from the tip of one middle finger to the tip of your other middle finger. This distance should be the same as your height.
- The length of your forearm from elbow to wrist should be the same as the length of your foot. Take off your shoe, rest it on your arm and see for yourself!
- Your body is seven head-lengths tall! Measure the length of your head and multiply this by seven. This should be the same as your height.

Fascinating fact
Some people can roll their tongue lengthways; other people can't and will never be able to learn. It's simply that people are all made a little bit different!

Introducing the subject: Anatomy and Physiology

Before you begin your study of the human body, it is worth considering what, exactly, you will be studying! Words like 'anatomy' and 'physiology' are used quite frequently by teachers and students and in books like these, but they are rarely given any explanation. Do you know what these words mean?

This preliminary section will define some of the key vocabulary you will come across in your studies. As you progress, you will develop a new way to describe the appearance and workings of the human body and its component parts. Many of the words used in science derive from ancient languages such as Latin or Greek and are difficult to pronounce, let alone remember – but don't be put off! There are some common prefixes, which are added to the beginning of words, and common suffixes, which are added to the end of words, which you will come across in several sections of the book as they are used in different systems. For example, the suffix -*cyte* at the end of a word means that word relates

different heights and sizes, we are basically the same shape. There is a good reason for this.

Every part of the human body is designed in a particular way in order to carry out a specific function. The human body consists of a central trunk and head with limbs attached. All of the heavy internal organs are squashed together in the abdomen, yet people carry these around all of their lives without falling over! Internally, human organs are linked together by a network of tubes, like the inside of any machine. This is what is called **human physiology**. Externally, people's bodies are very similar too and are designed in proportion, so that people look like people. This is known as **human anatomy**.

to a type of cell. So, while you might not know what the words *melanocyte*, *osteocyte*, *phagocyte* or *lymphocyte* mean just yet, you now know that they are all types of cell.

▼ Some words need to be explained before they make sense. This diagram illustrates the different types of cells found in blood.

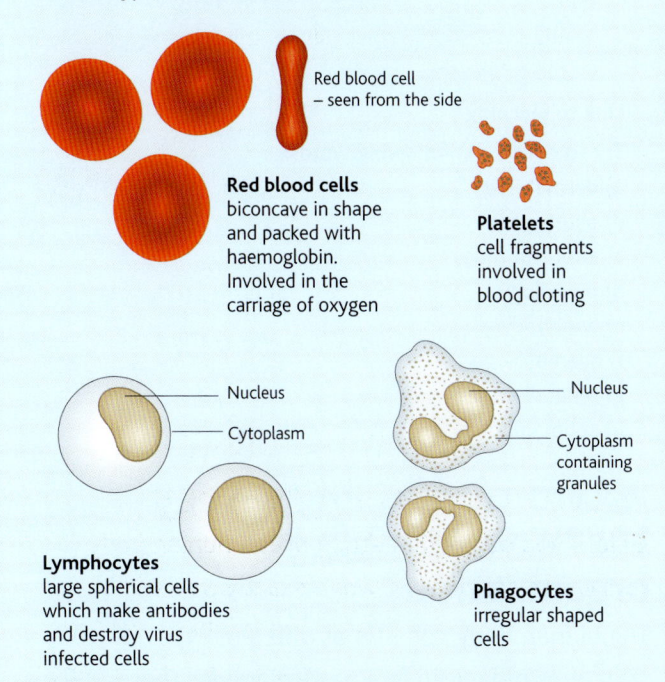

Red blood cell – seen from the side

Red blood cells biconcave in shape and packed with haemoglobin. Involved in the carriage of oxygen

Platelets cell fragments involved in blood cloting

Lymphocytes large spherical cells which make antibodies and destroy virus infected cells
- Nucleus
- Cytoplasm

Phagocytes irregular shaped cells
- Nucleus
- Cytoplasm containing granules

Students often ask why they need to learn all these difficult words borrowed from dead languages and the answer is this: it enables us to have a shared language with which to define, very specifically, the structure and function of the human body. The human body is an intricate piece of equipment. It consists of over 200 bones and more than 600 muscles, as well as cells and tissues, organs and systems, fluids, hormones and enzymes, so it is vital that people learn to speak and understand the same language of the human body.

> **Link to learning**
>
> Use an A–Z address book to make your own Anatomy and Physiology dictionary. Each time you learn a new word you can add it to the book, including a brief definition.

Definitions in anatomy and physiology

Science

Knowledge based on information which can be supported through testing. As our world is always changing, some people choose to think of science as a 'best guess' at a particular time in history and in a particular situation. After all, it is now accepted that the world is round which scientists once thought of as ridiculous!

- The 'natural sciences' explore animals, plants, chemicals and the Earth, and include biology, chemistry and physics.
- The 'social sciences' explore behaviour and interaction in humans and animals and include sociology and psychology.

Biology

The natural science which studies all kinds of living organisms including plants, animals, humans and micro-organisms. People interested in biology usually specialise in one particular area such as human biology.

Anatomy

An aspect of human biology which involves studying the structure of living things. In human anatomy this involves looking at the framework of the body – things like bones, joints and muscles. People interested in human anatomy explore how these structures are formed and how they work.

Physiology

An aspect of human biology which involves studying the function of living things. In human physiology this involves looking at the inside of the body and its system including the circulatory, respiratory, digestive and reproductive systems. People interested in human physiology explore how the systems are structured and how they work.

Common prefixes and suffixes

Prefixes (word beginnings)

Anti-: added to the beginning of a word to show something working against something else, e.g. an *antidepressant* drug may be used to treat the effects of depression, i.e. it works against them.

Derm-: added to the beginning of a word to mean something to do with the skin, e.g. *dermatitis* is a skin disorder.

Erythro-: added to the beginning of a word to define it as red in colour, e.g. an *erythrocyte* is a red blood cell.

Gastro-: added to the beginning of a word to mean it has something to do with digestion, e.g. *gastroenteritis* is a disorder characterised by diarrhoea and vomiting; a fabulous meal might be described as a *gastronomic* feast!

Haem-: added to the beginning of a word to mean it has something to do with blood, e.g. *haemoglobin* is a protein found in blood.

Leuco-: added to the beginning of a word to define it as white in colour, e.g. a *leucocyte* is a white blood cell.

Neur-: added to the beginning of a word to mean it has something to do with nerves, e.g. a *neurone* is a nerve cell.

Ost-: added to the beginning of a word to mean it has something to do with bone, e.g. *osteoporosis* is a bone disorder usually associated with ageing.

Peri-: added to the beginning of a word to mean it is located around another structure, e.g. the *pericardium* is a membranous sac which is located around the heart.

Phago-: added to the beginning of a word to mean it engulfs another organism, e.g. a *phagocyte* is a type of blood cell which engulfs bacteria and debris.

Renal: added to the beginning of a word to mean it has something to do with the kidneys, e.g. the *renal cortex* is the outer layer of the kidney.

Sub-: added to the beginning of a word to illustrate that its location is below another structure, e.g. the *subclavian vein* is located below the clavicle.

Supra-: added to the beginning of a word to illustrate that its location is above another structure, e.g. *suprarenal glands* is an alternative name for the adrenal glands as they are situated above the kidneys.

Suffixes (word endings)

-cyte: added to the end of a word to mean a type of cell, e.g. *leucocyte* and *erythrocyte* are blood cells.

-itis: added to the end of a word to mean a disorder of a structure e.g. *tonsillitis* is inflammation of the tonsils

-ology: added to the end of a word to mean the study or knowledge of a particular area of interest, e.g. *myology* is the study of muscles.

Link to learning

Try to define the following words:
a) dermatology
b) osteocyte
c) antihistamine
d) neurology
e) lymphocyte
f) haematology
g) renal disease
h) submandibular

Levels of biological organisation

The human body consists of different types of structures organised in a particular way. These structures all work together to maintain healthy functioning. From tiny cells to large organs, each structure has a special job to do and relies on another structure to support its function. This is what is meant by the term 'holistic' – working together as a whole. The arrangement of structures, from small to large, is called biological organisation.

Cell	Smallest biological structure which is able to exist independently
Tissue	Groups of cells with a shared structure and function
Organ	Specialised structure which consists of different types of tissues organised in a specific way
System	Group of organs which work together
Organism	The whole being – human, animal or plant

All about Anatomy and Physiology

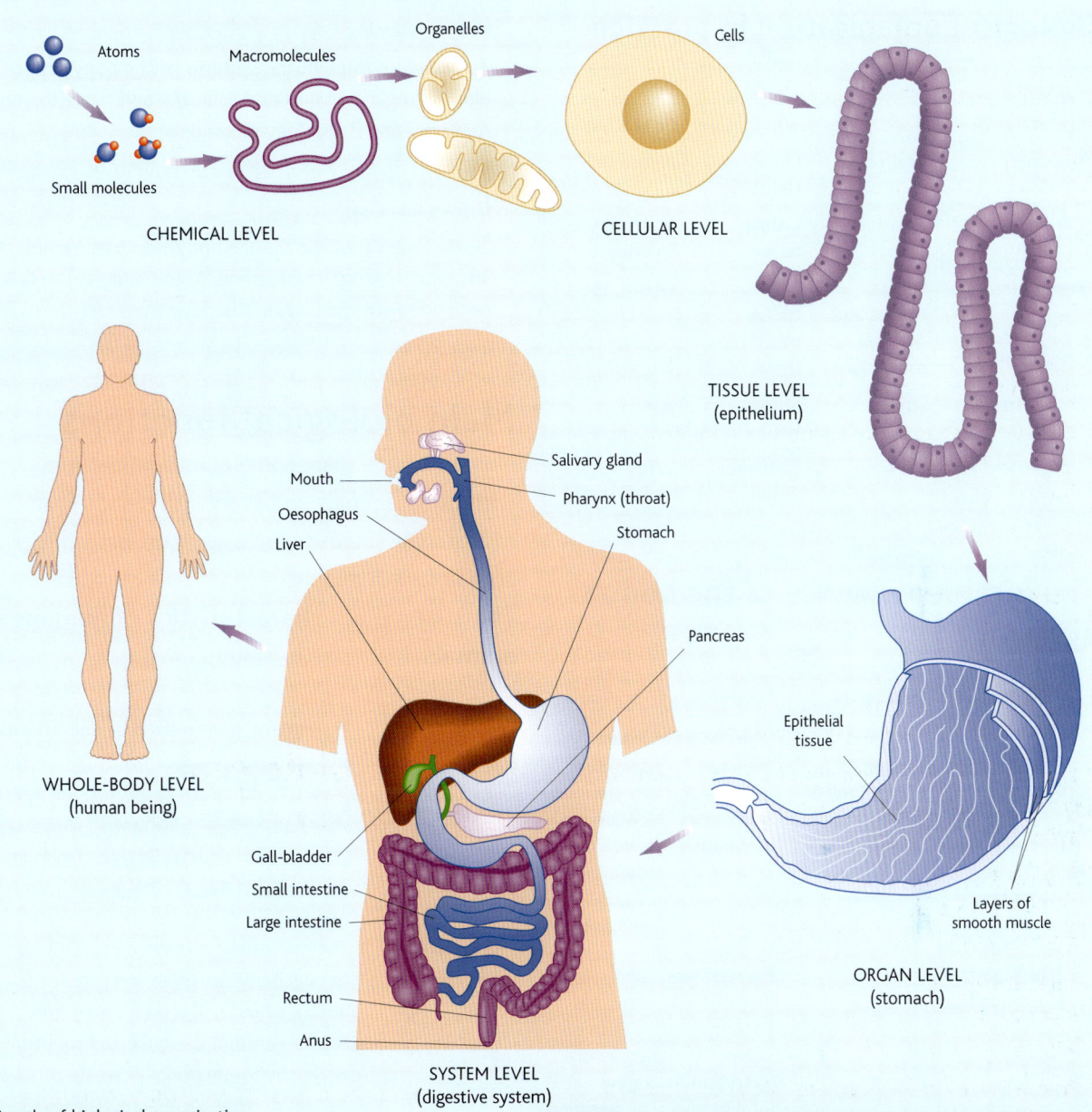

Levels of biological organisation

CHEMICAL LEVEL
- Atoms
- Small molecules
- Macromolecules

CELLULAR LEVEL
- Organelles
- Cells

TISSUE LEVEL (epithelium)

ORGAN LEVEL (stomach)
- Epithelial tissue
- Layers of smooth muscle

SYSTEM LEVEL (digestive system)
- Mouth
- Salivary gland
- Oesophagus
- Pharynx (throat)
- Stomach
- Liver
- Pancreas
- Gall-bladder
- Small intestine
- Large intestine
- Rectum
- Anus

WHOLE-BODY LEVEL (human being)

Fascinating fact
Cells are so small that the finger of a newborn baby contains about 10 billion individual cells.

Fascinating fact
The largest human cell is the female egg (ovum) and the smallest human cell is the male sperm.

▶ A human ovum and sperm

PAGE 5

SECTION 1

Biological organisation in practice

System	Organ	Tissue	Cell
Skeletal	Bone	Bone tissue	Osteocyte
Nervous	Brain	Nervous tissue	Neurone
Cardiovascular	Heart	Cardiac tissue	Erythrocyte, leucocyte
Reproductive	Female uterus and ovaries: male testes	Epithelial tissue, muscle tissue	Ovum, sperm
Respiratory	Lungs	Muscle tissue	
Integumentary	Skin	Epithelial tissue	Keratinocyte, melanocyte

The interdependence of the body's systems

	Circulatory	Digestive	Nervous	Endocrine
Circulatory		Glucose obtained from food is transported in the blood	Sympathetic nervous activity stimulates circulation	Insulin secreted by the endocrine system maintains blood glucose
Digestive	The digestive system has a rich blood supply		Sympathetic nervous activity slows secretion of digestive juices	The pancreas is both an accessory organ of digestion and an endocrine organ
Nervous	Parasympathetic nervous activity slows circulation	Parasympathetic nervous activity stimulates digestion		Both systems are involved in the co-ordination of the body
Endocrine	Hormones are transported in blood	Glucose from food is regulated by insulin	Both systems maintain homeostasis	

Link to learning

As you work through the systems of the body, try to identify organs, tissues and cells and add these to your Anatomy and Physiology dictionary.

Link to learning

Never forget that the human body works as a whole. As you work through the systems of the body, try to link each one with the body's other systems.

Main biological functions

Human beings share some common features with other animals and even with plants. Even microscopic single-celled organisms have things in common with people.

The seven main characteristics of humans and animals

Movement: Movement is permitted by the actions of voluntary muscles which act on the skeleton. Bones and joints act as levers which provide the body with mobility. (Link to The Skeletal System, page 54 and Muscles and the Muscular System, page 63)

Respiration: The process of respiration facilitates the exchange of gases in each of the body's cells. Oxygen is inhaled from the air through the nose and mouth while the by-product (or waste product) carbon dioxide is exhaled. (Link to The Respiratory System, page 115)

Sensation: The ability to sense changes in the external environment is an important function as it makes us aware of our surroundings and helps us to recognise potential harm. The body picks up signals via the five senses of sight, smell, taste, hearing and touch. (Link to The Nervous System, page 128)

Growth: People start to grow and develop from the moment of conception. Some parts of the human body, such as the skeleton, continue to grow into adulthood

All about Anatomy and Physiology

while others, such as the eyes, remain the same size from birth. (Link to development and ageing in all chapters)

Reproduction: Animal species reproduce sexually to ensure that the species grows and continues. Reproduction occurs when one male sperm and one female ovum become fused together during the process of fertilisation. (Link to The Reproductive System, page 186)

Excretion: Chemical processes in the body create waste products which would cause harm if they were not eliminated. The process of excretion rids the body of waste substances including sweat, urine and faeces. (Link to The Digestive System, page 156 and The Excretory and Urinary Systems, page 173)

Nutrition: Living organisms require nourishment in order to survive and develop. Humans require seven different nutrients which are obtained from a balanced diet. These are carbohydrates, proteins, fats, fibre, vitamins, minerals and water. (Link to The Digestive System, page 189)

> **Link to learning**
>
> The seven main characteristics of living things can be remembered by using the mnemonic M-R-S-G-R-E-N (MRS GREN).

Anatomical terms and features

Anatomical terms and features enable us to be exact when describing particular areas of the human body or specific structures within it. This is necessary, for example, when identifying specific locations on a bone for the attachment of muscles, or when locating the site of an injury in a client's medical history and understanding its nature. In this way, anatomical terms and features add to our vocabulary and enable us to communicate effectively.

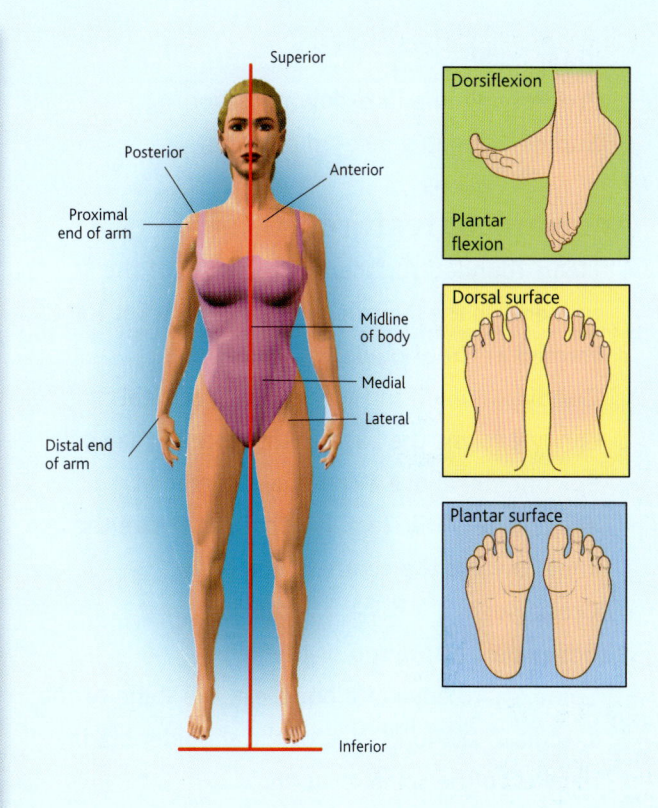

▲ Anatomical positions.

Anatomical terms

- **Aspect**: relates to the particular view of the body, e.g. anterior aspect (front view)
- **Anterior**: front of the body
- **Posterior**: back of the body
- **Medial**: nearest to or towards the midline of the body, e.g. medial rotation of leg (rotation towards the body)
- **Lateral**: sides of the body
- **Proximal**: nearest to the point of attachment of a limb
- **Distal**: furthest away from the point of attachment of a limb
- **Superior**: a structure which is above another or higher in the body, e.g. the superior vena cava is a vessel which returns blood to the heart from the upper body
- **Inferior**: a structure which is below another or lower in the body, e.g. the inferior vena cava is a vessel which returns blood to the heart from the

lower body
- **Prone**: lying in a face-down position
- **Supine**: lying in a face-up position

Anatomical features
- **Head**: rounded surface, e.g. the head of the humerus is the 'ball' of the ball and socket joint formed at the shoulder.
- **Condyle**: curved surface, e.g. the occipital condyle forms the base of the back of the skull.
- **Epicondyle**: above a condyle, e.g. medial epicondyle of the femur is the area above the knee towards the centre of the body.
- **Crest**: ridge of a bone, e.g. the iliac crest is the ridged part at the top of the pelvis.
- **Spine**: sharp edge of a bone, e.g. the spine of the scapula is the long edge of the shoulder blade parallel to the spinal column.
- **Tuberosity**: large rounded bump on a bone, e.g. the greater tuberosity of the humerus is the 'ball' at the top of the arm which forms the shoulder joint.
- **Foramen**: hole in a structure to allow nerves and vessels to pass through, e.g. the infra-orbital foramen is the hole below the eye socket in the cheek bone.
- **Sinus**: space filled with air, e.g. nasal sinuses.
- **Greater**: if there are two structures sharing the same name, this relates to the largest, e.g. the greater trochanter is the larger prominence at the head of the femur.
- **Lesser**: if there are two structures sharing the same name, this relates to the smallest, e.g. the lesser trochanter is the smaller prominence at the head of femur.

Movement at joints
Joints permit particular movements according to their structure and location. These can be specifically defined using the following terms:

Anatomical term	Definition	Illustration
Flexion	Reducing the angle between two bones at a joint	
Extension	Increasing the angle between two bones at a joint	
Abduction	Moving away from the midline of the body	
Adduction	Moving towards the midline of the body	
Rotation	Moving a body part on its axis	
Circumduction	Moving a body part round in a circle	
Supination	Outward rotation away from the body.	
Pronation	Inward rotation towards the body	
Inversion	Turning a body part inwards to the body	
Eversion	Turning a body part outwards away from the body	
Elevation	Lifting a body part	
Depression	Lowering a body part	

Link to learning
Try to locate the following anatomical features on the diagrams below:

a) Spine of scapula	▶ Anterior view of scapula
b) Vertebral foramen	▶ Superior view of single vertebra
c) Medial aspect of femur	▶ Anterior view of left femur
d) Iliac crest	▶ Anterior view of pelvis
e) Lateral arch	▶ Lateral view of foot

Assessing the client

An important aspect of the therapist's job is to assess the client's suitability for treatment and make suggestions and recommendations. With practice, you will learn to observe the physical, physiological and psychological characteristics of your clients during the preliminary consultation. You will also need to consider the benefits of treatment across these three categories and their effect on health, ageing, healing and success of treatment.

- **Physical**: relating to the body's features, either normal or abnormal. For example, an assessment of the client's skin may reveal indications for treatment such as cellulite or comedones, or contra-indications such as ringworm.
- **Physiological**: relating to the body's functions, either normal or abnormal, such as the systems of the body. For example, a preliminary consultation could highlight possible physiological contra-indications such as high blood pressure or diabetes.
- **Psychological**: relating to mental states and processes, either normal or abnormal. For example, a preliminary meeting with a client will help you to make an informed decision about his or her psychological well-being and may highlight concerns such as anxiety, stress, emotional confusion or depression.

Proving the point
Imagine that you are about to take your driving test or sit an exam. Think about the physical, physiological and psychological changes that would be occurring in your body and mind at that time. Share your ideas with others.

- **Health**: state of mental and/or physical well-being which is assessed in the preliminary consultation. Any signs of ill health such as diseases, disorders or medications may have implications for treatment.
- **Ageing**: natural process which occurs in all living organisms and involves the gradual slowing down and deterioration of cells and structures. Many of your clients may be concerned about the physical signs of ageing, such as lines and wrinkles, or the physiological effects, such as the menopause. It is part of the therapist's job to understand the physical, physiological and psychological implications of ageing in both genders.
- **Disorder**: abnormality of the body or mind

which is undesirable but usually non-contagious, such as scarring, dandruff or forgetfulness. Disorders are not usually contra-indications and may benefit from holistic or beauty therapy treatment. They may also require referral for other kinds of treatment.

- **Disease**: abnormality of the body which can be caused by a viral, fungal or bacterial infection, such as measles, athlete's foot or meningitis. Diseases are often contagious and are therefore a contra-indication to treatment and should be referred to a medical professional. Disease-causing micro-organisms can be eliminated by maintaining high standards of hygiene.
- **Contra-indication**: a condition which prevents treatment, usually for one of the following reasons.
  – It could cause harm to the client or the therapist. For example, an infectious skin disorder such as ringworm could be spread to a different area of the body or passed to the therapist.
  – It could be made worse by the treatment. For example, any area of broken skin, such as a cut, scratch or recent scar tissue, should be avoided as treatment could hinder the natural healing process.
  – It could cause discomfort to the client. For example, a bruise in an area where pressure would be applied, perhaps during massage treatment, should be avoided.
  Clients with suspected contra-indications should be treated sensitively and referred to their GP.
- **Contra-action**: undesirable though not uncommon condition which occurs following treatment, such as skin redness or sensitivity. Clients should be advised if contra-actions are likely to occur and should be given appropriate advice on dealing with them.
- **Indication**: condition which presents as a reason for treatment; for example, superfluous hair growth is an indication for depilation or epilation treatment.

> **Link to practice**
> Remember – it is not your job to diagnose a condition.

Your adventure has begun...

People study human anatomy and physiology for many different reasons but, as holistic and/or beauty therapists, you may have a few things in common as you come to the end of this introductory section. You may be feeling nervous as you embark on this difficult new subject. You may also be feeling excited by what you have heard from others who have experienced this subject before you and by the fascinating things you have read so far. You have taken the first important steps to success by reading this section and recognising the unfamiliar but ancient language of anatomy and physiology. And even though you are still a relative newcomer to the subject, you have learnt many things already which will help you as you continue through your studies.

> **Knowledge check**
> 1. Explain the meaning of anatomy.
> 2. Explain the meaning of physiology.
> 3. Name the levels of biological organisation.
> 4. List the seven characteristics which are shared by all living things (MRS GREN).
> 5. Give a definition of contra-indication.
> 6. What name is given to a reaction which occurs following treatment?
> 7. Give a brief definition of physical, physiological and psychological.
> 8. How should you react if a client presents a possible contra-indication to treatment during the consultation?
> 9. What would you do if you suspected that your client had chickenpox?
> 10. Why is it important to ascertain a client's mental and physical health prior to treatment?

SECTION 2

CHAPTER 1 Cells and Tissues

Fascinating fact

There are 26 billion cells in a newborn baby and 50 trillion cells in an adult.

Link to practice

It is really important that, as a therapist, you understand the structure and function of cells and the subsequent tissues they become. This is because all the activities which take place in the body are a direct result of what happens within cells. Understanding bodily functions at a cellular level will also help you to understand the functions of the body's organs and systems. This will enable you to understand why disease occurs and how you can help clients to maintain health.

The smallest living unit in the human body is the **cell**, and it is the basic building block of the human body. The body is composed of trillions of cells and although they all have a similar structure, they may have different jobs, functions and special qualities. When cells of the same type combine together they form **tissues**. Tissues form **organs** and also line the inside and outside of the body. Organs are part of **body** systems. Body systems allow the human body to function, exist and maintain life (see also page 193).

If you imagine a house, it requires the following: basic materials to build it (foundations, bricks, cement and timber); pipes, plumbing and electricity to allow it to function effectively; insulation for warmth; paintwork to protect surfaces; flooring for comfort; telephones and intercoms to communicate with the outside world; locks, alarms and smoke detectors, for safety. Similarly, the human body requires:

- a basic framework – the skeleton
- **connective tissues** to hold things together and provide insulation
- a **nervous system** to co-ordinate everything
- a **digestive system** to provide energy and warmth
- a **blood circulatory** system to pipe blood around the body
- a **urinary system** to remove waste products from the body
- tissues to line the interior and the exterior
- an **immune system** to protect the body from invaders
- a **respiratory system** to ventilate the body.

You will learn

In this chapter you will learn about:
- the structure and properties of cells
- cell metabolism and nutrition
- the basic principles of homeostasis
- types and functions of epithelial tissue
- types and functions of connective tissue
- types and functions of bone tissue
- types and functions of muscle tissue
- types and functions of membranes
- disorders and diseases of cells and tissues
- cells and tissues and the ageing process.

The structure and properties of cells

- **Cell membrane:** this encloses the cell and allows substances to pass in and out of it.
- **Cytoplasm:** this is a gel-like substance which fills the cell from the membrane to the nucleus. It is composed of about 80 per cent water, contains mini-organs and helps keep the cell contents in place.
- **Nucleus:** this is a membrane-bound structure that contains the cell's

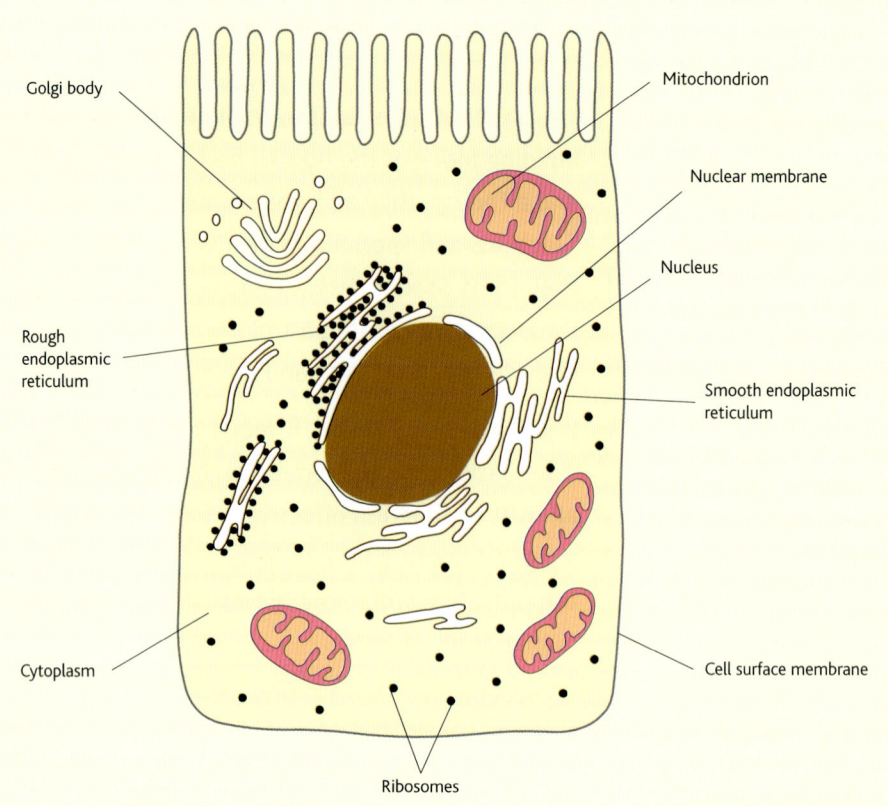

The structure of a human cell

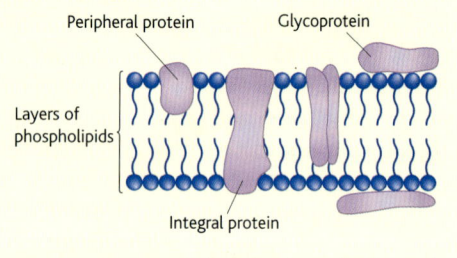

The structure of cell membrane

genetic information (**DNA**) and controls the cell's growth and reproduction.

— The nucleus is encased by a double membrane called the nuclear envelope. This membrane separates the contents of the nucleus from the **cytoplasm**. The envelope helps to maintain the shape of the nucleus.

— The nucleus also contains nucleolus.

- Nucleolus: this produces proteins called ribosomes, which allow **RNA** to translate the genetic code into proteins.

- Organelles are mini-organs which are situated inside the cell, in the cytoplasm. They can be thought of as miniature factories for the body.

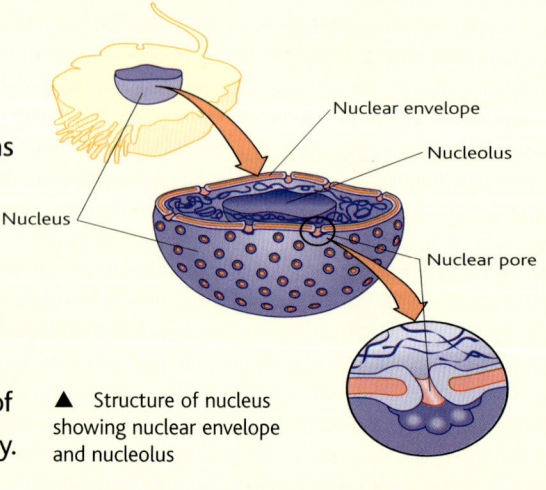

Structure of nucleus showing nuclear envelope and nucleolus

DNA (deoxyribonucleic acid)

DNA provides the genetic blueprint for the physical characteristics of all living organisms. It is arranged in long, spiralling molecules and organises the cell's daily operations. When made up of two strands, the strands intertwine like a spiral staircase to form a structure called a double helix. Subunits, called bases, form the rungs of the 'staircase'.

CHAPTER 1 Cells and Tissues

There are several different types of organelle:
– *Mitochondria*: these organelles are responsible for producing energy and cellular respiration.
– *Golgi body/apparatus*: an organelle present in cells that functions as a collection and/or packaging centre for substances, especially protein, that the cell manufactures for transport.

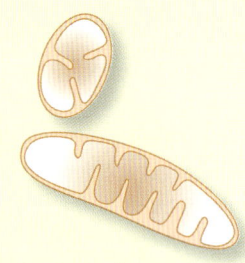

▲ Structure of organelles

Fascinating fact
DNA can be thought of as one big anatomy and physiology book, with each rung of the spiral staircase one chapter in the book! The entire chemical code for each person is over 3 billion letters long so the book would be 169 metres high.

Link to learning
When body cells are irritated, no matter where they are found in the body, they are likely to become inflamed. Inflammation is defined as the body part being red, hot, raised and sore. The inflammation occurs because of an external stimulus, over-stimulation or infection within the body.
To describe a body part which is inflamed, the suffix *-itis* is added to the name of the body part. For example, tonsillitis is inflammation of the tonsils and dermatitis is inflammation of the skin. Can you think of more examples?

The properties of cells
All cells show characteristics of life:
- Activity: movement takes place within the cell and some cells can move externally, e.g. muscle cells.
- Respiration: substances pass in and out through the cell membrane.
- **Metabolism**: cells utilise energy from food and produce waste products.
- Excretion: waste is excreted via the cell membrane.
- Growth: cells grow to a pre-determined size and then divide.
- Reproduction: known as mitosis, cells divide and produce 'daughter' cells.
- **Irritability**: cells have the ability to respond to an external stimulus – physical, chemical or thermal.

Link to learning
If you imagine a cell as a 'mini-you', it can be easier to understand how the cell is structured and how it functions.
- You have an outer covering of skin for protection (equivalent to the cell membrane).
- Your body contains various organs – the stomach and heart, for example (in the cell, these are the organelles).
- You are made up of approximately 60 per cent water and have mechanisms to hold the organs in place (a similar function to cell cytoplasm).
- You function in the same way as a cell:
  – you produce energy from the food that you eat (metabolism and respiration)
  – you are able to get rid of waste products (excretion)
  – you can move externally and things are able to move inside you, such as blood (movement)
  – you have the ability for growth and repair (growth)
  – you are able to respond to external stimulus (irritability)
  – you have the potential to produce offspring (reproduction).

Cell metabolism and nutrition
The continued life of the cell is only possible due to the cell membrane. Substances which are essential for the maintenance and development of the cell (for example, **oxygen**, water and nutrients) pass through the cell membrane. The cell utilise these products in two ways:

PAGE 13

> **Link to learning**
>
> If skin cells are constantly rubbed, or excessive heat is applied, or acid is accidentally dropped onto the skin, how does the skin react?

- **Catabolism** – this is when the useful products, such as nutrients, are broken down into useable units.
- **Anabolism** – this is when the units are used by the cell to build, repair and produce energy so that the cell can sustain its life cycle. As a result of anabolism, waste products are produced and these pass out of the cell via the cell membrane.

Homeostasis

A cell works best when the environment inside it remains constant. The term **homeostasis** describes the state of being the same. If this balance is not maintained, the body's cells cannot function effectively and the body falls ill. Examples of homeostasis are:

- the regulation of body temperature (mainly a skin function)
- the regulation of the quantity of water and minerals in the body. This is known as **osmoregulation** and it occurs in the kidneys
- the removal of waste products from metabolism. This is known as **excretion** and is carried out by organs such as the kidneys and lungs
- the regulation of **blood glucose**. This is mainly regulated by the **hormone** insulin, which is secreted by the pancreas, and the liver.

> **Proving the point**
>
> Where might you have heard about anabolism before? Anabolic steroids are a type of drug – what do they do and who would take them?

> **Link to practice**
>
> Although 37°C (98.6°F) is recognised as being normal body temperature, several studies have shown that this may vary from 36.1–37.8°C (96.9–100.0°F). Where the thermometer is placed in the body has an effect:
> - In the mouth, normal core body temperature registers at 37°C (98.6°F).
> - The axillary (underarm) area and the ear are the least accurate, typically registering 36.4°C (97.5°F).
> - The rectum is the most accurate at 37.6°C (99.7°F), but is probably not the most comfortable place to take a reading!

> **Fascinating fact**
>
> The rate at which a body metabolises nutrients varies slightly from person to person. If someone has a fast metabolism they expend energy more quickly. A person with a slower metabolism will store more energy and therefore tend to put on weight. (Link to The Digestive System, page 149)

Homeostasis is an important to survival because it means that people can adapt to live in different environments. For example, homeostasis enables a person's body temperature to remain constant whether living in a hot climate or a very cold one. The processes and activities that help to maintain homeostasis are termed **homeostatic** mechanisms. In addition to the body temperature regulation, other examples of homeostasis are:

- the control of sugar levels in the blood (Link to The Endocrine System, page 135)
- the maintenance of water balance in the body. (Link to The Endocrine System, page 137 and Excretory, and Urinary Systems, page 168)

Although the body will attempt to maintain a constant internal state, this

CHAPTER 1 Cells and Tissues

> **Fascinating fact**
> The human body must maintain a temperature of close to 37°C (98.6°F). If body temperature falls below 30°C (86°F) or rises above 41°C (105.8°F), immediate medical attention is essential to avoid death.

is only possible within reasonable limits. When the body is put into extreme conditions, for example, severe cold leading to hypothermia, the mechanism which controls homeostasis can fail. If this occurs, death can result unless medical care is forthcoming to help resume normality.

> **Link to practice**
> Understanding homeostasis in the body is important in a number of ways when treating clients, particulary if the client is on a weight-loss programme. For example, homeostasis enables you to understand why drinking the correct amount of fluid is important when dieting:
> - Excessive water intake can affect the salt balance in the body and lead to conditions which may cause seizure and coma.
> - Insufficient water intake can cause dehydration.
>
> You can therefore advise clients on why drinking a recommended intake of water is important whilst dieting.

Homeostasis and the pH scale

The **pH** scale measures **acidity** and **alkalinity** (pH stands for percentage of Hydrogen). The scale ranges from 0 (strongly acidic) to 14.0 (strongly alkaline), with 7.0 as neutral (neither acidic or alkaline). The pH scale is used to test all sorts of cosmetic, household and industrial products, and is particularly relevant to therapists for:

- ensuring that beauty products used are compatible with the pH of the skin
- maximising the correct skin conditions to repel bacteria.

Body fluids need to be maintained at a pH of 7.4 (very slightly alkaline). This is controlled by several systems acting together:

- Buffer systems: buffers are substances which prevent sharp changes in the concentration of hydrogen ions. They include bicarbonates, phosphates and proteins such as haemoglobin.
- Kidney function: the kidneys are responsible for reabsorbing or excreting

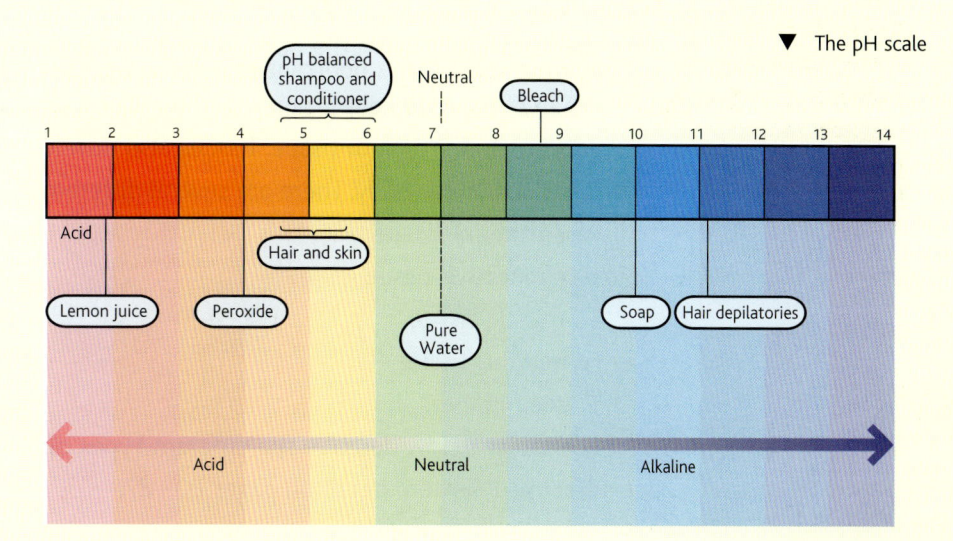

> **Link to learning**
> It will be necessary to reconsider homeostasis throughout your learning of physiology as it will arise in other chapters.

▼ The pH scale

PAGE 15

SECTION 2

> **Link to practice**
> To test pH, you can use **litmus paper** to test the pH of salon products and products belonging to your clients. Clients may be quite surprised to find that certain cosmetic preparations (particularly perfume) have the same pH as some bathroom cleaners! Also, soap tends to be more strongly alkaline (than skin).

hydrogen ions as required. This controls the pH of body fluids over the long-term.

- Respiration: the rate of respiration adjusts pH in the short-term. Releasing carbon dioxide makes the blood more alkaline.

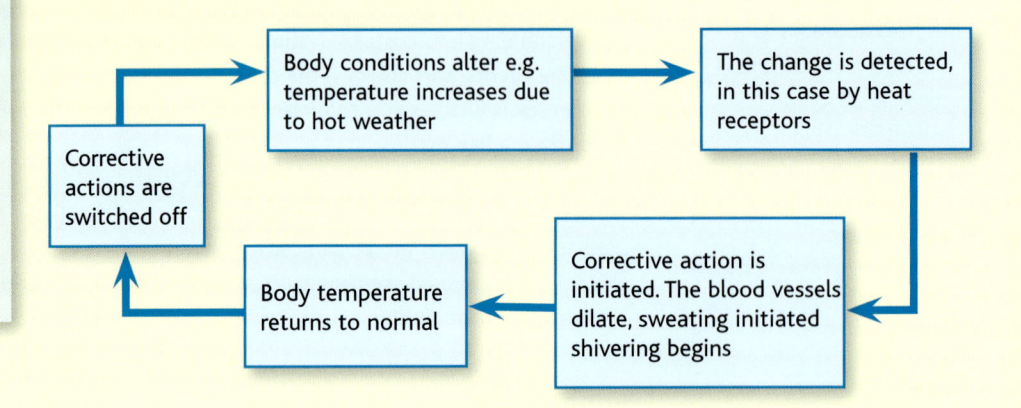

```
Body conditions alter e.g. → The change is detected,
temperature increases due    in this case by heat
to hot weather               receptors
       ↑                            ↓
Corrective                   Corrective action is
actions are                  initiated. The blood vessels
switched off                 dilate, sweating initiated
       ↑                     shivering begins
       ← Body temperature  ←
         returns to normal
```

▲ An example of homeostatic temperature regulation.

> **Link to practice**
> Certain diets that require you to eat more or less of a particualr nutrient, i.e. low carbohydrate or high protein diets, can cause changes in the pH of body fluids. This can lead to physical changes such as higher **cholesterol levels**, decreased minerals and potential damage to the liver and kidneys. With an understanding of homeostasis and the pH scale, you are in a better position to advise clients why eating a balanced diet is a healthier way to lose weight.

Tissues of the body

Every cell carries a 'blueprint' inside its nucleus, which determines what kind of cell it will be. This means that each cell becomes **specialised** to carry out a particular function in the body. This specialisation is known as **differentiation**.

When specialised cells group together, they form tissues – the type of cell will determine the type of tissue. Tissues also develop in order to carry out specific functions in the body. There are several different types of tissue. These include:

- **epithelial tissue**
- connective tissue
- muscle tissue
- nervous tissue
- membranes.

The tables below describe the different types of tissues, which are then described in more detail on pages 20–27.

Epithelial tissue

Function	Type	Structure	Illustration
Lining and covering	Simple	Single row of cells	Simple epithelial cells
	Stratified	Several layers of cells	Stratified epithelial cells (Squamous cells, Basement membrane, Columnar basal cells)
Glands	Exocrine glands	Ducts carry the secretions from the gland, e.g. sebaceous glands	Exocrine gland (Tubular, Duct)
	Endocrine glands	Do not have ducts but secrete the substance directly into the blood supply, e.g. the hormone thyroxine from the thyroid gland.	Endocrine gland (thyroid gland)

Connective tissue

Function	Type	Structure	Illustration
Joins other tissues together	Loose (areolar) connective tissue	Collagen and elastin fibres	Elastic fibre; Connective tissue cell; Fat cells; Collagenous fibres — *Loose connective tissue*
	Adipose (fatty) tissue	Fat filled cells	Collagenous fibres; Elastic fibres; Fat cells — *Fatty or adipose tissue*
	Fibrous (dense connective) tissue: • collagen fibres • reticular fibres • elastic fibres.	Very strong fibres; tendons and ligaments	Fibroblast nuclei; Collagen bundles — *Fibrous connective tissue (tendon)*
	Cartilage: • hyaline • fibrocartilage • elastic	Fibrous and hard connective tissue	Pure cartilage; Cartilage cell — *Cartilage*
	Bone: • compact • cancellous	Collagen impregnated with minerals, mostly calcium	Channel (for nerves and blood vessels); Bone cells — *Cancellous bone*
	Blood	Corpuscles and plasma	Red blood cell – seen from the side; Red blood cells; Platelets; Lymphocytes (Nucleus, Cytoplasm); Phagocytes (Nucleus, Cytoplasm containing granules) — *Blood*

Muscle tissue

Function	Type	Structure	Illustration
Contracts and can produce movement	Skeletal	Striped or striated fibre	Skeletal muscle.
	Smooth	Smooth fibres	Smooth muscle.
	Cardiac	The heart muscle	Cardiac muscle.

Nervous tissue

Function	Type	Structure	Illustration
Receives stimuli and conveys impulses	The brain, spinal cord and nerves		Neuron (nerve cell)

Membranes

Function	Type	Structure
Covering, lining, dividing, anchoring	Serous	Lines body cavities and outer layer of organs
	Mucous	Lines tubes which lead to the outside of the body; secretes mucus
	Cutaneous	The skin; consists of an outer layer of epithelium
	Synovial – a connective tissue membrane	Lines the joint cavity; produces synovial fluid to allow for ease of movement

Epithelial tissue

Epithelial tissue (or epithelium) is a **lining** tissue which lines and protects areas and organs of the body, such as the skin, the respiratory tract, the inside of blood vessels and the body's cavities, to provide smooth surfaces. Epithelium is also the tissue which lines the sebaceous, sweat and endocrine glands.

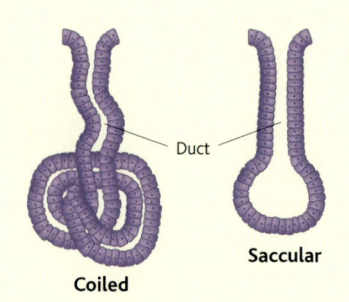

▲ Sweat gland and sebaceous gland

Classification of epithelial tissue

Epithelium is classified according to how the cells within the tissue are arranged, either in a single row, simple epithelium or in layers, stratified epithelium. Epithelium is also classified according to the shape of the specific cells.

- squamous epithelium cells are flat, like scales
- cuboidal epithelium cells are square cubes
- columnar epithelium cells are tall and rectangular.

Further classifications describe the specialist functions of epithelial tissue. For example, epithelial cells may possess fine hair-like structures called cilia, which assist with the movement of substances across the surface of the tissue. In the lining of the respiratory tract, the cilia help move mucus upwards and out of the lungs.

The table below summarises the classification of epithelial tissue.

Link to practice

Epithelial tissue cells reproduce more rapidly when you sleep. This is one way in which sleep helps the body to grow and repair tissues. When helping your clients with their skincare, you should advise them of the benefits of plenty of sleep for their skin.

Type of epithelial tissue	Illustration
Simple squamous • Lines the blood vessels and air sacs (alveoli) in the lungs • Allows for the exchange of nutrients, gases and waste products	Squamous epithelium
Simple cuboidal • Lines the tubules of the kidney and some glands • Secretes and absorbs water and small molecules	Cuboidal epithelium
Simple columnar • Lines most of the organs of digestion • Absorbs nutrients and produces mucous	Ciliated columnar epithelium Simple epithelium
Stratified squamous • Found in the epidermis and the mouth • Protects against friction, dehydration and bacterial invasion	Squamous cells
Stratified cuboidal • Lines the ducts of sweat glands • Secretes water and mineral salts	Basement membrane / Columnar basal cells
Stratified columnar • Lines the mammary glands and the larynx • Secretes mucous	Stratified epithelium

CHAPTER 1 Cells and Tissues

> **Fascinating fact**
> The word strata is a Greek word which means layer.

> **Fascinating fact**
> Stratified epithelium can be **keratinised** or non-keratinised. Keratinisation (hardening) occurs in skin, hair and nails, and provides a tough, impermeable barrier. Non-keratinised tissues are found on moist areas of the body, for example, the lining of the mouth.

Type of epithelial tissue	Illustration
Transitional epithelium • This is a specialised type of epithelial tissue. It lines organs that have the ability to expand, such as the bladder. • The cells are rounded not flat and overlap each other in layers. When the organ is distended (expanded), for example, as in a full bladder, it appears as if there are only a few layers of cells. When the organ is contracted, for example, as in an empty bladder, it appears as if there are several layers of cells.	Transitional epithelium

Connective tissues

There are several types of connective tissues in the body, and their job is to support or bind structures of the body together. The connective tissue cells themselves are separated by a matrix or mesh of tissue which is non-cellular. Some of this tissue contains fibres, whilst other tissues are without fibres.

Below is an overview of the types of connective tissue in the body. The way in which their matrix is structured determines the tissue type – whether it will be fluid, soft, firm or rigid.

Type of connective tissue	Functions
Loose (areolar) connective tissue	Collagen and elastin fibres provide strength and resilience
Adipose (fatty) tissue	Insulates; protects; stores energy
Fibrous (dense connective) tissue	Very strong fibres; tendons and ligaments
Yellow elastic tissue	Has ability to stretch and recoil
Reticular connective tissue	Tissue fibres form the framework of lymph nodes, the bone marrow and the spleen
Cartilage	Supports and cushions joints
Bone	Supports soft tissue
Blood	Transports particles suspended in a fluid

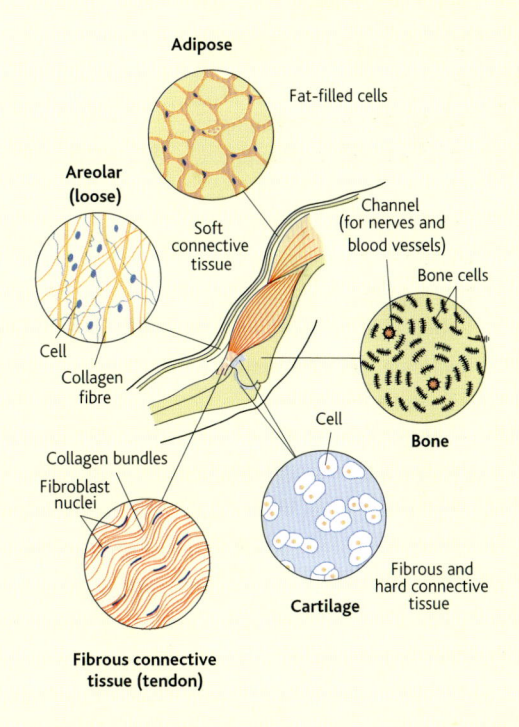

▲ Types of connective tissue

PAGE 21

> **Link to practice**
>
> Collagen fibres give the skin resilience and strength, while elastic fibres help it to recoil back into shape. Both of these fibres reduce and degenerate with age, which is why the skin sags and loses elasticity. Exposure to the sun speeds up the destruction of collagen, thus forming wrinkles prematurely and making them more pronounced. So, remember to tell your client to wear sunblock and avoid the sun!

> **Link to practice**
>
> If a person takes in more energy (calories) than he or she expends, the body will store this excess energy as fat in the fat cells. The fat will remain there until it is needed as energy for the body – for example, during exercise. However, if the person continues to consume excess calories, the body will keep storing fat and the fat cells will get larger and larger. Fat cells will not multiply, just get bigger. Therefore, if a client wishes to lose some stored fat, he or she will have to reduce the quantity of calories going in and burn more calories during exercise.

Loose (areolar) connective tissue

This is the most common of all the connective tissues. Areolar tissue supports organs and structures which are mobile, for example, the skin, the digestive organs and muscles. The tissue is situated between the muscles, the blood and lymph vessels, and nerves. It binds them together as well as binding them to the surrounding structures.

Loose connective tissue is actually semi-fluid and forms a matrix or network containing fibres (white **collagen** and yellow elastic) which are very fine but that offer resilience and strength. In between the network spaces there is room for several types of cell. These are mainly cells known as fibroblasts and it is their job to form the fibres of the connective tissue.

Loose and dense connective tissue differ according to the proportion of fibres in their tissue (collagen, elastin and reticular). An example of dense connective tissue is the **dermis** of the skin, and an example of loose connective tissue is the submucosa tissue underlying the epithelial tissue, which lines the oral cavity (mouth).

Adipose tissue

This consists of areolar tissue whose spaces are filled with large fat cells. The fat cells or adipocytes have thin walls and are swollen with liquid fat.

Adipose tissue is found in most areas of the body, but it is not found in both the nervous system and the lungs. It is commonly found in the subcutaneous tissues (under the skin) and often in large amounts. It is also found in significant amounts surrounding the abdominal organs. Its job is to store energy and provide cushioning for the body.

Fibrous (dense connective) tissue

This type of connective tissue is very dense. It contains white collagen fibres in large amounts (which is why it is also known as white fibrous tissue) and the matrix is tightly packed together, which binds the fibres. The main feature of this tissue is its strength – it can withstand considerable tension and, importantly, does not stretch (is inelastic). It forms tendons and ligaments, and sheaths which surround certain muscles.

Yellow elastic tissue

This type of tissue only occurs in certain situations in the body. It is found in the walls of arteries and in some (spinal) ligaments in the body. Its main feature is that is has the capacity to stretch and then return to its former shape and size. The fibres within the tissue responsible for its special feature are composed of the protein elastin.

Reticular connective tissue

This type of connective tissue contains a network of fibres (the word reticular means network). It is found in internal organs such as the liver, spleen and lymph nodes. It provides an internal framework to support the insides of the organ.

Cartilage

Cartilage is a type of connective tissue which consists of a tough matrix. It is a firm, tough tissue which is also flexible. There are two basic types: hyaline and fibro-cartilage. There are two varieties of fibro-cartilage: white and yellow elastic.

- **Hyaline**: this type of cartilage is smooth and tough, yet flexible. It is mainly found covering the ends of long bones (also known as articular cartilage) and it prevents the bones fusing together and provides a smooth surface to minimise friction. Hyaline also forms the costal cartilages, the rings around the trachea and the nasal septum. It is also found in the developing foetus, before the bones have formed and hardened. It is what you might recognise as gristle.
- **White fibro-cartilage** is found between bones that form slightly moveable joints, such as the vertebrae. Its job is to provide support and cushioning. The pads of fibro-cartilage between the vertebrae act as shock absorbers.
- **Yellow elastic fibro-cartilage** is so-called because it contains numerous yellow elastic fibres, which are embedded in the matrix. It is found in areas where it would not be possible to have bone, for example, the upper part of the outer ear. Its job is to give shape and some support, the elastic fibres making it flexible but resilient.

Bone

Bone is in fact a specialised type of cartilage in which the collagen has been impregnated with minerals (mainly calcium). The collagen fibres make the bone tough and the minerals make it rigid. This means that bone can give full support to soft tissues. The cells between the collagen fibres are known as osteocytes.

Bone is the hardest and heaviest tissue of the body. It is designed to bear weight – for example, the pelvis and lower legs, and to protect delicate structures like the brain and spinal cord.

Blood

Blood consists of a suspension of cells in a fluid called **plasma**. Although blood is classified as a connective tissue, it has no connective or physically supportive function.

> **Link to learning**
>
> Cartilage is found in some places of the body instead of bone for reasons of practicality. Imagine if the very tip of your nose or your ears were made out of bone – you would have broken these body parts many times over by now!

Proving the point

Suck in your cheeks and carefully grasp the inside of your cheeks with your back teeth. Now pinch the skin on your cheeks with your finger and thumb and try to move the outer layer of skin over the inner layer (submucosa). Which of the two tissue types moves the furthest? The amount of collagen in the tissue will determine how far it can move.

Link to practice

Botox™ is a poisonous substance which when injected into muscle tissue prevents it from contracting. Many women and some men now use Botox™ to paralyse the muscles of the forehead and between the brow, to prevent the formation or reduce the appearance of wrinkles. Although the treatment is effective in reducing wrinkles, it means that these muscles cannot contract and expressions of the upper part of the face are not possible. The effects of the long-term use of Botox™ are not known at this stage.

Muscle tissue

All muscle tissue has four characteristics – the ability to:
- shorten or contract
- stretch when relaxed
- return to its original shape after contracting (elasticity)
- respond to a stimulus from a nerve impulse.

There are three types of muscle tissue: skeletal, smooth and cardiac. (Link to Muscles and the Muscular System, page 62)

Skeletal muscle tissue

There are over 600 **skeletal muscles** in the body, most of which are attached to the skeleton (hence the name!). Some skeletal muscle is attached to the skin, for example, the muscles of the face. Skeletal muscle tissue is attached to the bones (by tendons) and allows the body to move, by moving the joints. It also provides the means to produce facial expression. Skeletal muscles tire easily.

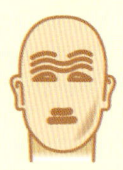

FRONTALIS — Amazement, wonder, shock
DEPRESSOR ANGULIORIS — Dislike, disapproval
ORBICULARIS ORIS — Pouting, smoking, kissing

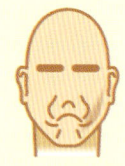

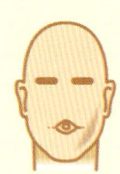

▲ Sketelal muscle tissue in the face provides the means to produce facial expression.

Skeletal muscle is also known as **voluntary muscle** because it is under the control of the will, and **striated muscle** because under a microscope the fibres show up as being striped or striated (see page 62).

Smooth muscle tissue

Smooth muscle tissue is so-called because under a microscope the fibres show up as being smooth (see page 62). It is also known as **involuntary muscle** as these muscles are not under conscious control but are regulated by the **autonomic nervous system** and by the hormone adrenalin. For example, the muscle in blood vessels, which constricts to help blood through the vessels is smooth muscle tisue.

Smooth muscle tissue is also referred to as visceral muscle because it is found in the viscera of the body (the abdominal organs).

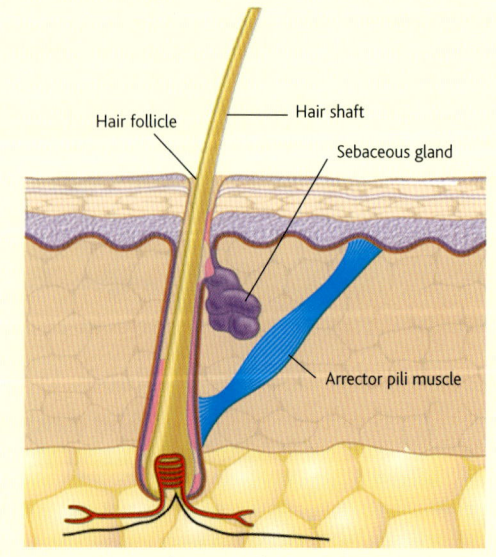

Hair follicle — Hair shaft — Sebaceous gland — Arrector pili muscle

▲ Smooth muscle tissue in the skin

For example, smooth muscle is found in the digestive tract where it contracts to produce wave-like motions known as **peristalsis** that push food through the tract. (Link to The Digestive System, page 154)

Smooth muscle tissue is also found in the walls of blood vessels and at the base of each hair follicle. This muscle contracts slowly and does not tire.

Cardiac muscle tissue

Cardiac muscle is the tissue of the heart. It contracts rhythmically throughout life and does not tire. It is found only in the wall of the heart, and is completely involuntary. (Link to Muscles and the Muscular System, page 62)

The heart is often described as the hardest working muscle in the body, but the power output of the heart is much less than the maximum power output of other muscles; for example, the quadriceps in the thigh provides far greater bursts of 'high energy' over a far shorter period. However, the heart works continuously over a whole lifetime and in that respect it works far harder than some skeletal muscles.

Membranes

Membranes are types of tissues that have different functions according to how they are formed. These include: lining body cavities and certain organs; dividing regions of the body; facilitating movement; the protection and support of parts of the body.

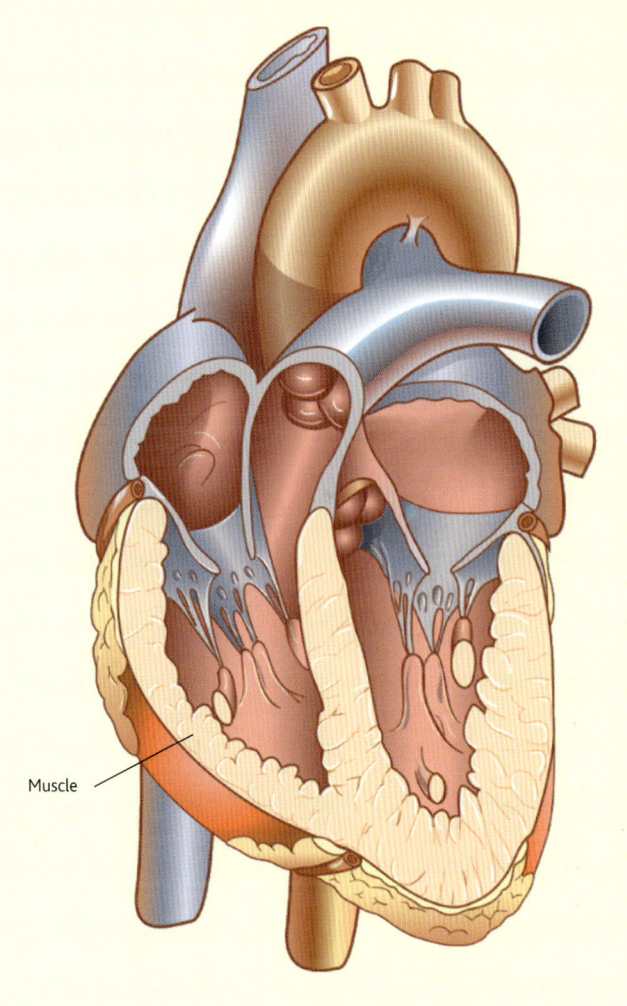

▲ Cardiac muscle tissue is found only in the heart

Membranes are composed of connective tissue and elastic fibres. They may be epithelial membranes (a layer of epithelium and a layer of connective tissue) or connective tissue membranes.

Epithelial membranes

There are three basic types of epithelial membrane:

| Serous membrane | - This type of membrane exists only inside the body – it does not come into contact with the outside of the body.
- It lines the cavities of the body, e.g. the lung cavity, the sac enclosing the heart, and the abdominal walls and organs. It also covers organs in the cavities to allow a smooth, sliding motion.
- It consists of a thin layer of areolar connective tissue, covered by epithelial layer. A watery fluid oozes through these layers |
|---|---|
| Mucous membrane | - This type of membrane lines the body cavities that open to the outside, e.g. the digestive and respiratory passages.
- These membranes secrete mucus – a fluid which lubricates surfaces. This provides a smooth passage for substances passing through various tubes. The mucus is secreted by specialist goblet cells in the epithelial layer.
- Some mucous membranes also have tiny hairs (cilia) with wave-like motions which ease the passage of matter, mainly to rid the body of unwanted particles. |
| Cutaneous membrane | Commonly known as the skin, this is an intricate epithelial membrane. (Link to The Skin, Hair and Nails, page 31) |

Connective tissue membranes

There are four basic types of connective tissue membrane:

Synovial	These are thin membranes which line the joint cavities and secrete a thick fluid known as synovial fluid. This lubricates joints and nourishes the cartilage. Regular exercise stimulates the production of synovial fluid.
Meninges	These layers of connective tissue membranes cover the brain and the spinal cord.
Fascia	Sheets or bands of tough, fibrous tissue which hold muscles in place and support subcutaneous tissue.
Membranes which surround	These membranes include:
- periosteum: a thin covering around bones
- pericardium: the sac enclosing the heart
- perichondrium: surrounds cartilage.

> **Proving the point**
>
> Your heart beats about 100,000 times a day – that's about 3.5 million times a year. If you live to be 100 years old, how many times will your heart muscles have contracted in a lifetime?

Nervous tissue

This type of tissue forms the nervous system, which includes the brain, spinal cord and nerves (Link to The Nervous System, page 121). It co-ordinates all the processes in the body and creates harmony and order. Its job is to receive messages from internal and external stimuli and send electrical impulses within the body to command the various body parts to respond. For example, the feeling of cold on the skin results in shivering and the decision to put on an extra layer of clothing.

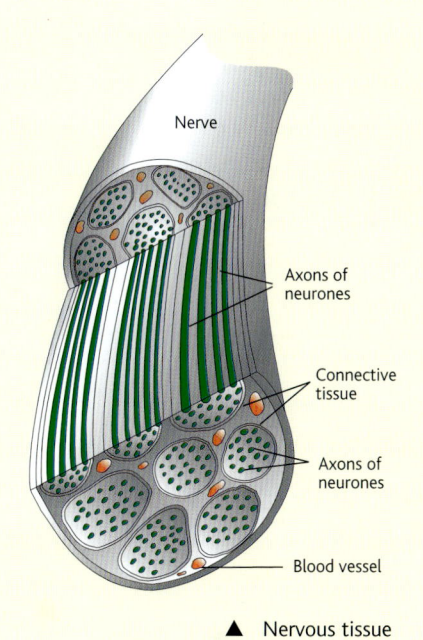

▲ Nervous tissue

Nervous tissue consists of:
- **Neurones** – these are the basic tissues of the nervous system. They are very specialised nerve cells, which transmit messages (see page 122).
- **Neuroglia** – this is connective tissue which supports the neurones by insulating and protecting them.

Disorders and diseases of cells and tissues

Acidosis
A condition where the body fluids become too acidic. It is caused by disorders such as diarrhoea, diabetes mellitus and kidney failure, or by being on a low carbohydrate diet.

Alkalosis
A condition where the body fluids become too alkali. It may be caused by excess vomiting and taking excessive amounts of antacids (indigestion remedies).

Arthritis
This is where the hyaline cartilage of the joints has been lost. There are two basic types:
- Osteoarthritis is where the cartilage has been worn away due to wear and tear. It normally affects older people and joints which have been over-used.
- Rheumatoid arthritis is a degenerative disease and may affect any age group.

Joint replacement is the only real solution although drugs can help with inflammation and pain.

Cellulitis

This is an inflammation of body tissue mainly below the dermis, caused by an infection of the skin and its underlying connective tissue. It is characterised by fever and swelling, redness and pain. (Cellulitis is not related to the condition known as cellulite.)

Oedema

This is the term for excess fluid surrounding the tissue. It can be caused by standing up for too long, being immobile on long flights, or pregnancy (this can cause **oedema** of the ankles). Oedema can also be the result of more complicated conditions such as kidney failure, heart failure, blockages in blood or lymph vessels, or a lack of protein in the blood.

Tumours

When cells divide and do not reproduce exactly, they mutate. Abnormal cells which group together are known as **tumours**. Tumours can be benign and (usually) harmless. Abnormal cells which spread may die or be destroyed by the immune system, and if this is the case the body functions as normal. However, if cells mutate, spread and continue to survive, the tumour is known as malignant and cancer occurs. When this occurs, the malignant tumour dominates other cells and prevents normal tissue functioning.

> **Proving the point**
> Take a tennis ball in your hand and give it a good squeeze. That is the same force that your heart uses to squeeze the blood out every time it contracts.

> **Fascinating fact**
> When the meninges are inflamed, this is known as meningitis.

> **Fascinating fact**
> The prefix *peri-* is a Greek word meaning 'around'

> **Fascinating fact**
> The term 'cellulite' originated in France (and should actually be pronounced cell-u-leet). Other names for cellulite include orange peel effect, cottage cheese skin, the mattress phenomenon, and gravel bags.

Link to practice

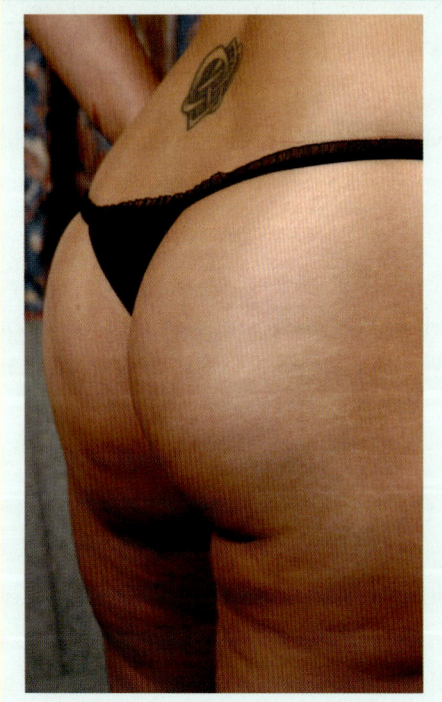

▲ Cellulite created a dimpled 'orange peel' appearance on the skin.

Cellulite

Cellulite is neither a medical or a scientific term, nor is it a medical condition. The word describes the appearance of adipose tissue beneath the skin's surface (see page 22). When adipose tissue stores energy (as fat), it grows in size. These cells push against the supporting matrix of fibres and create an effect similar to orange peel.

Cellulite occurs mostly on the thighs and buttocks. Women suffer from cellulite more than men, probably because women store more fat around the lower body and their adipose tissue lies closer to the skin. Cellulite is not necessarily related to being overweight; people who are otherwise quite slim may have cellulite. It may be pre-disposed by genetics.

The beauty industry offers many solutions to cellulite – mostly ineffective. Dieting may not erradicate cellulite but healthy eating, regular exercise and massage help.

CHAPTER 1 Cells and Tissues

Link to practice

Water – How much is enough?

The body is a remarkable machine fitted with exceptionally clever pieces of equipment that work harmoniously to ensure its health and survival. These include osmoregulators that sense when the concentration of water in the blood drops below 2 per cent. When this happens, the body responds by creating the sensation of thirst.

The body needs water to function and without it the body would survive for only a few days. It is generally accepted that people should drink around 8 glasses (4 pints or 2 litres) of pure water a day. Food contains water and it is estimated that about 20 per cent of fluid intake comes from food. Research shows that even the fluid within tea and coffee and other caffeinated drinks counts towards our daily water intake.

Drinking large volumes of water does not necessarily contribute to health and can actually be harmful. Water intoxication can occur if the kidneys cannot excrete sufficient quantities, and there are documented cases of death occurring when vast amounts of water have been ingested. Of course, if you exercise strenuously, carry out heavy work or are in a hot climate, you need to increase your fluid intake accordingly, as you lose more water through sweating.

Cells and tissues and the ageing process

The body's cells age at different rates:

- Some cells are replaced on a regular basis; for example, skin cells are replaced approximately every 28 days.
- Some cells, like brain cells, are not replaced at all.
- As a person grows older, the rate at which cells reproduce diminishes and the body is unable to manufacture cells quite so efficiently.

Case study

Level 2

Premature ageing

A client is booked in for a course of facial treatments. Whilst completing a full consultation, she states that her main concern is that she is ageing faster than her friends of a similar age. Left is some of the information from consultation sheet. What advice would you give her?

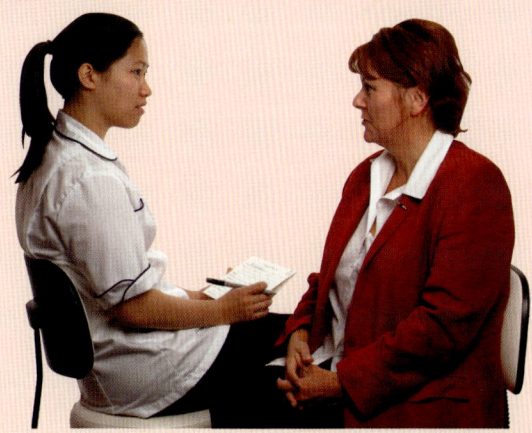

Age: 43
Occupation: Nurse
Hobbies: Gardening, sailing, walking
Diet: Usually good, eating more snacks than before (recently stopped smoking)
Alcohol: Consumes most days.
Fluid intake: Tea and coffee only during the day.
Sleep patterns: Only gets about 5 hours a night as she stays up late and then doesn't feel tired until about 2am. Also, dog wakes her several times during night (wanting to get on the bed). She does night shifts occasionally.
Skin care routine: Uses baby lotion.

Knowledge check

1. Describe the basic structure of a cell.
2. State the function of the cell membrane.
3. How would you describe cell metabolism?
4. Why do red blood cells not reproduce?
5. What is cytoplasm?
6. What are organelles?
7. Name the types of epithelial tissue.
8. Epithelial tissue can be described as simple or stratified. Explain what this means.
9. State a specialised type of epithelium and its function.
10. Name the types of connective tissue in the body.
11. Which tissue type stores energy?
12. What is the function of areolar tissue?
13. Name the types of membranes and state their functions.
14. State the three types of cartilage and list their functions.
15. How many types of muscle tissue are there? Name them.
16. What does voluntary and involuntary mean?
17. Which tissue performs peristalsis? Where do you find this type of tissue?
18. Which tissue is found around the heart?
19. Name the tissue of the nervous system.
20. What special job does nervous tissue do?

SECTION 2

CHAPTER 2 The Skin, Hair and Nails

Fascinating fact

The skin is the largest **organ** in the human body, covering an area of approximately 2 square metres (3,000 square inches) in the average adult. It weighs approximately 4 kilograms (9 pounds) and accounts for 7 per cent of total body weight.

The skin is an **epithelial tissue** that forms a tough waterproof covering to protect the body from the environment as well as protecting all the underlying structures from injury. It also plays an important role in ensuring that body temperature is maintained at 37°C (98.6°F), the optimum temperature for the perfect functioning of all the cells of the body.

The skin is the first thing that people notice about each other and it gives information about health, emotions and well-being. As a therapist, you can assess clients as soon as they come into the salons, based on the appearance of their skin. A client's skin condition can tell you whether they are dehydrated or stressed, whether they have a good diet, and if they are looking after their skin properly.

As a therapist, you need to understand the structure of the skin so that you can advise clients about the best products for their skin type and how to protect the skin from the harmful rays of the sun. The skin begins to age as soon as a person stops growing (around 16–17 years in women and 18–19 years in men) and as a youthful appearance is considered highly desirable, many older clients will worry about the way their skin is ageing and will be looking for ways to slow down this process. A course of facials or the clever use of make-up might help clients to achieve a more youthful appearance. Also, the skin is covered with tiny hairs that need to be examined in detail for electrolysis.

Fascinating fact

Epidermis literally means 'a covering for' (*epi-*) the 'true skin' (*dermis*).

The skin is associated with other structures or appendages; these include the hair and the nails. Together they form the **integumentary system**. Good grooming is not limited to the skin: nail care and manicures are becoming increasingly popular and profitable for salons.

You will learn

In this chapter you will learn about:
- the structure and functions of the skin
- the layers of the epidermis
- the structures found in the dermis
- the subcutaneous layer
- the structure of the hair
- the hair growth cycle
- the structure of the nail
- diseases and disorders of the skin, hair and nails
- skin and the ageing process.

SECTION 2

> **Proving the point**
>
> Look at your skin with a magnifying lamp. Can you see any fine blood vessels? What does this tell you about the epidermis?

The structure and functions of the skin

Skin structure

The skin is divided into three separate layers:

- The outer layer is called the **epidermis**. It is made up of layers of epithelial tissue (Link to Cells and Tissues, page 20) and has no blood vessels. It is the layer that is visible to the outside world and that is of most interest to therapists and clients.

> **Link to practice**
>
> Women are particularly prone to deposits of lumpy fat known as cellulite. Unfortunately, massage will not help to disperse cellulite but may improve its appearance.

- The true skin or **dermis** is composed of areolar connective tissue supported by **collagen** and **elastin** (Link to Cells and Tissues, page 22). The dermis contains blood vessels, nerve endings, sweat glands, hair, hair follicles and **sebaceous glands**.
- The **subcutaneous layer** is a protective layer consisting mostly of fatty or **adipose tissue** (Link to Cells and Tissues, page 22). It protects the body from injury and provides a store of energy.

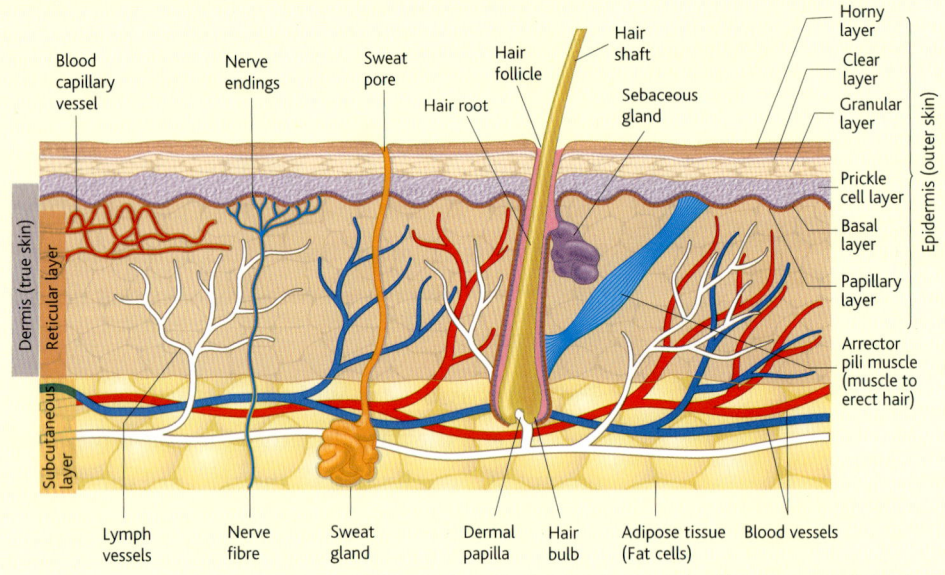

▲ The structure of the skin

> **Fascinating fact**
>
> Every square cm of the skin contains:
> - 70 cm of blood vessels
> - 55 cm of nerves
> - 100 sweat glands
> - 15 oil-producing glands
> - 230 nerve endings
> - 500,000 cells which are constantly dying and being replaced.

Skin functions

The main functions of the skin are to protect the body and to regulate body temperature. These functions can be further divided as follows, using the acronym SHAPES:

- Sensation
- Heat regulation
- Absorption
- Protection
- Excretion
- Secretion.

Sensation

The thousands of sensory nerve endings in the skin send vital messages, known as impulses, to the brain. These messages include information about changes

> **Link to practice**
>
> If sensory nerve endings are impaired, a person becomes very vulnerable to injury and treatments may be contra-indicated. For example, diabetics often lose sensation in their feet and are therefore contra-indicated for a pedicure treatment.

in sensation, for example, the sensation of temperature, pain, itchiness and pressure. This process ensures that a person is constantly aware of his or her external environment and can respond as necessary.

Some examples of sensory nerve endings in action include:
- if your hand touches a very hot surface, nerve endings will send information to the brain to move the hand away before a serious burn occurs
- touch is an important way to communicate feelings to others, for example, hugging somebody who is upset or holding on tight when afraid
- touch forms the basis of all 'hands on' treatments – therapists soon develop their own special 'touch' when performing treatments
- 'rubbing it better' is sometimes the first thing a person does after receiving a knock or other minor injury.

Heat regulation

Maintaining the body temperature at 37°C (98.6°F), the optimum temperature for the perfect functioning of all the cells of the body, is an essential part of homeostasis. Any variation from the norm can be very serious – even fatal.

> **Link to practice**
>
> The pleasant sensation of a massage is caused by the soothing of the skin's nerve endings, muscular relaxation and improved blood flow to muscles.

If the body temperature starts to rise, blood vessels in the skin become wider (dilate). This allows a greater volume of blood to travel to the skin's surface. Body heat from the blood is lost through the skin, causing the body to cool down. This process is known as **vasodilation**.

Similarly, when the body temperature starts to fall, the body can retain heat by closing down (constricting) blood vessels in the skin. This reduces the amount of body heat lost through the skin and helps to retain heat in the core of the body (the liver, heart, brain and other vital organs). This mechanism is known as **vasoconstriction**.

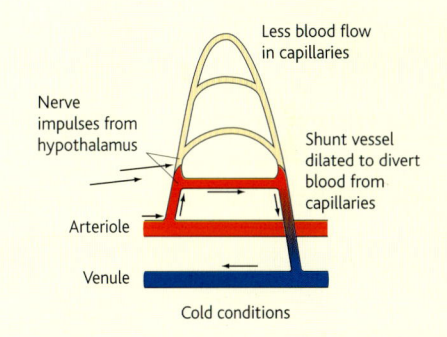

> **Proving the point**
>
> Bringing blood to the skin's surface allows heat to escape from the body. Can you think of ways of helping this cooling-off process when you are hot? For example, allowing your limbs maximum access to cool air. In what ways can you help your body to retain heat when you are feeling cold?

▲ Vasoconstriction

The production of sweat will also lower body temperature because the sweat evaporates and cools on the skin's surface.

Absorption

The absorptive properties of the skin are limited because its main function is to repel moisture and act as a waterproof covering. Most substances applied to the skin are composed of large molecules that are too big to penetrate through the outer layers, although treatments such as galvanic will help to dissolve large molecules to aid penetration.

> **Proving the point**
>
> Massage stimulates the flow of blood to the skin. Which massage movements are the most likely to increase blood supply to the skin?

> **Link to practice**
>
> Careful handwashing will remove a significant proportion of the bacteria that live naturally in the dead cells of the skin's horny layer. Gentle rubbing must be part of the handwashing routine – a simple rinse under the tap is not enough to remove the dead cells and the bacteria.

> **Link to practice**
>
> Dermatitis (inflammation of the dermis) is a disorder characterised by dry, flaking and cracked skin. It can be caused by sensitivity to chemical ingredients in cleaning or cosmetic products, or by excessive exposure to soap and water. Careful use of barrier creams and hand lotions can help to prevent this condition.

However, specialised cells in the skin called **melanocytes** absorb UV rays from the sun. This is essential for the **synthesis** of vitamin D in the body, so some exposure to the sun is essential for healthy functioning. However, overexposure to the sun must be avoided as this is linked to premature ageing and skin cancers.

Protection

The skin provides protection for the body in the following ways:
- The outer layer of the skin, or epidermis, contains a protein called **keratin** that gives the skin its leathery property, making it tough and difficult to penetrate.
- Nerve endings in the skin communicate the sensation of pain and in this way help to prevent serious injury.
- The fatty, subcutaneous layer of the skin provides a protective cushion.
- The **acid** mantle, a combination of sweat and **sebum**, slows the spread of bacteria on the skin.

Excretion

Small amounts of salts are **excreted** in sweat (although the main function of sweating is to maintain body temperature). The salts in sweat ensure that the fluid evaporates quickly on the skin, and this means that the cooling mechanism is effective. The sweating mechanism usually works with vasodilation.

Secretion

The production of oil called sebum from the sebaceous glands prevents the skin from cracking and splitting. Sebum also helps to form an acid mantle, which slows the spread of bacteria on the skin's surface.

The layers of the epidermis

The outer layer of the skin, or epidermis, is formed from a total of five layers (strata) of epithelial tissue which sit on a basement membrane. The epidermis is thinnest around the eyelids and the lips and at its thickest on the palms of the hands and the soles of the feet. It is also slightly thicker on the back of the body than on the front.

The layers of the epidermis are:
- the **basal layer** (stratum germinitavum)
- the **prickle cell layer** (stratum spinosum)
- the **granular layer** (stratum granulosum)
- the **clear layer** (stratum lucidum)
- the **horny layer** (stratum corneum).

The basal layer

The basal layer (stratum germinitavum) is the deepest layer of the epidermis. It is made from square cells that are living and constantly dividing all the time in a process called **mitosis**. The basal layer receives the nutrients it needs for mitosis from nearby blood vessels below.

Skin colour

One cell in ten in the basal layer is called a melanocyte. These cells are very important because they form a pigment called **melanin**. Melanin gives the skin its colour and provides protection from the sun's ultraviolet (UV) rays. The concentration of melanocytes in a person's skin will determine its colour: black skin contains larger, more active melanocytes in greater number than white skin.

Vitamin D

The cells of the basal layer are able to absorb UV from the sun and use it to synthesis vitamin D, or calciferol, from food. This vitamin aids in the absorption of calcium from the digestive system and is therefore important for building strong bones and teeth.

> **Link to learning**
>
> Remember the functions of the skin by remembering the acronym **S.H.A.P.E.S**! But don't forget Vitamin D synthesis, which is also an important function of the skin.

> **Proving the point**
>
> Why do you think the epidermis is thicker in some parts of the body than it is in others?

> **Proving the point**
>
> The more melanocytes there are, the darker the colour of the skin. How is this understanding important to your practice as a therapist?

> **Link to practice**
>
> As vitamin D is synthesised by the skin, it is essential to have some exposure to the sun for short periods during the summer months. Sunscreens with a high sun protection factor (SPF) will block the synthesis of vitamin D in the skin. Clients should therefore be advised that small amounts of UV are not harmful as long as the skin does not burn and sunbathing is kept to a minimum (using a sunscreen and never in the hottest part of the day). In addition, some nutritionists recommend increasing the intake of foods rich in vitamin D (milk and dairy products) during the winter months.

The prickle cell layer

As the basal cells reproduce they are forced upwards to the next layer and begin to change their shape, developing spindles or prickles – hence the name prickle cell layer (stratum spinosum).

The granular layer

The cells are constantly being pushed up from below and gradually they start to die. By the time they reach the third layer – the granular layer (stratum granulosum) – mitosis, or cell division, has stopped. Here the cells become filled with a granular protein called keratin. This protein forms a waterproof barrier for the skin and makes the skin tough and impenetrable. The granular layer is generally very thin, but on the soles of the feet and the palms of the hands a thicker layer is formed known as the clear layer, or stratum lucidum.

Fascinating fact

Lack of vitamin D causes a rare condition known as Rickets, a disorder which affects the long bones as they grow. The bones fail to develop properly and may become bowed. Fortunately, rickets is rarely seen today as most children have plenty of vitamin D in their diet.

Link to practice

Some fake tans contain a dye that colours the skin but most professional ranges contain a colourless sugar called dihydroxyacetoine (DHA). This reacts with the keratin to produce a brown colouring. It only lasts a few days because the cycle of cell renewal means that the surface cells are exfoliated taking the colour with them.

Link to practice

Moisturisers are formed from an emulsion of oil and water, which will usually only penetrate through the horny layer or stratum corneum as far as the granular layer or stratum granulosum. They work by penetrating the cells of the horny layer and preventing moisture loss. Some moisturisers also contain a UV-screen to protect the skin from the sun's ultraviolet rays.

The horny layer

By the time the cells reach this top layer, stratum corneum, they are very flat, flaky and keratinised. This means that they come off very easily in a process called **desquamation**. The horny layer of the epidermis is also visible and responds well to moisturisers and exfoliants. This layer is thicker in darker skins, giving them greater protection from the UV rays of the sun.

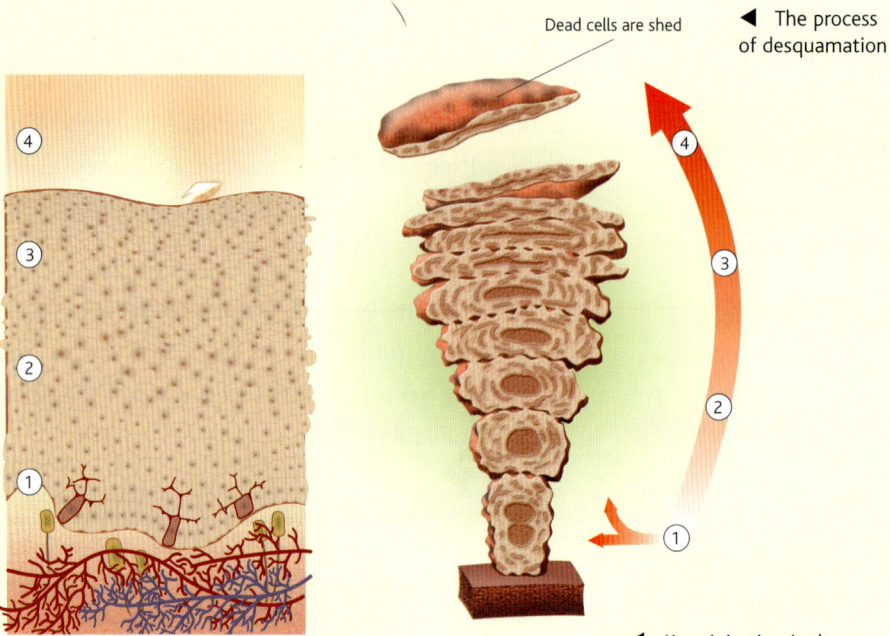

◀ The process of desquamation

◀ Keratinisation is the process by which the skin is continually renewing itself. New cells are made in the basal layer of the epidermis by mitosis. Slowly the cells are pushed up into the prickle cell layer where mitosis slows down. By the time the cells reach the horny layer they have become flat and scale-like, and eventually flake off

Link to practice

Psoriasis is a non-infectious skin condition found in 5 per cent of people with European skin (see also page 43). It is characterised by the over-production of epidermal cells, resulting in small red patches called plaques. The life cycle of the epidermal cells can be as short as 5 days instead of the usual 28 days. Psoriasis can become worse in times of stress but often improves when the skin is exposed to UV rays. Psoriasis can also cause thickening of the nails.

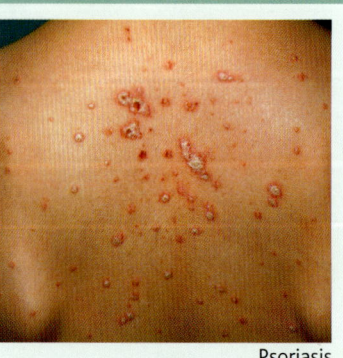

Psoriasis

> **Fascinating fact**
> It takes approximately 28 days for cells to travel from the basal layer to the horny layer. This process of keratinisation is faster in exposed parts of the body, such as the face and hands.

The structures found in the dermis

The dermis or true skin is made up of a loose jelly-like connective tissue called areolar tissue; this is supported and strengthened by fibres of elastin and collagen. The elastin fibres allow the skin to stretch and return to its original shape. Collagen is more 'rubbery' and gives the skin its structure.

The dermis is thinner around the eyes and mouth, and thickest on the soles of the feet and the palms of the hands. The dermis is arranged in ridges called **papillae**; these are clearly visible on the fingertips and are known as fingerprints.

The appendages of the skin

The appendages of the skin found in the dermis are:

- sweat glands
- sebaceous glands
- blood and lymphatic vessels
- nerve endings
- hair.

Sweat glands

Sweat glands or **sudoriferous glands**, are found all over the skin. They resemble coiled tubes with a passageway or duct that opens onto the surface of the skin. Their main function is to cool the body by producing sweat.

Factors which increase sweat production include:

- environmental temperature
- exercise
- hormonal activity, for example, during pregnancy and the menopause
- infectious illness
- spicy foods.

The two types of sweat gland are:

- **Eccrine glands**: These are found all over the body. They are constantly excreting small amounts of sweat in order to maintain optimum body temperature.
- **Apocrine glands**: These are confined to the underarm and pubic regions, and are activated at puberty. They produce a milky substance.

Sebaceous glands

Sebaceous glands are like tiny sacs wrapped around the hair follicle. They become active at puberty when they start producing an oily substance called sebum. Sebum is a natural oil or grease that helps to prevent the skin and hair from cracking or flaking.

Sebaceous glands are not evenly distributed around the body – they are more densely packed on the shoulders and chest, and on the 'T' zone of the face. Men usually have more sebaceous glands than women, and people with darker skins tend to have more sebaceous glands than people with fairer skins. Those with a greater number of sebaceous glands are more likely to have an oily skin type.

> **Proving the point**
> During a facial skin analysis, you may notice that a client has open pores. This may be caused by over-exposure to extremes of temperature, poor diet or neglect. What treatment advice would you suggest?

> **Link to practice**
> If sebum collects in sebaceous glands, blackheads or comedomes can develop. The collection of sebum will encourage the growth of bacteria and may result in spots or acne (see page 43). Sebum production is affected by hormone production and is not a result of a poor diet, as is often thought.

> **Link to practice**
> **Acne vulgaris**
> This condition is very common in teenagers and often clears up by the age of 25 years. It is defined as an inflammatory disorder of the sebaceous glands. Acne is closely linked to the activity of hormones and can flare up when a woman is pre-menstrual, for example. Acne is also brought on by stress and anxiety.

> **Fascinating fact**
> Body odour occurs when the secretions of the apocrine glands come into contact with the bacteria that live on the surface of the skin. The fluid contains a chemical called a pheromone that is attractive to the opposite sex.

> **Link to practice**
> **The acid mantle**
> The combination of sweat and sebum makes the surface of the skin slightly acidic (it varies from between **pH** 4.0 and pH 5.5). (see also Cells and Tissues, page 15) This means that bacteria are unlikely to reproduce on the skin's surface, creating a natural antiseptic effect. Astringent soaps will raise the pH of the skin (make it more alkaline), leaving the skin vulnerable to bacterial and fungal infections. Nourishing products such as moisturisers and massage creams tend to have a pH of 5.5, whereas cleansing products tend to be slightly alkaline.

Blood and lymphatic vessels

The dermis has a rich supply of blood vessels. **Arteries** bring oxygen and nutrients to the cells of the dermis and the basal layer of the epidermis, where they are released from the capillaries. Waste products from the skin are then returned in the capillaries to the **veins**.

Lymphatic vessels are present in the subcutaneous layer of the skin. They return excess tissue fluid to the bloodstream and help to fight infection.

> **Link to practice**
> **Disorders of the sweat glands**
> Anhidrosis – lack of perspiration
> Hyperhidrosis – excessive perspiration
> Bromhidrosis – foul-smelling perspiration
> Miliaria rubra – an itchy rash; also called heat rash or sweat rash

> **Link to practice**
> **Allergic reactions**
> Some people are sensitive to chemicals or allergens, and their skin will show an allergic reaction if they come into contact with these. The process of allergic reaction involves the release of a substance called histamine from mast cells, a type of white blood cell. Histamine often has a vasodilatory (reddening) effect but can cause other symptoms, such as skin itchiness, swelling of the affected area, or breathing difficulties. Histamine is released in response to an allergen; this may be pollen, nut-based products or chemicals found in cosmetic products. If symptoms persist, the sufferer should seek medical attention. Full details of any allergic reaction must be noted on the client's record card.

> **Link to practice**
>
> Massage will result in dilation of the small blood vessels in the dermis and the skin will appear red and feel warm – this is known as **erythema**.

> **Proving the point**
>
> Name the massage movements most likely to result in erythema.

> **Fascinating fact**
>
> There are no sebaceous glands on the palms of the hands or the soles of the feet. This means that water is readily absorbed here: you may have noticed that the ends of the fingers and toes become swollen with water if you stay in the bath too long.

> **Fascinating fact**
>
> Excessive production of sebum is called seborrhoea.

Nerve endings

There are many nerve endings in the skin. The sensations that can be felt through the skin are:

- touch
- pain
- temperature (hot and cold)
- pressure
- itchiness.

Sensory nerve endings carry information back to the brain so that the external environment can be interpreted and the body can respond accordingly, for example, scratching your back.

Some sensory nerve endings are very near the surface of the skin, so some sensations will be felt before others. For example, pain receptors are very close to the skin's surface whereas heat receptors lie deeper below.

Hair

Hair is covered in greater detail below, on pages 40–41.

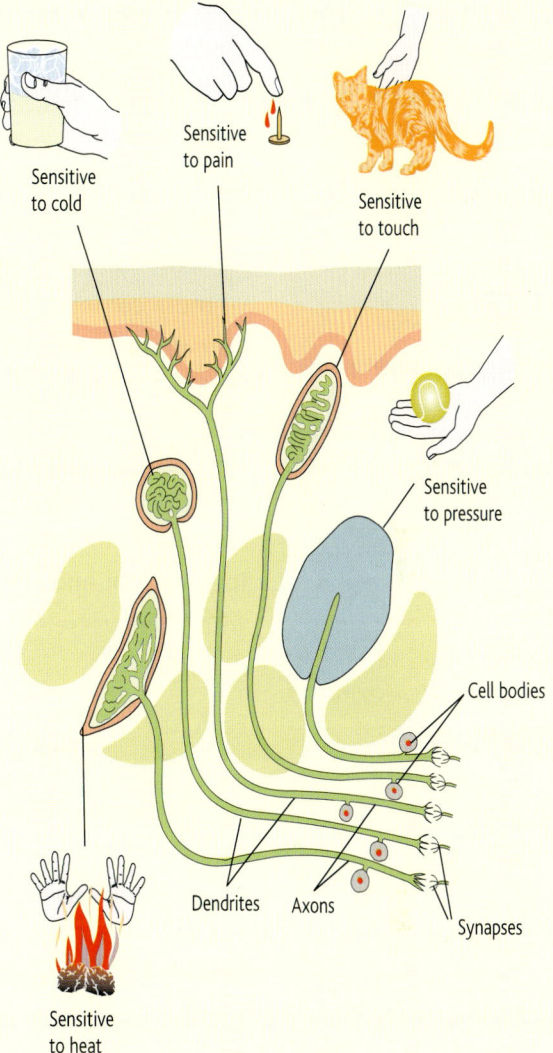

▲ Nerve receptors in the skin.

The subcutaneous layer

The subcutaneous layer is the adipose layer that separates the dermis from the underlying structures. It serves as a cushion, to protect the body from injury. The fat also forms a reserve supply for energy in times of famine, since excess calories can be stored here.

Fat is a very poor conductor of heat so the subcutaneous layer has excellent insulating properties. It keeps warmth in the body and protects against cold. Female skin tends to retain more moisture in the subcutaneous layer than male skin, giving a softer, more rounded appearance.

Proving the point
Ask your tutor for some litmus paper so that you can check the pH of some well-known beauty products. How will these affect the skin's pH? You may be surprised by the results!

Proving the point
What would happen to the skin and hair if the sebaceous glands did not produce enough sebum?

The structure of the hair

Hair is found all over the body and is mostly soft and fine, although it tends to be thicker and more prevalent in other places such as the head and pubic regions. There are three types of hair found on the body:

- **Lanugo** – soft, downy hair present in foetal life shed just before or just after birth
- **Vellus** – short, downy, non-pigmented (colourless) hair found all over the body
- **Terminal** – stronger, coarser hair. It can occur anywhere on the body but is more common on the head, eyebrows, pubic area, legs and underarms.

Hair contains keratin to keep it waterproof.

The hair shaft, which is visible above the skin, is not living, but the hair root, is living and reproducing. The hair bulb is the enlarged base of the hair root and connects directly with blood vessels in the skin, which nourish it.

Each hair shaft is made up of:
- the inner layer or medulla
- the **cortex**, which contains the pigment of the hair
- the outer layer or **cuticle**.

▲ The structure of the hair in the follicle

The hair follicle

The hair follicle surrounds the root of the hair. It consists of:
- The inner root sheath. This has three layers: Henle's layer, Huxley's layer and the cuticle.
- The outer root sheath, which surrounds the inner root sheath.

The hair grows from the bottom of the hair follicle in an area known as the **papilla**. The papilla is filled with blood vessels that nourish the hair as it is growing.

Straight hairs grow from straight follicles, but if the hair is curled then

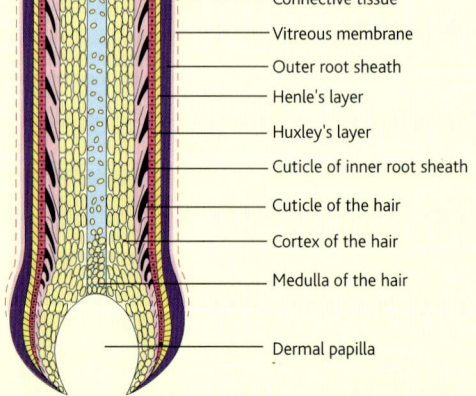

▲ Cross-section of the hair in its follicle

Link to practice
In electrolysis, the hair bulb is destroyed by an electric current applied through a probe.

the follicle is also curled. This can be important in electrolysis when a straight follicle is easier for probing.

Attached to each hair follicle is a smooth muscle called the **arrector pili** muscle (see page 61). This muscle keeps the hair at an angle. When the body temperature falls, or if a person feels frightened, these muscles contract, making the hair stand on end and giving the appearance of gooseflesh.

The hair growth cycle

Hair growth is not a continuous process; it has three phases known as the hair growth cycle.

- **Anagen** is the most active period when the cells in the dermal papilla reproduce rapidly. During the early anagen stage, the new hair begins to form and at the next stage grows out of the follicle. At any one time, approximately 90 per cent of the hairs on your head will be in the anagen stage.
- **Catogen** is the transitional stage, when the papilla separates from the **matrix** and the follicle begins to degenerate. Gradually, the hair becomes detached from the follicle.
- **Telogen** is the resting stage of the hair growth cycle, when the follicle is waiting to begin a new cycle. During this time the hair is not receiving any nourishment and will eventually fall out. On average, between 50 and 100 hairs are shed daily. The telogen stage can also last indefinitely, causing baldness.

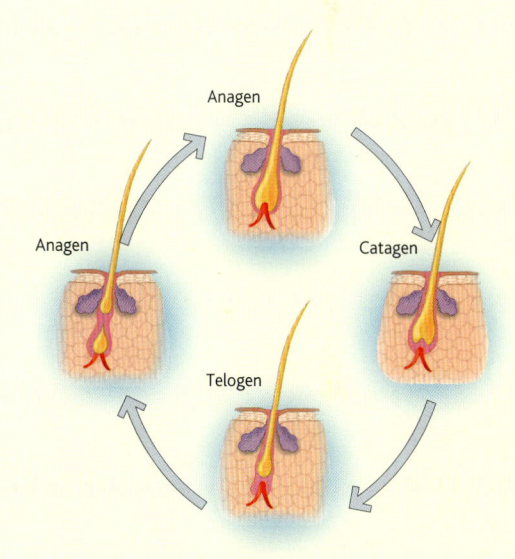

▲ The different stages in the hair growth cycle

The structure of the nail

Nails are hard, keratinised extensions of the epidermis. They protect the fingers and toes from damage and help with grasping small objects and performing intricate tasks.

- The nail plate is the part of the nail that is visible. The free edge is the part that grows beyond the end of the finger or toe.
- The nail cuticle is a band of epidermis growing over the nail plate. It protects the matrix from invading bacteria. The part of the cuticle at the

SECTION 2

Proving the point

Sensory nerve endings are referred to as tactile corpuscles. If someone referred to you as a tactile person, what would this mean?

Link to practice

White spots on nails are caused by knocks and bumps, not poor diet as is sometimes supposed.

Fascinating fact

The movement of hair by the arrector pili muscle does not play an effective role in the regulation of body temperature.

base of the nail is called the **eponychium** and the part at the side of the nail is called the **perionychium**.

- The nail matrix or nail bed is the living part of the nail, formed from the epidermis that provides the nail with its nourishment. If a nail is damaged, a new nail will grow in its place, but if the matrix is damaged, the new nail will be distorted.
- The lunule or half moon, is an area of incomplete keratinisation at the base of the nail plate. It is a different colour because it contains new cells, packed together very closely.

Diseases and disorders of the skin, hair and nails

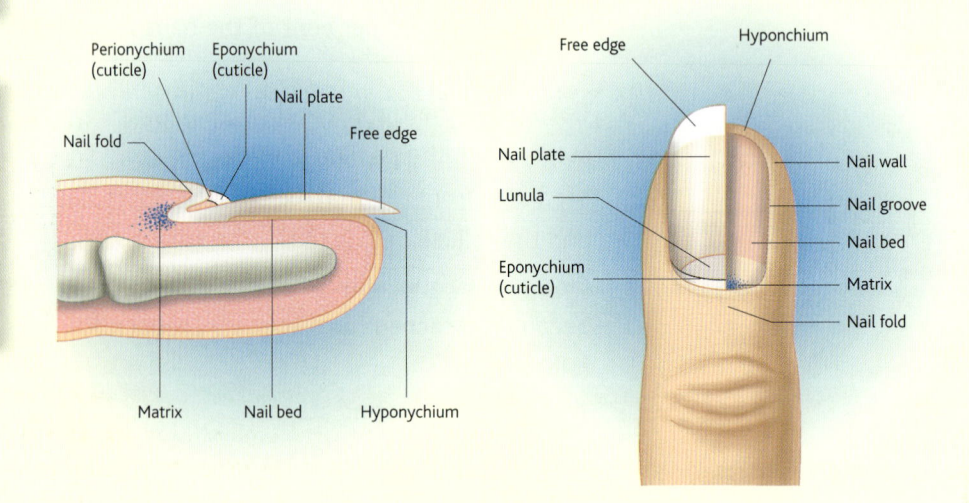

▲ Cross-section of the nail in its nail bed   ▲ The structure of the nail

Non-infectious skin conditions

Condition	Cause	Appearance
Dermatitis	Usually an adverse reaction to an external irritant	Dry, flaky, itchy skin
Eczema	A sequence of inflammatory changes triggered by the skin's intolerance to a sensitiser	Similar to dermatitis – dry, flaky, inflamed skin
Naevus (mole)	Usually congenital (inherited); may develop in puberty or increase with age	Flat, light to mid-brown in colour with smooth, even texture
Vitiligo	Under-production of melanin pigment	White patches; extra sensitivity, especially to UV light; more obvious in darker skins

CHAPTER 2 The Skin, Hair and Nails

Link to learning
The hair, the sebaceous gland and the arrector pili muscle work closely together and are often referred to as the pilo sebaceous unit.

Fascinating fact
You have approximately 100,000 hairs on your head. Each hair follicle will grow about 20 hairs during your lifetime.

Fascinating fact
As people grow older, they tend to lose pigment from the hair cortex. This means that new hairs are white. The onset of this process will vary from one individual to the next.

Link to practice
Eczema (meaning 'to boil out') is a type of dermatitis characterised by very dry skin (see also page 42). People who suffer from eczema often have highly sensitive skin and should be treated with great care.

Condition	Cause	Appearance
Chloasma	Over-production of melanin. Sometimes caused by sunburn as a reaction to light-sensitive ingredients or during pregnancy	Irregular patches of darker pigmentation; more obvious in darker skins
Psoriasis	Thought to be stress-related	Reddened skin with silvery, scaly patches
Sebaceous cysts	Cause unknown	Nodular lesions with smooth, shiny surface, situated in the dermis
Acne vulgaris	Build up of sebum	Congested skin with comedomes and pustules; can become inflamed
Milia	Hormonal changes typically during puberty; worsened by poor skin hygiene	Small white pearls beneath the skin
Acne rosacea	Weakened or broken capillaries over nose and cheeks caused by external or internal pollutants; more typical in male clients	Red 'spider-veined' skin (couperose)
Basal cell carcinoma	Usually over-exposure to UV light; rare before puberty	Moles typically have a raised edge and are dark brown or black in colour
Melanoma	Usually over-exposure to UV light; rare before puberty; can be benign (non-cancerous) or malignant	Moles are usually dark in colour and irregular in shape; may be flat or nodular

Link to practice
Melanoma
Melanoma is a skin cancer that forms in the melanocyte cells of the skin. It typically begins as a dark skin lesion and may quickly spread to other parts of the body (become malignant), although it is more commonly restricted to one site in the body.

The incidence of skin cancer is currently rising each year. It is reported that one in four Australians suffer or have suffered from skin cancer and that the numbers of those with melanoma is also on the increase in the UK. It can affect people of all ages but is more common in women, those with a pale skin and those with a family history of skin cancer.

The early signs of melanoma include changes to a mole, such as bleeding or spreading. The chances of recovery are better when treated in its early stages. The risk of melanoma can be significantly reduced by avoiding excessive exposure to the sun.

Ten of the most common infectious skin conditions

Condition	Cause	Appearance
Folliculitis	Bacterial infection of hair follicle; may be due to in-growing hairs or poor skin hygiene	Inflammation, erythema, discomfort
Furuncle (boil)	Staphylococcal bacterial infection of hair follicle due to fatigue	Red, swollen, painful, pus-filled nodule; commonly found in axilla, neck, back of thighs

PAGE 43

SECTION 2

▲ Dermatitis

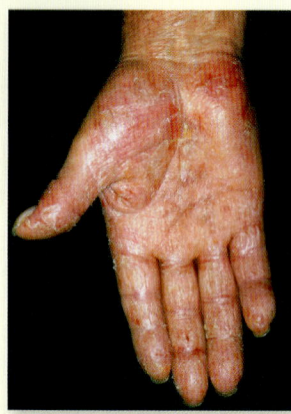

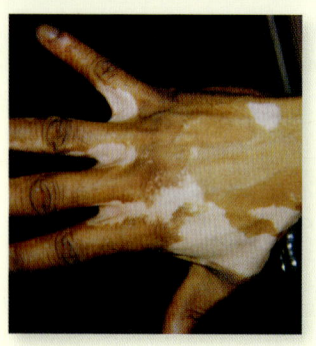

▲ Vitiligo

Proving the point

Electrolysis is more effective when performed in the anagen phase. Can you give an explanation for this?

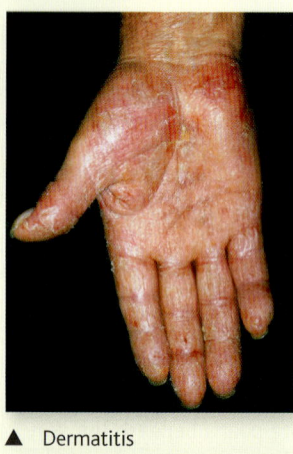

Condition	Cause	Appearance
Carbuncle	Staphylococcal bacteria	Group of boils
Impetigo	Streptococcal and staphylococcal bacteria spread by dirty fingers	Weeping or dry crust on inflamed skin; commonly found on facial areas
Wart	Virus	Raised, skin-coloured; can be smooth or rough; vary in size and are contagious
Plantar wart (verruca)	Virus	Painful in-growing wart on sole of foot
Herpes simplex (cold sore)	Virus; recurrent cold sores may be related to stress or illness	Usually found on face or lips; tingling, red, raised; may weep
Herpes zoster (shingles)	Virus related to chickenpox	Painful; erythema along nerve pathways; acute inflammation
Tinea (ringworm)	Superficial fungus	Typically red papules which resemble a ring
Scabies	Sarcoptes scabiei parasite ('itch mite')	Itchy rash, commonly found in warm folds of skin between fingers, axilla and palms

Diseases and disorders of the hair

Condition	Cause	Appearance
Alopecia (hair loss)	Age; illness; stress; self-harm	Loss of hair in defined places
Tinea capitis (ringworm of the scalp)	Superficial fungus	Round scaly patches on the scalp; hair breakage near root
Dandruff	Dry scalp or irritation from chemicals or detergents	White scales which shed from scalp; sometimes have an oily texture
Pediculosis capitis (head lice)	Contagious parasitic infection	Lice lay small, round, white eggs (nits) that attach to hair
Endocrine disorders	Inherited or acquired disorders which cause hormonal imbalance	Male hair growth pattern in women (hirsutism)

Disorders and diseases of the nail

Condition	Cause	Appearance
Beau's Lines	Slow nail growth caused by illness	Deep transverse ridges across the nails
Discolouration	Smoking; poor general health	Greyish yellow or blue tinges
Onycholysis	Trauma; injury; illness	Distal nail plate separation
Onycophagy	Acquired nail-biting habit	Chewed nail and cuticle, exposing the hyponychium
Hangnail	Dehydrated cuticle, distortion by biting	Curved nail with a split nail groove

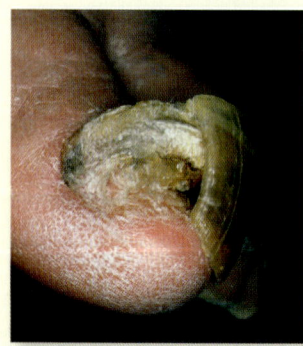

▲ Onychocryptosis (in-growing nail)

Fascinating fact

Fingernails grow at the rate of approximately 1 mm (0.04 inch) per week. The longer the digit, the faster the nail growth. Toenails grow at a slightly slower rate. A toenail will grow out in a year but a fingernail only takes 6 months.
Nails grow more rapidly in the summer than the winter.

Condition	Cause	Appearance
Onychocryptosis (in-growing nail)	Poorly fitting shoes, incorrect cutting and filing of toenails	Inflammation, bleeding
Pterygium	Poor circulation	Overgrowth adhering to nail plate
Paronychia	Cuticle becomes infected by bacteria	Painful weeping, swollen nail plate
Ringworm (Tinea ungium)	Fungal infection	Brown, thickened nails with 'crumbly' material under the nail plate; prone to shedding
Onychogryphosis	Poor circulation and fungal infection	Thickening of the nail with excessive curvature; common in the big toe

Skin and the ageing process

As soon as a person stops growing, the elastic tissue in the skin begins to degenerate. The first signs of ageing usually appear around the eyes during the mid-twenties.

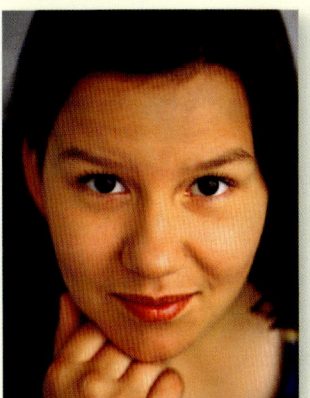

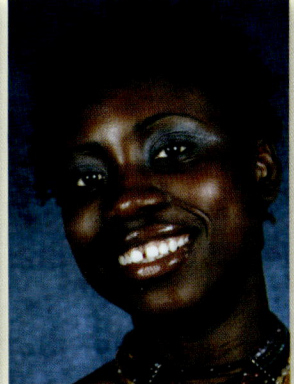

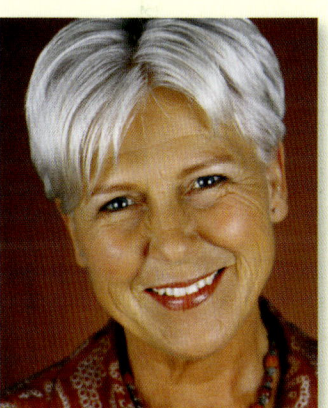

▲ Age is reflected in the face – but how accurate can estimations of age really be?

Link to practice

Care of the skin and nails

A large part of the work of the therapist involves looking after the client's skin, whether it is performing facials or recommending the right products for a particular skin type. Clients often ask how they can slow down the ageing process and enhance the appearance of the skin. Therapists will always recommend a thorough skincare routine and regular salon treatments. The client can help by eating a healthy diet and drinking plenty of water. Some foods that are particularly good for the skin include:
- carrots, broccoli and apricots – these help the production of sebum
- fresh figs prevent constipation, a condition often accompanied by a dull skin
- oat-based cereals, such as porridge, prevent the skin from drying out
- avocados and oily fish are rich in vitamins A, B, C and E, which have an **anti-oxidant** effect and slow down the ageing process
- linseed, oily fish, sesame and pumpkin seeds contain Omega 3 oils, which have an antioxidant effect and help in the production of sebum.

You should also recommend that clients avoid tea, coffee, refined sugars, excessive exposure to sunlight and smoking.

Nails will also benefit from a balanced diet, as well as the regular use of moisturisers.
- A lack of vitamin A may cause the nails to become brittle and dry; foods rich in vitamin A include oranges, liver, dark green vegetables and dairy products.
- Vitamin C in the diet will prevent hangnail; foods rich in vitamin C include citrus fruits, green vegetables and potatoes.

Remember that good grooming is not just for clients – you as therapist should set a good example and ensure that your follow your own advice!

Case study

Sylvia is 45 years old. In her teens and early twenties, she was a self-professed sun worshipper, taking every opportunity to top up her tan. With her partner, Sylvia has just bought a property in Spain and spends all her holiday entitlement there. She now realises that her skin is looking very lined and tired. She has come to the salon in search of a treatment that can slow down the ageing process. How would you plan Sylvia's treatment?

Proving the point

Make a list of the signs of ageing you might expect to see on clients in their:
a) twenties
b) thirties
c) forties
d) fifties and beyond.
What advice would you give to clients about delaying the ageing process?

Knowledge check

1. Name the type of tissue that forms the epidermis.
2. How does the epidermis provide protection from the harmful UV rays of the sun?
3. Give the names of the different layers of the epidermis in the correct order (starting from the top).
4. Name the layer of the epidermis that contains:
   a) keratin
   b) melanin.
5. Name the vitamin synthesised by the skin.
6. Where is the dermis thickest?
7. State the scientific name for sweat glands.
8. Where is sebum produced?
9. Describe the acid mantle.
10. Define erythema.
11. Name and briefly describe the hair growth cycle.
12. Name the sweat gland responsible for body odour.
13. Explain how the skin regulates body temperature.
14. Describe three non-infectious skin conditions.
15. Describe three infectious skin conditions.
16. Explain why infectious skin conditions are always a contra-indication to treatment.
17. Identify two types of capillary found in the dermis.
18. State four structures that comprise the hair follicle.
19. Name the layers of the hair shaft.
20. Give the location for fat cells.
21. Describe two ways in which the skin provides protection from injury.

SECTION 2

CHAPTER 3 The Skeletal System

Fascinating fact

Although everybody has a skeleton, you will probably never even see it during your lifetime!

In this chapter you will discover that the skeleton is a truly amazing construction, which provides the body with shape, support and movement. It is the main framework of the body and provides attachments for and protection of many other structures. It is strong enough to carry around the weight of the internal organs, body fluids, excess fat and even a developing baby, yet light and flexible enough to enable walking, dancing and jumping. It allows a great range of movement, for example, turning of the head, shrugging of the shoulders, writing a letter, pedalling a bike, lifting heavy objects. This is because the bones which make up the skeleton are strong yet lightweight, and vary in shape to suit their location.

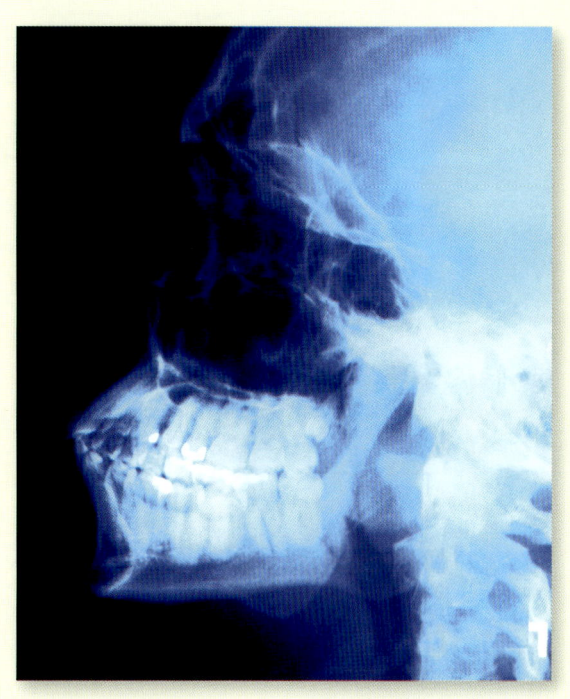

▲ The skeleton is a truly amazing construction.

Like all human structures, the skeleton can deteriorate with age or because of homeostatic disorders, but it can be kept in good condition by regular exercise and proper nutrition. As a therapist, it is important to understand the structure of the skeleton, as well as normal and abnormal functioning of bones and joints, in order to carry out body treatments such as Swedish massage to a safe, commercial standard.

You will learn

In this chapter you will learn about:
- the structure of the skeleton
- functions of the skeleton
- ossification and growth
- types of bone tissue
- classification of bone
- types of joints
- the structure of synovial joints
- movement at joints
- cartilage, ligaments and tendons
- disorders of bones and joints
- effects of ageing on the skeletal system

PAGE 47

The skeleton

The structure of the skeleton

The human skeleton consists of 206 individual bones which can be divided into different parts.

- The **axial skeleton** consists of 80 bones and incorporates:
  - the skull (cranium and facial bones)
  - the vertebral column
  - the thorax.
- The **appendicular skeleton** consists of 126 bones and incorporates:
  - the shoulder girdle
  - two upper limbs
  - the pelvis
  - two lower limbs.

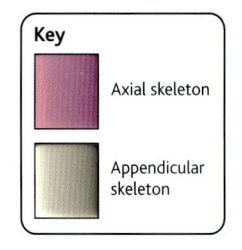

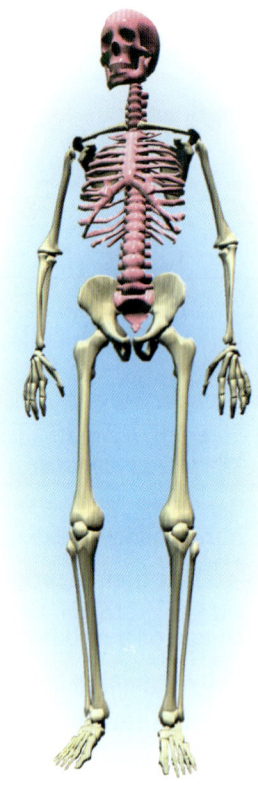

▲ The axial and appendicular skeletons

Key
- Axial skeleton
- Appendicular skeleton

The axial skeleton

The skull

Frontal x 1	Nasal x 4
Parietal x 2	Vomer x 1
Temporal x 1	Maxilla x 1
Occipital x 1	Mandible x 1
Ethmoid x 1	Zygomatic x 2
Sphenoid x 1	Palatine x 2
Lacrimal x 2	Hyoid x 1

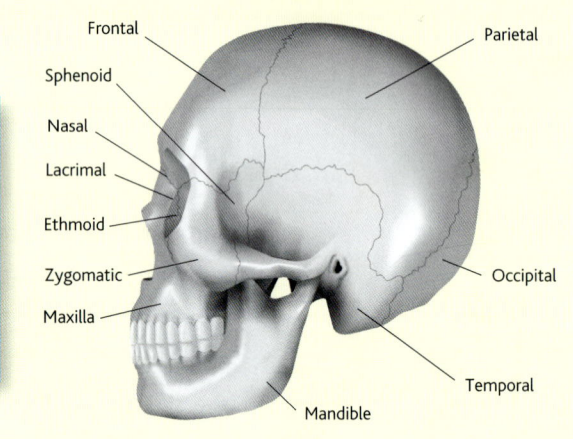

▲ The bones of the skull

The vertebral column

Cervical vertebrae x 7	Coccyx x 4 fused vertebrae
Sacrum x 5 fused vertebrae	Lumbar vertebrae x 5
Thoracic vertebrae x 12	

▼ The bones of the vertebral column.

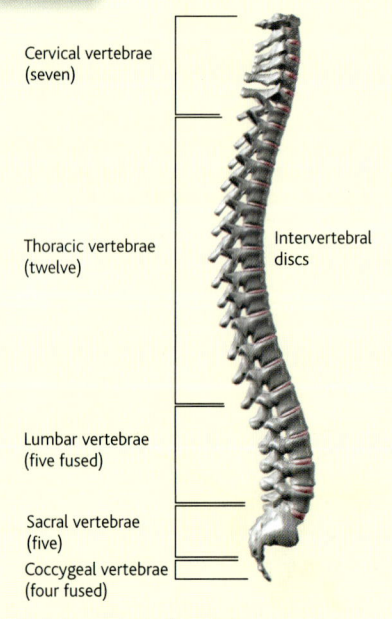

The thorax

Ribs x 12 pairs
Sternum x 1

▼ The bones of the thorax.

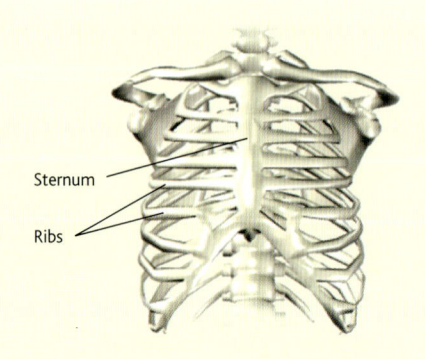

Cervical vertebrae (seven)
Thoracic vertebrae (twelve)
Intervertebral discs
Lumbar vertebrae (five fused)
Sacral vertebrae (five)
Coccygeal vertebrae (four fused)

CHAPTER 3 The Skeletal System

The appendicular skeleton

The shoulder girdle

| Scapula x 2 |
| Clavicle x 2 |

▼ The bones of the shoulder girdle

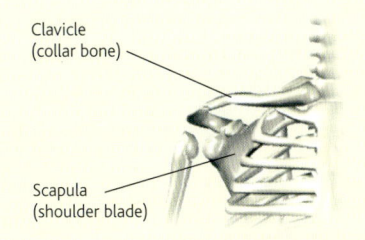

Clavicle (collar bone)
Scapula (shoulder blade)

The pelvis

| Pelvic bone x 2: |
| each pelvic bone is a fusion of three individual bones: ilium, ischium and pubis. |

▼ The bones of the pelvis

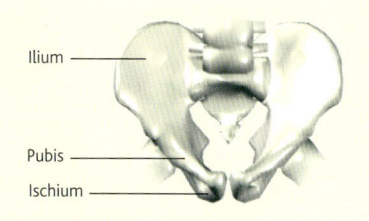

Ilium
Pubis
Ischium

The upper limbs

Two upper limbs, each with:	
Humerus x 1	Metacarpals x 5
Carpals x 8	Ulna x 1
Radius x 1	Phalanges x 14

▼ The bones of the upper limbs

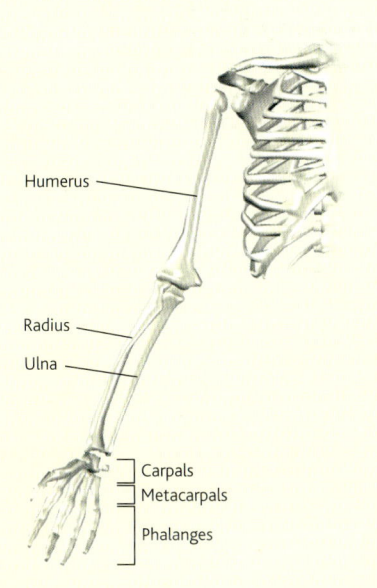

Humerus
Radius
Ulna
Carpals
Metacarpals
Phalanges

The lower limbs

Two lower limbs, each with:	
Femur x 1	Tibia x 1
Tarsals x 7	Phalanges x 14
Patella x 1	Fibula x 1
Metatarsals x 5	

▼ The bones of the lower limbs

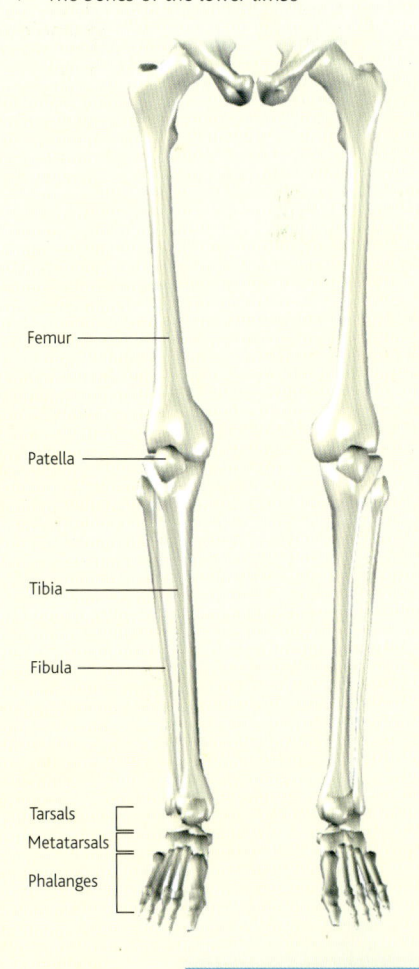

Femur
Patella
Tibia
Fibula
Tarsals
Metatarsals
Phalanges

Fascinating fact

The human body has more bones at birth than as an adult. This is because some bones become fused together, such as the sacrum, coccyx and pelvis.

PAGE 49

Arches of the foot

Medial longitudinal arch	Lateral longitudinal arch
Anterior transverse arch	Posterior transverse arch

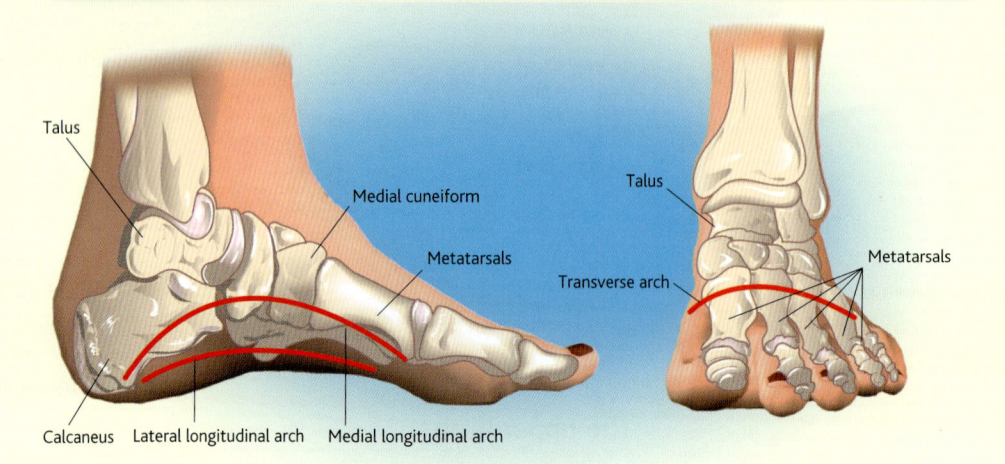

▲ The arches of the (right/left) foot. Arches help the foot support and distribute the weight of the body and provide leverage during walking

Functions of the skeleton

- **Support**: the human skeleton is an upright frame which gives the human body its characteristic shape. It is arranged to provide a means of support for the body and its component parts.
- **Protection**: Bones form protective containers for the internal organs. For example, the flat bones of the skull surround and protect the brain; the bones of the thorax protect the heart and lungs; the pelvic girdle protects the reproductive organs.
- **Movement**: muscles attach to bones, enabling them to act as levers. This allows a range of movement at joints and provides mobility.

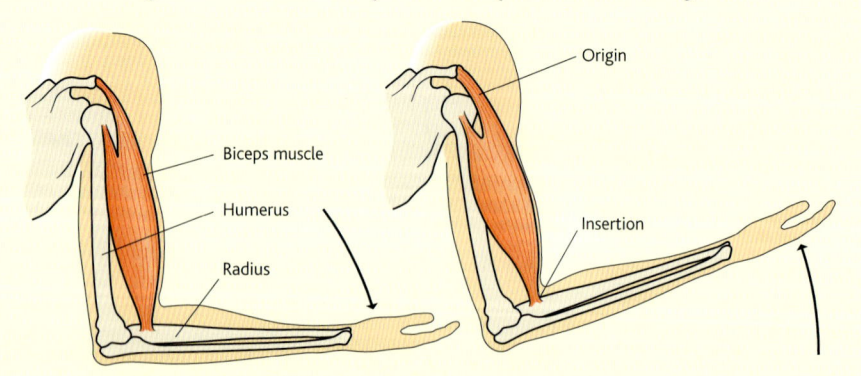

▲ Muscle attaches to bone to facilitate movement.

- **Development of blood cells**: many bones in the human skeleton are hollow, with cavities containing bone marrow. In adults, this bone marrow is the site for the production of red blood cells.
- **Mineral reservoir**: approximately 97 per cent of the mineral calcium is

stored in bones. If this store is diminished, for example, during pregnancy or the menopause, or because of a poor diet, the bones become more brittle. This can lead to a condition known as **osteoporosis**, which occurs when bone mass diminishes. People suffering from osteoporosis are more prone to suffer breaks or fractures as their bones become weaker (see also page 58).

Bone formation and types

Ossification and growth

Bone formation begins in the seventh week of development in the womb, when flexible **cartilage** is gradually replaced by hard bone tissue in a process called **ossification**. Areas of incomplete ossification, such as the soft spots on the skull and some small bones in the wrist, continue to develop through infancy. Nearly all cartilage is eventually replaced by hard bone tissue, although some remains on the surfaces of most bones in the form of articular cartilage. Development of the skeleton continues until about the age of 25 years by which time the final size and shape of the skeleton has been established. However, growth, destruction and repair of bone tissue continues throughout life, to maintain the strength and health of the skeletal system.

Fascinating fact

One of the greatest influences on skeletal development in infancy is nutrition. Vitamin A influences osteoblast and osteoclast activity while vitamin D is required to aid the absorption of calcium from the intestines. Vitamins C and B12 are also essential to bone growth.

Ossification depends on a delicate balance between the construction and destruction of bone tissue, which is maintained by specialist cells called **osteoblasts** and **osteoclasts**. This is known as bone **homeostasis**.

Osteoblasts make new bone tissue. They secrete collagen which forms a strong yet flexible framework. Mineral salts, especially calcium, are then deposited within this framework to provide hardness in a process called **calcification**.

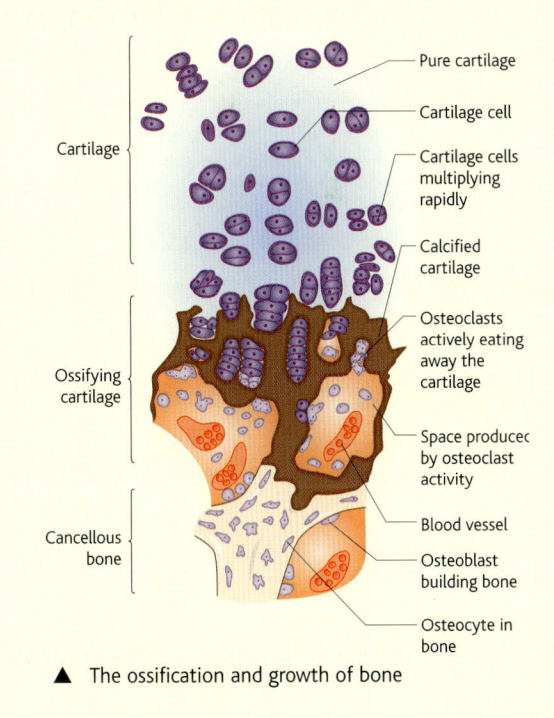

▲ The ossification and growth of bone

Osteoblasts become trapped in the framework of bone tissue and develop into **osteocytes** (mature bone cells), which release further calcium ions that become part of the bone tissue. Osteoclasts contain enzymes that digest

> **Fascinating fact**
> Bone is as strong as cast iron but only about a third of its weight.

protein and break down minerals in old bone tissue. In this way the skeleton is maintained as osteoclasts destroy old tissue while osteoblasts construct new tissue. This process also allows bone tissue to act as storage for calcium. An imbalance in the activity of osteoblasts and osteoclasts can result in disorders of the skeleton (see page 58).

Types of bone tissue

Bone tissue is rigid and non-elastic, consisting of about 67 per cent calcium and 33 per cent organic matter, mainly collagen. There are two types of bone tissue:

- **Compact tissue** is hard and strong and forms the outer casing of many bones.
- **Cancellous tissue** is less tightly structured and so is more lightweight. It has the appearance of a sponge under the microscope and is therefore referred to as spongy bone tissue. The spaces in cancellous tissue contain bone marrow, which is where blood cells are formed.

> **Proving the point**
> Talk to people of different ages who have suffered a broken bone or fracture and compare their experiences of recovery. Think about the implications for treatment.

Classification of bone

There are five different types of bones, which are classified according to shape, as follows:

- long bones
- short bones
- flat bones
- irregular bones
- sesamoid bones

Each type of bone has a different structure, which suits its location and function.

Long bones

If you were asked to draw a cartoon-style bone, it is likely that your illustration would resemble a long bone. They consist of a shaft, or **diaphysis**, and two ends called **epiphyses** (singular: epiphysis).

- The diaphysis is a hollow tube with walls of strong compact bone tissue, arranged like plywood for strength. If excess force is placed on the diaphysis it can fracture or break. Young bones contain less calcium than fully mature bones, and

> **Proving the point**
> Think of examples of each classification of bone.

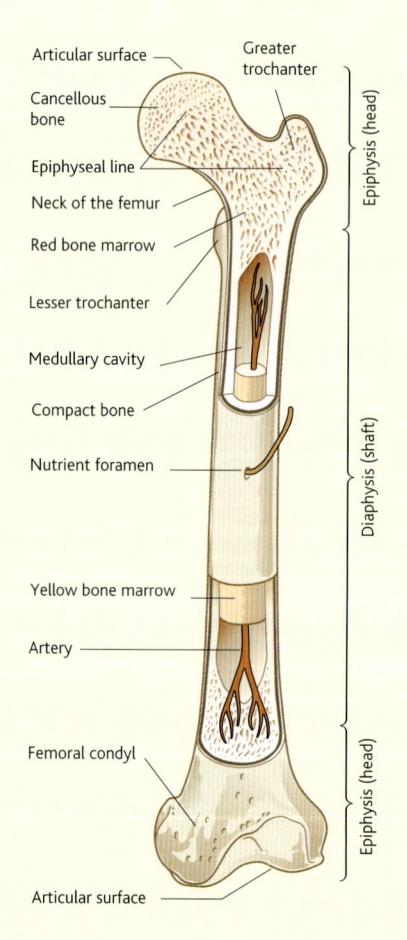

▲ Structure of a long bone.

this influences the type of break as well as the healing process. The hollow shaft of long bones contains bone marrow, which is where red blood cells are formed.
- The epiphyses consist of softer cancellous bone tissue, to allow for growth and attachment at joints.

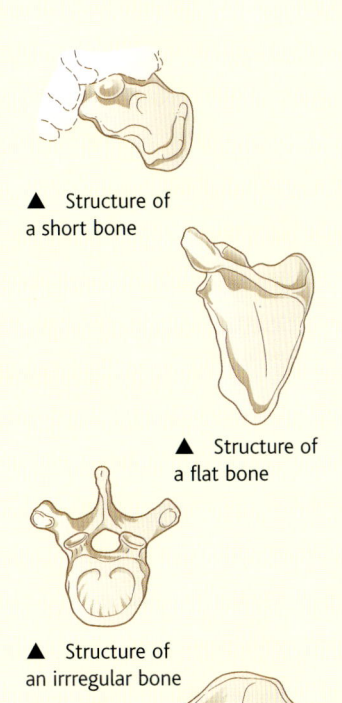

Short bones
Think of a sweet with a hard shell and a soft centre and you will begin to understand the structure of short bones. The shell consists of compact bone tissue while the centre is made of cancellous bone tissue. Short bones have no shaft and tend to be cuboidal in shape. They are small, strong and articulate (jointed), to allow a larger range of movement than joints formed by long bones.

▲ Structure of a short bone

Flat bones
Flat bones are plate-like in structure. They consist of a sandwich of bone tissue, with cancellous tissue acting as the filling between two layers of compact bone. These bones are usually curved to fit their location. They also have a protective function as they are often situated around delicate organs, such as the brain.

▲ Structure of a flat bone

Irregular bones
Irregular bones are small and strong with a structure similar to short bones. However, unlike short bones, they do not have a regular shape.

▲ Structure of an irrregular bone

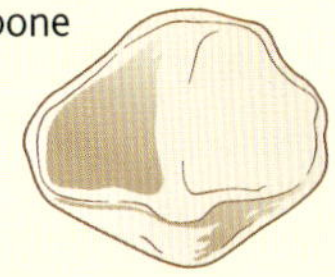

Sesamoid bones
Sesamoid bones are situated in tendons. This means that they are protected from the friction in a joint.

▲ Structure of an sesamoid bone

Types of joint
A **joint** is formed where two or more bones meet. There are three groups of joints, which permit different types of movement; some allow no movement. The groups are:
- fibrous joints
- cartilaginous joints
- synovial joints.

Fibrous joints
Fibrous joints are found where two bones dovetail together. They are bound together with thin bands of fibrous tissue called sutures. Fibrous joints do not permit any movement and are therefore also known as fixed or immovable joints. Examples of fibrous joints are found between the bones of the skull (cranium).

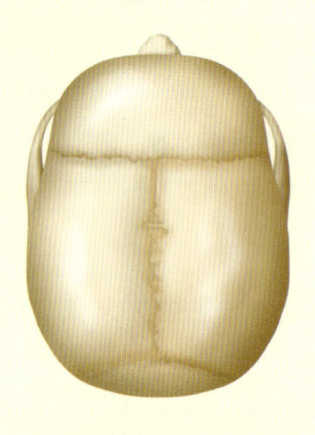

▲ Fibrous joint in the cranium.

Cartilaginous joints

Cartilaginous joints permit limited movement and are therefore also known as slightly moveable joints. They are formed where two bones are connected by a pad of fibrocartilage, which acts as a shock absorber. They are also surrounded by fibrous connective tissue which holds the joint in place. Examples of this type of joint are between the vertebrae and between the pubic bones (pubic symphysis).

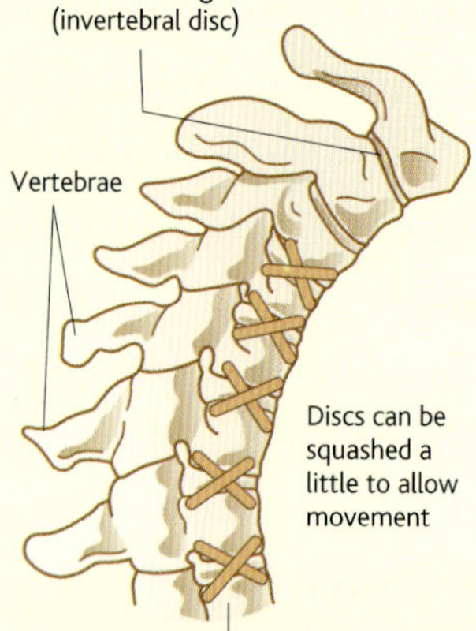

▲ Cartilaginous joint in the vertebral column.

Synovial joints

Synovial joints are formed where two or more bones meet. They are freely moveable and are named according to the movements they permit. Movements at synovial joints are dependent on the shape and size of the bones which form them as well as muscle tone. There are about 70 synovial joints in the body in total.

> **Proving the point**
> Try to locate the 70 synovial joints in your body. In what ways do the joints differ from each other?

The ends of the bones which form synovial joints are covered with fibrous connective tissue called articular or hyaline cartilage. This helps to reduce friction between bones. Synovial fluid is contained in the connective tissue which enables free movement and nourishes the cartilage cells. The bones of a synovial joint do not meet but instead form a synovial cavity. The cavity is lined with a synovial membrane, except over the ends of the bone. The entire cavity, including the ends of the bones, is enclosed within a fibrous capsule which protects the joint.

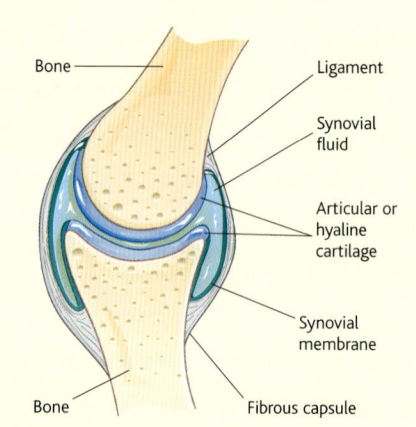

▲ The structure of a synovial joint

Movement at joints

There are three types of movement possible at synovial joints:
- angular movements
- rotary movements
- gliding movements.

Angular movements

Angular movements include flexion/extension and abduction/adduction.

> **Link to practice**
>
> As a body therapist you must be able to describe movements at joints for the purpose of making accurate records, prescribing exercise and monitoring client progress.

- Flexion at the elbow would bring the hand up towards the shoulder, decreasing the angle at the joint. Extension, which is the opposite movement, would return the arm to an outstretched or 'extended' position, increasing the angle at the joint. Weight training to strengthen the biceps muscle is a good illustration of flexion and extension.
- Abduction means 'to take away', so abduction of the leg would involve swinging the leg away from the body at the hip, increasing the angle at the joint. Adduction, which is the opposite movement, would return the leg to its normal position, decreasing the angle at the joint.

Rotary movements

Rotary movements include rotation (pronation and supination) and circumduction.

- Rotation means turning on an axis; for example, rotation of the forearm changes the position of the hand so that the palm is either facing upwards (supination) or facing downwards (pronation).
- Circumduction is the rotary movement of a part of the body, such as the arm, hand, leg, foot or finger, at the joint. This can be illustrated by imagining that the extremity was drawing a circle in the air. Another example is a cricketer's over-arm bowling action.

Gliding movements

Gliding movements are those in which one part of the joint slides across another, and they provide very small movements. An example of a gliding joint is found where the foot meets the ankle. Movement here can be illustrated by lifting the toes and arches off the floor.

There are five types of synovial joint, each of which has a different structure and function.

Type of synovial joint	Example	Movement
Gliding	Clavicle/scapula	Small, versatile gliding movements
Hinge	Phalanges	Flexion, extension; in one plane only
Pivot	Radius and ulna	Rotation including pronation and supination
Ball and socket	Pelvis/femur	The widest range of movement: flexion, extension, adduction, abduction, circumduction and rotation (including pronation and supination)
Condyloid	Carpals	Movement in two planes; adduction, abduction, flexion, extension, limited circumduction

SECTION 2

Proving the point

Identify the location and type of synovial joints illustrated in the following activities. What movements are being permitted?

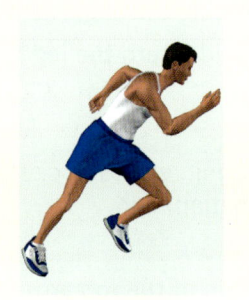

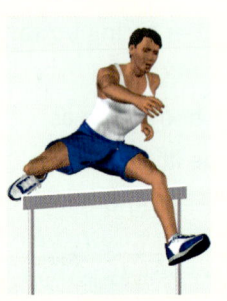

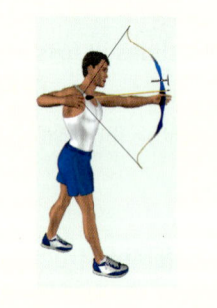

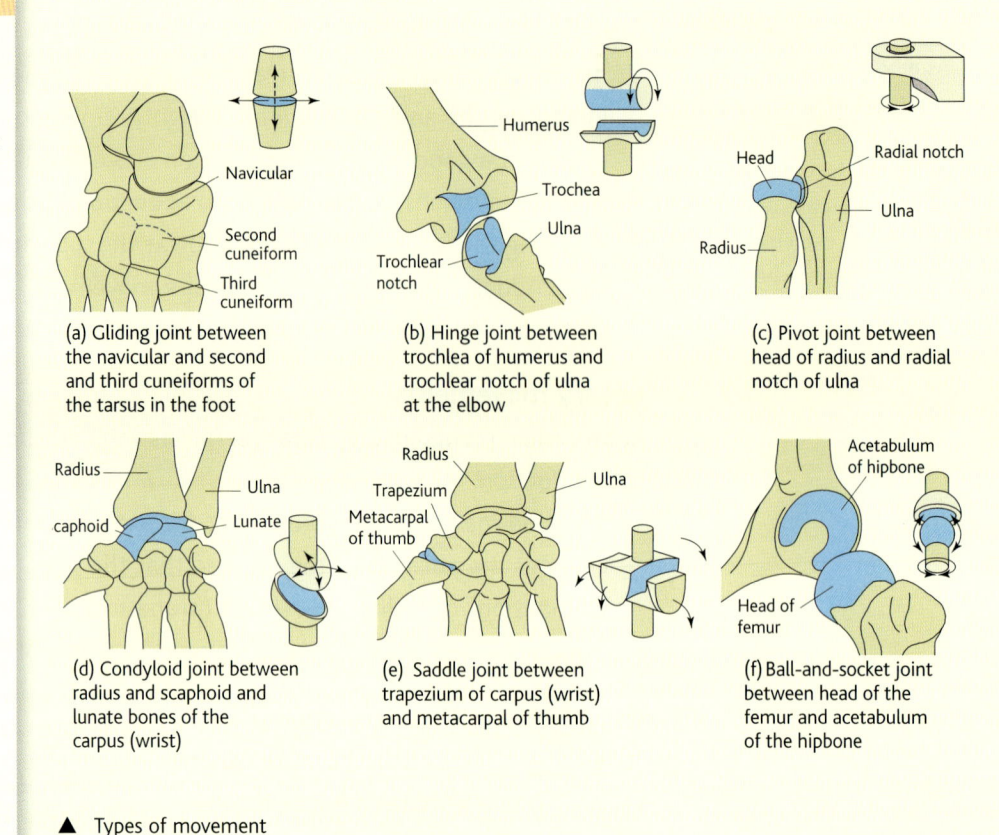

(a) Gliding joint between the navicular and second and third cuneiforms of the tarsus in the foot

(b) Hinge joint between trochlea of humerus and trochlear notch of ulna at the elbow

(c) Pivot joint between head of radius and radial notch of ulna

(d) Condyloid joint between radius and scaphoid and lunate bones of the carpus (wrist)

(e) Saddle joint between trapezium of carpus (wrist) and metacarpal of thumb

(f) Ball-and-socket joint between head of the femur and acetabulum of the hipbone

▲ Types of movement at a synovial joint.

Cartilage, ligaments and tendons

- **Ligaments** are bands of strong, fibrous connective tissue which hold bones together across joints and stretch to allow movement.
- **Tendons** are strong, fibrous bands of connective tissue which attach muscles to bones. They are almost inelastic. It is the contraction of a muscle through a tendon which causes the movement of a bone at a joint. An example of a tendon is the Achilles tendon which attaches the calf muscle (gastrocnemeus) to the heel of the foot (calcaneum).
- An **aponeurosis** is a flattened sheet of tendinous fibres. Examples are the palmar aponeurosis on the palm of the hand, and the inguinal ligament in the groin.
- Cartilage is a type of firm connective tissue with a dense network of collagen and elastin fibres. Cartilage is unusual in that it contains no blood vessels or nerves. Hyaline cartilage is a particular type of cartilage which covers the end of long bones and also forms the nose, larynx, trachea and bronchi. Fibrocartilage provides both strength and rigidity and is located in the intevertebral discs. Elastin cartilage, on the other hand, provides strength and support. It helps to maintain the shape of the internal organs.

Fascinating fact

In an upright position, the amount of force exerted on the hip joint is about six times a person's body weight, due to the gravitational pull of muscles.

PAGE 56

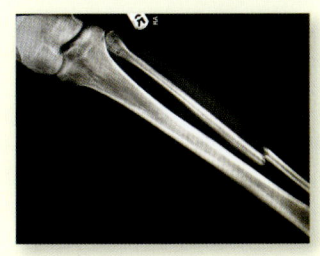

CHAPTER 3 The Skeletal System

Disorders of bones and joints

Broken bones

Bone tissue is able to heal itself in a process which is an amplification of the normal process of cell renewal. The initial response to a break in the bone is pain, swelling, inflammation and localised heat, which is a sign of increased blood flow to the area. The fractured bone severs blood vessels in the area and, to prevent continued blood loss, a clot is formed. Before a broken bone is set in plaster, the ends of the bones are aligned manually so that they can mend and remodel in place. The activities of osteoblasts and osteoclasts play an important part in restructuring bone when it becomes injured. Osteoclasts remove cellular and bony debris while osteoblasts produce spongy bone tissue which eventually develops into compact bone tissue.

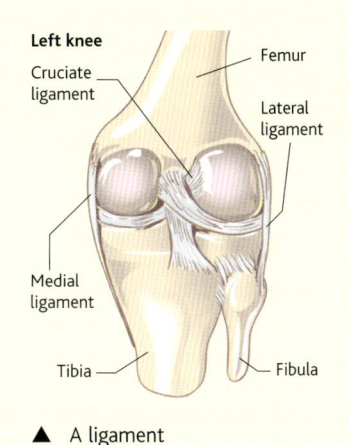

The bones of children are still quite flexible as they are not yet fully formed. A break in this type of bone tissue is called a 'greenstick fracture' because the broken bone resembles a green, flexible piece of wood with one side breaking and the other side bending. Bone healing occurs quicker in young people and is retarded by age. This may be due to poor blood supply or a reduced capacity for repair due to a general slowing down of metabolism. Poor nutrition may also be a factor.

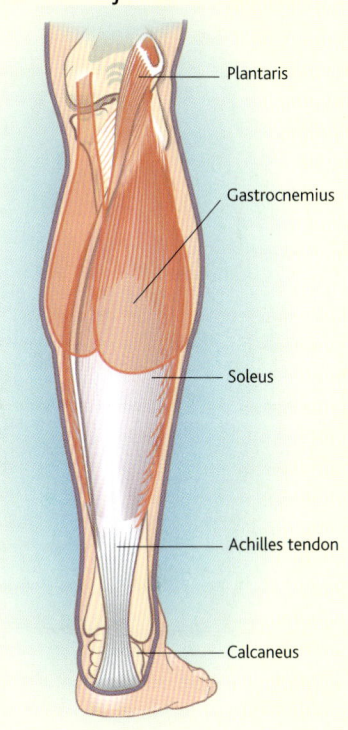

▲ A broken bone

Left knee
Cruciate ligament
Femur
Lateral ligament
Medial ligament
Tibia
Fibula

▲ A ligament

Plantaris
Gastrocnemius
Soleus
Achilles tendon
Calcaneus

▲ A tendon

Summary of bone tissue repair after injury

Timescale	Physiological response	Physical response
Immediate	Bone fractures or breaks; blood vessels are severed	Pain; internal and/or external bleeding
Within hours	Increased blood flow to area: formation of a blood clot	Heat, swelling; inflammation prevents further blood loss
Within weeks	Increased activity of osteoclasts	Removes cellular and bony debris
Within 3-4 weeks	Increased activity of osteoblasts and osteoclasts	Formation of a pad of spongy bone tissue which is replaced with compact bone tissue; trims away excess bony tissue

Link to practice

Pressure should not be applied in the area of a break, fracture or recent injury until the area has fully healed as internal healing can take several months. Check with a GP if you are unsure.

PAGE 57

> **Case study**
> **Level 2**
> Rhiannon has been looking forward to the manicure a friend booked for her as a present. During the consultation she tells you that she broke her wrist recently after falling from a horse. Describe the problem and what treatment advice you would give.

> **Case study**
> **Level 3 and holistic**
> Sanjay suffered a broken ulna when he fell awkwardly on his arm during a football match four months ago. X-rays show that his arm is fully healed. However, he still has limited movement and cannot extend his arm fully. Describe the problem and what treatment advice you would give.

Bone formation disorders

Disorders of bones can occur when osteoblast and osteoclast activity becomes imbalanced.

- Excessive osteoblast activity could result in bones becoming thick and heavy or lumps forming, which could affect joint activity and movement.
- Excessive osteoclast activity could result in bones becoming thin, weak or brittle.

Osteoporosis

One of the most common disorders of bones is osteoporosis. This occurs when bone mass falls below a certain level and the bones become more prone to fractures and breaks. This condition is usually associated with age and tends to affect women more than men. This is because women tend to have a lower bone mass than men at maturity and so the further reduction in mass causes them more of a problem. Treatment with the hormone oestrogen has been found to have a positive effect on calcium metabolism, which in turn reduces loss of bone density and reduces the risk of osteoporosis.

Disorders of joints

Rheumatism

Rheumatism is the term given to a variety of disorders of the joints and related tissues which are characterised by pain, swelling and limited mobility.

Arthritis

Arthritis is inflammation of one or more joints which is characterised by pain, swelling and restricted movement. In some forms of arthritis the articular cartilage breaks down, causing painful friction between bones.

Spondylosis

Spondylosis is a degenerative disease of the intevertebral discs of the spine which typically causes pain in the cervical and lumbar regions of the back.

> **Proving the point**
> Consider the implications of these disorders, and any others you can think of, for a client seeking body treatment.

Bursitis

Bursitis is an inflammation of the bursa, the small pads of tissue which reduce friction. The largest bursa is found in the knee, which can produce excess fluid if the joint undergoes severe stress (water on the knee). Bursitis is characterised by pain, swelling and restricted movement.

Tendinitis

Tendinitis is inflammation of a tendon usually caused by over-use and is also known as repetitive strain injury (RSI). Tendinitis can also be the result of unaccustomed exertion or failing to warm up adequately before sport.

Sprains

Sprains are injuries to ligaments, cartilage or muscle in the locality of a joint which occur when the joint is over-stretched. A sprain causes localised pain and swelling.

Dislocation

Dislocation can occur as a result of sudden or unnatural movements. The bones of a joint become disconnected causing damage to the ligaments and surrounding joint capsule.

Effects of ageing on the skeletal system

Bone weakness

As the body ages, compact bone tissue is lost more quickly than it can be replaced. Also, cancellous bone tissue loses some of its internal structure due to the breakdown of collagen fibres and so there is a reduction in bone mass and the bones become weaker.

> **Fascinating fact**
> During middle age, bones start to shrink, height decreases and the skin can become saggy as it fits less snugly.

> **Case study**
> **Level 3 and holistic**
> Lilia is a 54-year-old woman who comes for treatment and advice due to joint pains. She has a family history of arthritis and is in the later stages of the menopause. What treatment advice would you give her?

Age-associated changes in the digestive system can radically affect the condition of the skeleton. As a person ages, less calcium is absorbed from the diet. This appears to affect post-menopausal women more than men of the same age, adding to the tendency towards osteoporosis. Changes in the digestive system also affect the absorption of vitamin D, and changes in the skin slow down the production of vitamin D activated by natural sunlight. As the function of vitamin D is to transport calcium from the digestive system to the bones, a deficiency means that new bone tissue is produced more slowly than existing tissue is destroyed.

Link to practice

Advice for the maintenance of healthy bones

- Maintain regular gentle exercise, which prevents loss of bone mass.
- Get outside to encourage the production of vitamin D in the skin via sunlight. This aids the absorption of calcium from the intestines.
- Drink one pint of skimmed milk daily to ensure an adequate intake of calcium.

Proving the point

Compare your own height when you get up in the morning with your height just before bed. Try to explain any differences with reference to the anatomy of joints.

Stiffening of joints

It is sometimes difficult to separate age-associated changes in the joints from mechanical strain or injury. The repetitive actions of joints due to occupation, sporting activities or strain caused by poor posture can influence the stability of joints as a person ages. Also, cold weather and inactivity during sleep cause the body's circulatory system to slow down, which can lead to a build-up of fluid at the joints, resulting in swelling or discomfort.

An age-associated joint problem is the loss of water from cartilage. The intevertebral discs, for example, contain fluid which is squeezed out by the pressure of gravity over time. This makes the joints less flexible and can cause problems with lifting and bearing heavy weight. As the discs lose water they become flatter, which also explains why a person's height diminishes with age.

Knowledge check

1. List and briefly describe the main functions of the human skeleton.
2. Describe the process of ossification.
3. Compare and contrast the two types of bone tissue.
4. List and briefly describe the different classifications of bone.
5. Name and locate the bones of the skull.
6. Name and locate the bones of the shoulder girdle.
7. Name and locate the bones of the vertebral column.
8. Name and locate the bones of the thorax.
9. Name and locate the bones of the limbs.
10. Name and locate the bones of the pelvis.
11. Name and locate the arches of the foot.
12. Draw and label a long bone.
13. Compare and contrast the three types of joints.
14. Describe the different types of synovial joints and the movements they permit.
15. Give an example in the body of each type of synovial joint.
16. Briefly describe, with examples, the different types of connective tissue, including: cartilage, tendons, aponeurosis and ligaments.
17. Describe five disorders of joints and the implications for treatment.
18. Explain the meaning of homeostasis in relation to maintenance of the skeleton.
19. Explain the physiological changes which occur in the skeleton due to ageing.
20. Provide suitable homecare advice for a mature client concerned about the effects of ageing on bones and joints.

CHAPTER 4 Muscles and the Muscular System

SECTION 2

Fascinating fact
There are over 600 individual muscles in the human body – three times the amount of bones. Each muscle has its own name and specific function, but don't panic – you won't be expected to know them all!

Link to practice
When performing treatments on the face and body, it is important to be aware of the underlying structures. Treatments such as manual massage, electrical muscle stimulation (EMS) and microcurrent depend on a good working knowledge of the muscular system in order to be effective.

The muscular system is closely related to the skeletal system, so these areas of human anatomy are sometimes linked together and referred to as the muscular–skeletal system.

The study of muscles is called **myology** and is concerned with the structure and function of muscle tissue. There are different types of muscular tissue each of which have a unique structure and function in the human body. Some types of muscle work without conscious control, such as the muscles in the heart which function automatically throughout our lifetime. Other types of muscle require conscious effort in order to function, such as the muscles in the hand, which can pick up a pen, or the muscles in the legs, which enable walking.

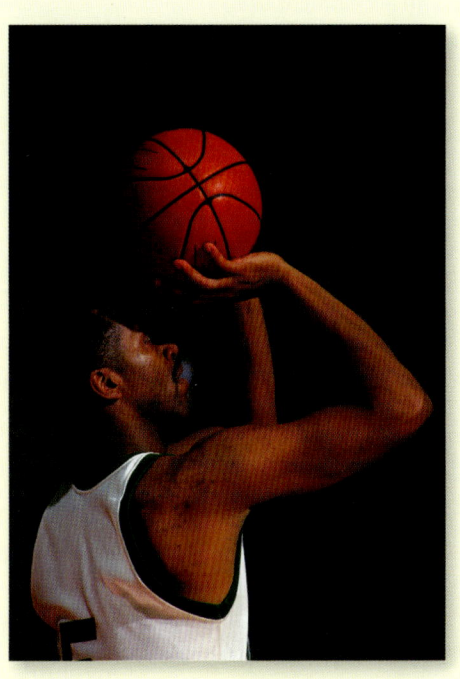

▲ An athlete playing basketball

Muscle function can be affected by different internal and external factors, such as health, body temperature and the ageing process. Because muscles work so hard they are susceptible to injury and may be prone to certain disorders. These disorders can in turn affect muscle performance and, in some cases, may prove a contra-indication to treatment.

You will learn
In this chapter you will learn about:
- types of muscles tissues: voluntary, involuntary, cardiac
- the functions and structure of voluntary muscle
- the structure and function of tendons
- chief muscles of the head and neck
- chief muscles of the shoulders
- chief muscles of the upper and lower limbs
- chief muscles of the anterior and posterior aspects of the trunk
- muscle contraction
- muscle fatigue
- variations in muscle performance
- effect of treatments on muscle performance
- diseases and disorders of muscles
- effects of ageing on the muscular system.

SECTION 2

> **Fascinating fact**
>
> In a treatment like electrical muscle stimulation (EMS) it is important to work groups of muscles with similar functions and avoid padding antagonistic muscles.

Types of muscle tissue

Muscle type	Structure	Function
Cardiac muscle	Short, striped cylindrical cells which are branched	Rhythmic beating of the heart
Involuntary muscle	Spindle-shaped smooth cells	Contracts walls of blood vessels and internal organs
Voluntary muscle	Long, striped cells	Contracts strongly when stimulated to provide voluntary movement

Cardiac muscle

Cardiac muscle is a specialist type of muscle tissue found only in the wall of the heart. The muscle cells are short, cylindrical and branched, and have a striped appearance. Individual muscle fibres are bound together by connective tissue, which allows nerve impulses to pass through them. Cardiac muscle functions without conscious effort, producing rhythmic **contractions** of the heart from before birth until the last moments of life.

Involuntary muscle

Involuntary muscle is not under conscious control – and you might not have even realised it exists until now! This type of muscle is supplied by automatic nerves (Link to The Nervous System, page 129), which means that it functions automatically to provide slow contractions over long periods of time. It is found in areas of the body where movement occurs throughout life without conscious thought. These areas include:

- the pupils of the eye which dilate and contract in response to light
- the eyelid which blinks automatically
- the internal organs such as the lungs, bladder and stomach, which expand and contract as their volume changes
- the walls of the blood vessels, which expand and contract to allow for **vasodilation** and **vasoconstriction**. When the blood vessels are constricted, blood pressure is higher as there is less space inside the vessels for blood to pass through.

Involuntary muscle cells are spindle-shaped and are bound together by connective tissue. They are smooth in appearance and therefore this type of muscle is sometimes known as smooth or unstriped (unstriated) muscle.

Voluntary muscle

When you think of muscles in the human body, you probably tend to think about those muscles you can see or feel – for example, the defined 'six pack' or sculptured limbs of a well-toned body, or the aches and pains after a hard day's work or session at the gym. These are **voluntary muscles** which are attached to bones and are sometimes called skeletal muscle. This type of muscle is under conscious control and enables movement.

Some muscles work together in groups. For example, what is commonly referred to as 'the hamstrings' is actually a group of three muscles at the back of the thigh which work in conjunction with one another. Similarly, the gluteal muscles which form the buttocks are a group of three individual muscles which overlap each other, adding to their strength and supportive function. Other muscles, instead of working together, work against each other. These are called **antagonists**. A good example of a pair of antagonistic muscles is the biceps on the inner aspect of the upper arm and the triceps on the outer aspect of the upper arm. When the biceps contracts it pulls the lower arm up towards the shoulder; the triceps has the opposite action of pulling the arm back down so that it becomes straight again. However, voluntary muscle has several other functions, which may not be controlled consciously.

The functions and structure of voluntary muscle

Functions of voluntary muscle

The functions of voluntary muscle are:
- to facilitate movement
- to maintain posture
- to maintain body temperature
- to aid venous return and lymph flow.

Facilitating movement

The most obvious function of skeletal muscle is to facilitate movement. Muscle is attached to bones via **tendons** at the point of **origin** and the point

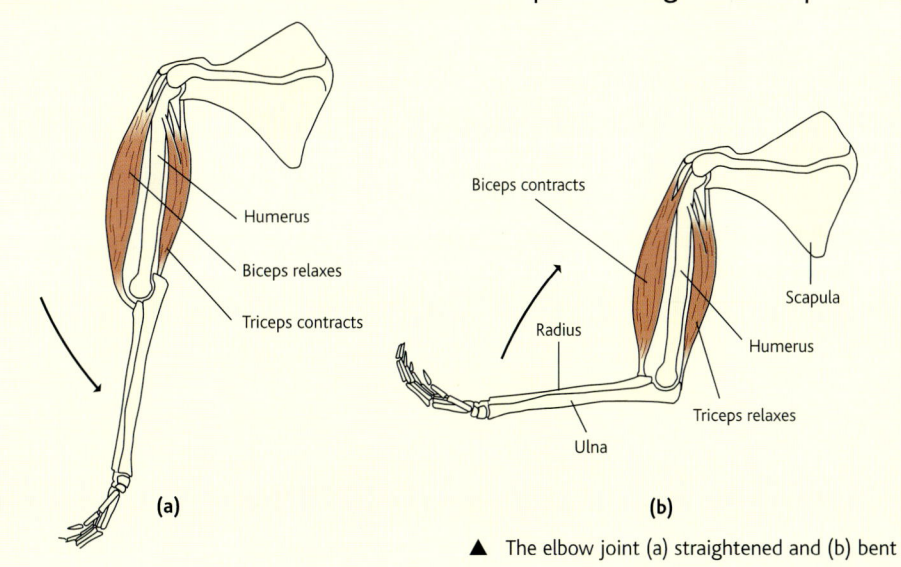

> **Fascinating fact**
> A single bone may be surrounded by up to 650 layers of muscle tissue.

> **Link to learning**
> Contraction of muscles creates skeletal movement by reducing or increasing the angle at a joint.

▲ The elbow joint (a) straightened and (b) bent

Link to practice
Posture depends on the partial contraction of certain muscles. It can be improved by relaxing certain muscle groups using massage techniques, and toning other muscle groups through exercise and weight training.

Link to practice
People who stand for long periods at a time, perhaps due to their occupation, may have weak valves in their blood vessels, causing the blood to flow back down and accumulate in the vessels, thereby stretching them. These stretched blood vessels, characterised by enlarged, bumpy blood vessels close to the skin's surface, are called **varicose veins**.

Fascinating fact
Voluntary muscle tissue is mostly water. It is composed of:
- 75 per cent water
- 20 per cent actin and myosin
- 5 per cent mineral salts, **glycogen** and fat.

of **insertion**. When a muscle contracts, the origin remains fixed while the insertion moves towards it, thus reducing the angle of the joint. For example, flexing the lower arm is achieved by contraction of the biceps muscle. The muscle becomes shorter and fatter and the insertion, near the elbow, is pulled towards the origin, near the shoulder. All skeletal movements happen in this way.

Maintaining posture
As well as enabling movement, skeletal muscle is responsible for maintaining posture, which is achieved by the same process of muscle contraction. Under normal, resting circumstances, the muscles are in a state of partial contraction which is known as **muscle tone**. If the muscles were completely relaxed all the time, the body would not be able to hold itself upright – the weight of the bones and internal organs would pull the body over! Not surprisingly, the muscles with the greatest **tonicity** in humans are found in the neck and back. Postural muscles do not require conscious effort to carry out their function, although they can be affected by bad habits and improved through training.

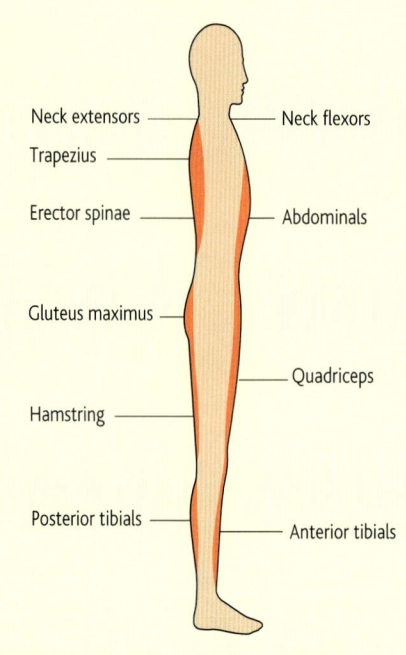

▲ The muscles of postural alignment.

Maintaining body temperature
Another action of skeletal muscle which does not require conscious effort is shivering. When the body feels cold, either because of external temperature or due to illness, the muscle contracts and relaxes very quickly to produce a shiver. This shivering action produces heat which is absorbed into the bloodstream and transported around the body to increase its temperature.

Aiding venous return and lymph flow
Skeletal muscle also plays a part in returning blood from different parts of the body to the heart, which is known as **venous return**. This is achieved by the 'milking action' of skeletal muscle surrounding blood vessels, which squeezes blood along as it contracts and relaxes. Inactivity for long periods, perhaps due to illness, can halt this milking action. The milking action of skeletal muscle also plays an important function in the movement of lymphatic fluid around the body.

CHAPTER **4** Muscles and the Muscular System

> **Link to learning**
>
> When you feel cold, a good way of warming up is to get moving. The same principle is true of an individual muscle which produces a shiver when cold.

> **Link to learning**
>
> Imagine holding an ice pop which has melted so that all the juice sits at the bottom of the bag. If you squeeze the bag the juice moves upwards and you can suck it out of the top. This illustrates the milking action of muscles and the effect it has on the flow of blood and lymph around the vessels.

> **Link to practice**
>
> Over-exertion can lead to inflammation of a tendon known as **tendonitis** or repetitive strain injury (**RSI**). Gentle massage can ease the pain and swelling but should only be administered with prior medical approval.

Structure of voluntary muscle

Muscle tissue consists of relatively large, elongated cells which have a striped appearance. Another term for this striped appearance is **striated**, which is an alternative name for voluntary muscle.

Running the length of voluntary muscle cells are filaments of two types of protein: **actin** and **myosin**, which form **fibrils** or 'little fibres'. Filaments of actin are thinner and more transparent than the thicker, darker bands of myosin, which is why muscle tissue appears to be striated. It is therefore these fibrils of protein that give muscle its characteristic striped appearance.

The fibrils are bound together either in bundles or sheets by connective tissue called fascia. This connective tissue contains collagen fibres, which give muscle its strength and elastin fibres which provide elastic properties, or 'stretchability'. (Link to Cells and Tissues, page 22) Collagen and elastin are types of protein. Within the bundles of muscle fibres there is also a rich supply of blood vessels and nerve attachments.

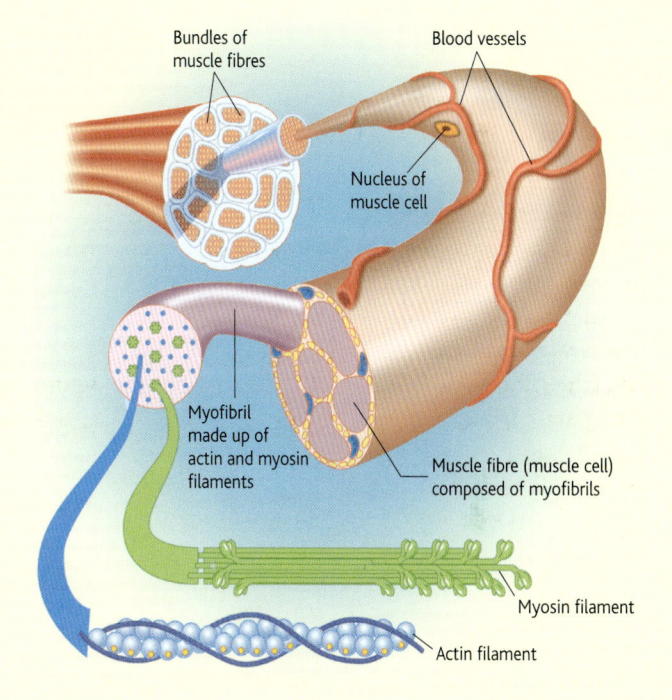

▲ The internal structure of skeletal muscle

The structure and function of tendons

Voluntary muscle is attached to the skeleton by tendons. These are like strong cords made up of thinner strands of strong collagen fibres. Tendons are connective tissue and do not stretch. The most well-known tendon is the Achilles tendon, which connects the calf muscles to the heel bone.

Where muscles attach to each other, the fibres of one muscle interlace with the fibres of the other. Some tendons are flat and these are called **aponeuroses**. An example of an aponeurosis is in the palm of the hand.

PAGE 65

SECTION 2

Proving the point

With a partner, perform each of the actions listed (in the third column of the table below) in an attempt to locate each muscle of the head and neck.

The chief muscles of the human body

Chief muscles of the head and neck

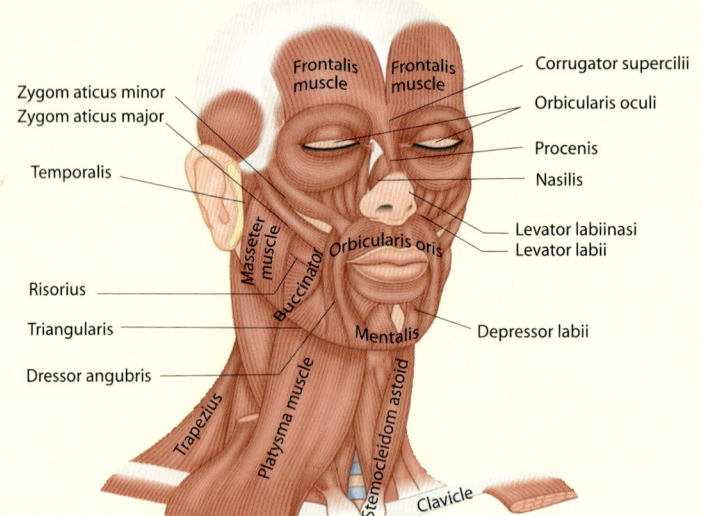

▲ Facial muscles

Link to practice

The sternocleidomastoid muscle can be damaged by whiplash, for example, following a car crash. Medical approval should be sought prior to treatment.

Link to practice

Electrical muscle stimulation (EMS) is an electrical facial treatment which artificially stimulates facial muscles in order to improve muscle tone. It relies upon the exact placement of electrodes on individual muscles.

Muscle	Position	Action
Frontalis	Covers forehead	Raises eyebrows, wrinkles forehead
Temporalis	Covers temporal bone at sides of head to jaw	Raises, retracts lower law; aids mastication
Corrugator	Inner corner of eyebrow on socket line	Draws eyebrows together
Buccinator	Angle of jaw to corner of mouth	Compresses cheeks, aids mastication
Risorius	Supports buccinator	Retracts mouth
Masseter	Fleshy part of cheeks	Raises lower jaw, aids mastication
Orbicularis oculi	Forms sphincter around eye	Closes eyelid
Zygomaticus	Covers cheek bone	Raises corners of mouth (smiley face)
Mentalis	Centre of chin	Wrinkles the chin
Orbicularis oris	Forms sphincter around mouth	Closes mouth
Sternocleidomastoid	Tendinous muscle at sides of neck	Flexion of neck
Platysma	Covers the neck	Draws down lip and jaw in yawning; wrinkles neck
Occipitalis	Covers occipital at back of head	Draws scalp backwards
Nasalis	Sides of nose	Compresses and dilates the nostrils
Triangularis	Lower corner of mouth to jaw	Draws down corners of mouth (sad face)
Digastric	Under the chin	Aids swallowing
Procerus	Bridge of nose	Wrinkles across bridge of nose

PAGE 66

CHAPTER **4** Muscles and the Muscular System

> **Case study**
> **Level 2**
> Alexis has just turned 40 years old and is worried about the visible signs of ageing. She is particularly concerned about crow's feet around the eyes, lines on the forehead and a double chin. Alexis does not like electrical treatments. Design a treatment plan for this client with specific details of massage adaptations.

> **Case study**
> **Level 3**
> Fatima has just turned 40 years old and is worried about the visible signs of ageing. She is particularly concerned about crow's feet around the eyes, lines on the forehead, naso-labial folds and a double chin. Design a treatment plan for this client with specific details for electrical muscle stimulation.

> **Proving the point**
> Design a series of facial exercises which concentrate on common client concerns such as a double chin. This could be used as a facial aftercare leaflet.

> **Link to practice**
> A dislocated shoulder will cause damage to supraspinatus. Medical approval should be obtained prior to treatment.

> **Link to practice**
> Most clients and therapists complain of aching shoulders from time to time because certain muscles are prone to being too tight (**hypertonic**). Manual massage can be of great relief when specific muscles, such as the trapezius, rhomboids and levator scapulae are manipulated.

Chief muscles of the shoulders

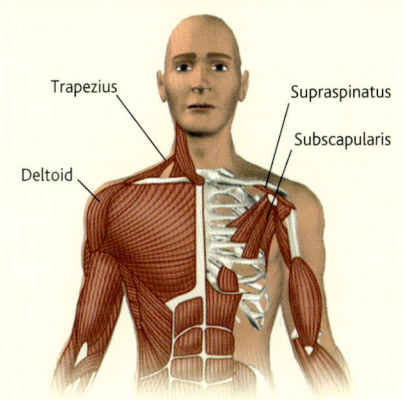

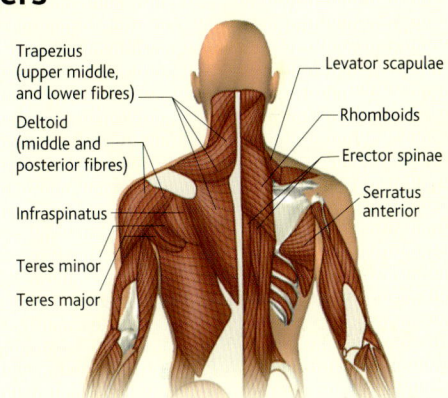

▲ Chief muscles of the shoulders

Muscle	Position	Action
Trapezius	Large triangular muscle at top of back	Elevates and braces shoulder; rotates scapula
Deltoid	Forms cap of shoulder	Abduction of shoulder
Serratus anterior	Covers sides of ribs	Stabilises shoulder; forward rotation of scapula
Rhomboids	Four-sided muscle between scapula and spine	Adducts scapula towards spine
Teres major	Small muscle between scapula and humerus	Adducts arm, rotates inwards
Teres minor	Small muscle between scapula and humerus	Rotates arm outwards
Levator scapulae	Tendonous muscle from base of skull to scapula	Elevates shoulder, rotates scapula
Subscapularis	Relatively large muscle under scapula	Inward rotation of humerus
Supraspinatus	Small muscle above scapula	Abduction of shoulder; keeps shoulder in place
Infraspinatus	Below spine of scapula	Stabilises shoulder socket; outward rotation of humerus

Chief muscles of the upper limbs

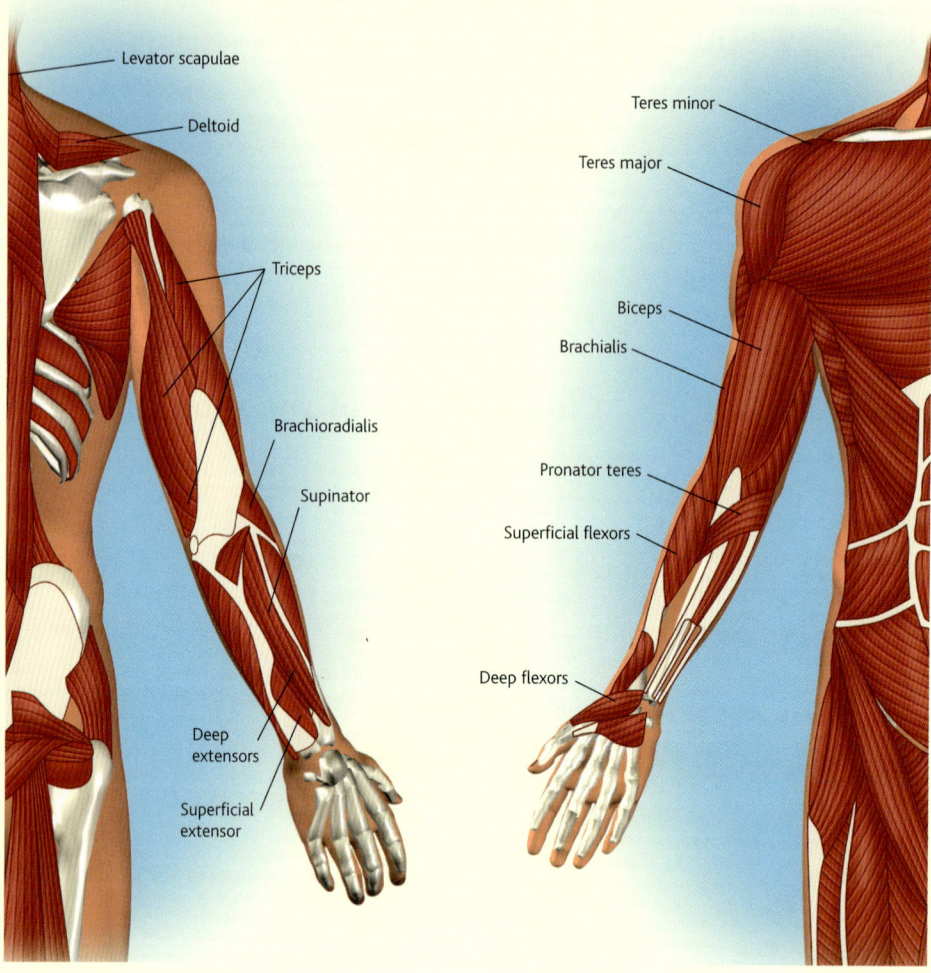

▲ Chief muscles of the arm: posterior view.

▲ Chief muscles of the arm: anterior view.

Muscle	Position	Action
Biceps	Inside of upper arm	Flexion of arm at elbow, supination of forearm
Brachialis	Deep to biceps	Flexion of arm at elbow
Triceps	Outside of upper arm	Extension of arm at elbow
Pronator teres	Crosses lower forearm	Pronates forearm and hand
Superficial extensors	Lower arm from elbow to digits	Extension of wrist and fingers
Deep extensors	Lower arm from elbow to thumb and forefinger	Extension of thumb and forefinger
Superficial flexors	Lower forearm across palm to fingers	Flexion of wrist and fingers
Deep flexors	Lower forearm across palm to fingers	Flexion of thumb and forefinger

Link to practice

If a client has difficulty gripping an object, this could indicate damage to the flexors and/or extensors, perhaps caused by falling onto the hands.

CHAPTER 4 Muscles and the Muscular System

Chief muscles of the lower limbs

Link to practice

The adductor muscles can stretch and tear if over-exerted. This is what is known as a groin strain injury, which is common in footballers.

Link to practice

Tensor fascia lata has a tendency to be over-tense (hypertonic) and therefore benefits from deep manual massage to relax the muscle fibres.

Link to practice

Walking in high heels can strain the gastrocnemius and soleus muscles. Heavy walking or jumping on hard surfaces can cause aches and pains to tibialis anterior.

Link to practice

During a figure analysis, you might notice that a client has 'knock knees' caused by a weak sartorius and biceps femoris (medial hamstring). Or you might observe 'bow legs', which are caused by a weak tensor fascia lata and semimembranosis and/or semitendinosis (lateral hamstring muscles).

▲ Chief muscles of the lower limbs: anterior view.

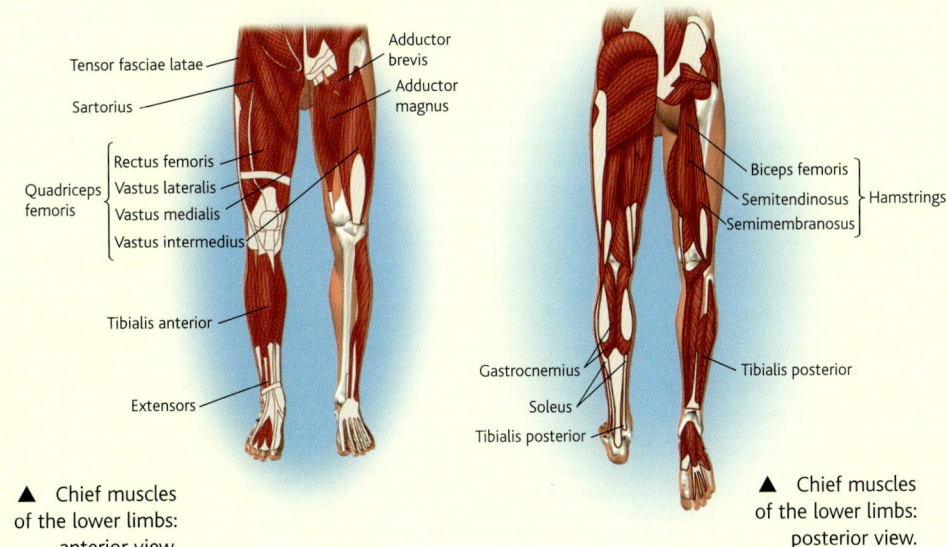

▲ Chief muscles of the lower limbs: posterior view.

Muscle	Position	Action
Hamstrings: – biceps femoris – semitendonosus – semimembranosus	Group of muscles at back of thigh	Extension of hip; flexion of knee; lateral rotation of femur when semi-flexed
Quadriceps femoris: – rectus femoris – vastus lateralis – vastus intermedius – vastus medialis	Group of muscles at front of thigh	Extension of knee and flexion of hip
Adductors	Inner thigh	Adduction; lateral rotation of femur
Tensor fasciae latae	Outer thigh	Abduction of thigh and hip; extension of knee; medial rotation of femur
Sartorius	Crosses thigh from outer hip to inside of knee	Flexion and abduction of hip; flexion of knee; lateral rotation of femur
Tibialis anterior	Front of tibia on lower leg	Dorsiflexion and supination of ankle; inversion
Tibialis posterior	Back of tibia on lower leg	Plantarflexion and inversion
Gastrocnemius	Large calf muscle	Flexion of knee; plantarflexion of ankle
Soleus	Deep to gastrocnemius	Plantarflexion

Case study

Level 3

Shakina used to be a dancer. Now aged 33 years, she is concerned about the poor muscle tone in her legs, especially the inner and outer thighs. There are also signs of cellulite. Design a treatment plan with aftercare for this client.

SECTION 2

Link to practice
Women's breast tissue is mostly fat. However, by maintaining good tone in the pectoral muscles, the breasts are better supported and less likely to droop. This helps maintain good posture and improve body shape. Exercise using a rowing machine can help to tone the pectoral muscles as well as the muscles of the upper back and arms.

Link to practice
As well as maintaining posture, abdominal muscles support the internal organs so poor muscle tone can be linked to digestive disturbances.

Link to practice
Anterior and posterior muscles work together to stabilise the trunk. A weakness in one area or the other creates imbalance, which can result in pain and injury to muscles and/or joints.

▼ Chief muscles of the chest and abdomen

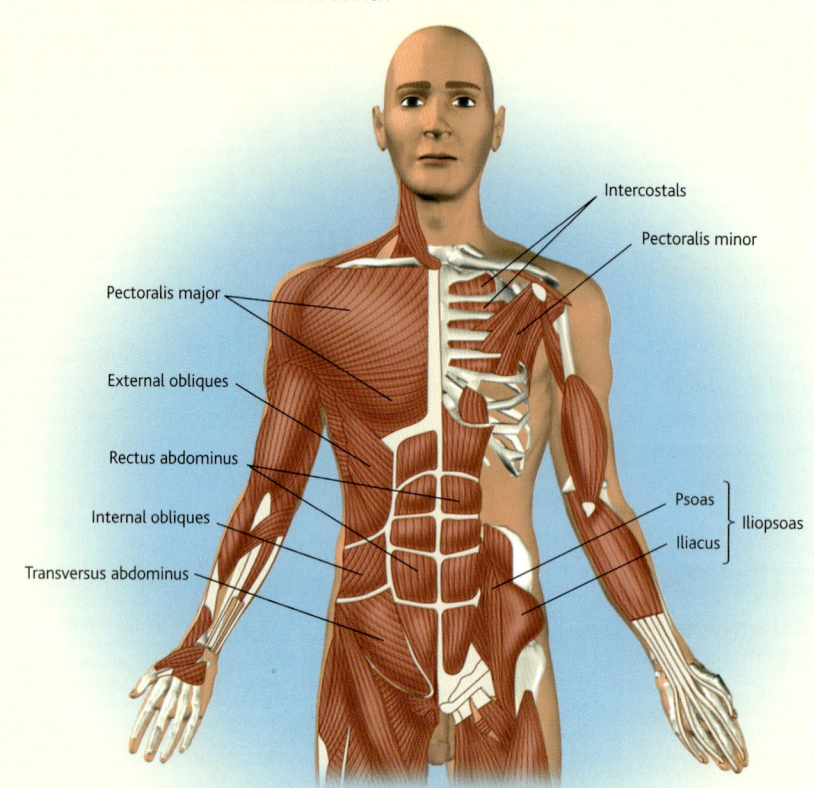

Labels: Intercostals, Pectoralis minor, Pectoralis major, External obliques, Rectus abdominus, Internal obliques, Transversus abdominus, Psoas, Iliacus, Iliopsoas

Muscle	Position	Action
Pectoralis major	Large chest muscle	Adduction, inward rotation of the arm
Pectoralis minor	Thin chest muscle, deep to pectoralis major	Depression of scapula
Diaphragm	Dome-shaped muscle beneath ribcage	Flattens to create more room in thorax during inhalation
Intercostals	In between ribs	Pulls ribs up and out during inhalation; maintains shape of thorax
Rectus abdominus	'Six-pack' muscle running down abdomen	Ventral flexion of trunk
External obliques	Forms waist by crossing with internal obliques	Flexes trunk ventrally; rotation of trunk
Internal obliques	Forms waist by crossing with external obliques	Flexes trunk ventrally; rotation of trunk
Transversus	Across the abdomen	Forced expiration; defecation; vomiting

Case study
Level 3
Emma has gone from a size 18 to a size 12 by carefully controlling her calorie intake. While Emma is delighted with the weight loss, she feels 'saggy' and comes to the salon for advice about toning treatments. Design a treatment plan with specific pad layout for EMS and suitable homecare advice.

CHAPTER 4 Muscles and the Muscular System

Chief muscles of the back and buttocks

▼ Chief muscles of the back and buttocks

Proving the point

Why are the hamstrings so often injured by footballers?

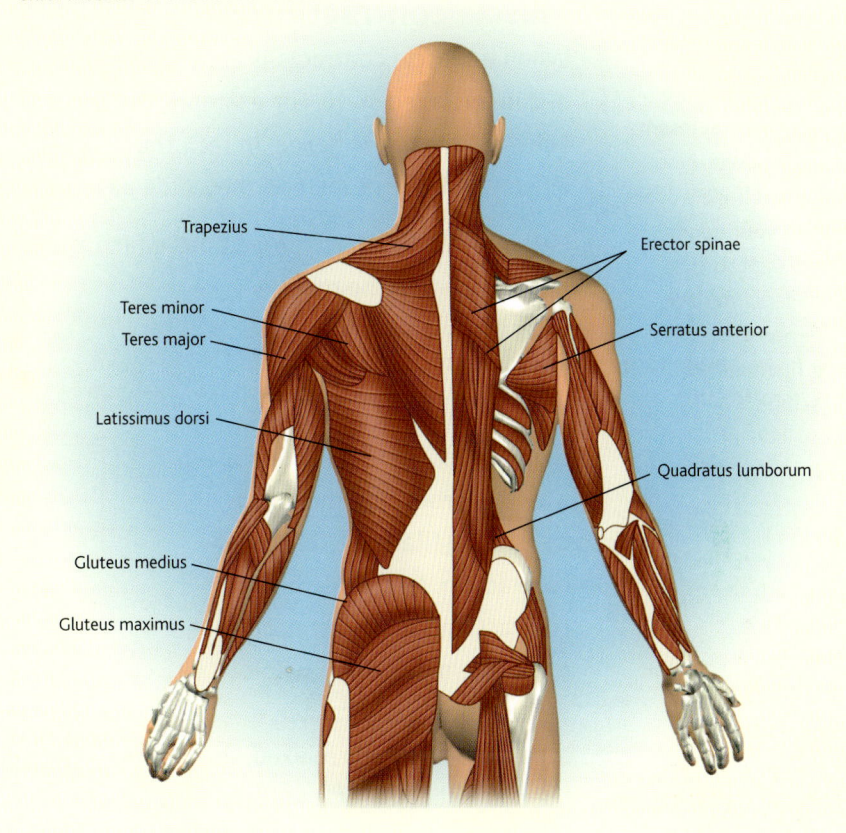

Link to practice

Problems in the lower back and hip can be the result of tension in iliopsoas (two muscles: psoas and iliacus). Clients may display either an exaggerated or reduced lumbar curve and are likely to suffer from lower back pain.

Link to practice

The gluteal muscles maintain posture and stability. Weakness can cause complaints in other areas such as the hip and/or knee joints. A weak gluteus maximus can cause excess curvature in the lumbar region (hollow back).

Muscle	Position	Action
Erector spinae	Long muscle running either side of spine	Extension of spine, lateral flexion of trunk, pulls head back, erect posture
Latissimus dorsi	Covers back of lower ribs	Adduction of arm at shoulder, depression of shoulder
Quadratus lumborum	Relatively square muscle of lower back	Extension and lateral flexion of trunk, steadies 12th rib
Iliopsoas: – psoas – iliacus	Extends from pelvis to top of femur	Flexion of hip, stabilises lower back
Gluteus maximus	Large muscle on buttocks	Adducts hip, outward rotation of thigh, extension of knee
Gluteus medius	Medium sized muscle at side of hips	Abduction and rotation of hip
Gluteus minimus	Smaller muscle deep to gluteus medius	Abduction and rotation of hip

Case study

Level 3

Thomas is a stay-at-home dad in his late thirties who looks after two boys aged 3 and 5 years. Thomas is suffering from lower back pain and pain in his right hip and leg. Design a treatment plan and homecare for this client.

PAGE 71

> **Proving the point**
>
> Place your hands flat on the table facing each other so that the two middle finger tips are touching. This represents a relaxed muscle. Now spread your fingers apart and push your hands towards each so that your fingers interlace. This demonstrates the sliding filament theory of contraction.

The actions of muscles

Muscle contraction

When a muscle contracts it appears to become shorter and fatter than when it is in a relaxed state. For example, the contracted biceps muscle appears to bulge as the arm is flexed. In fact, the filaments within a muscle do not change in length at all but instead they slide past each other.

Myosin filaments have projections which allow them to move along actin filaments when the muscle is excited by a stimulus. The filaments of actin and myosin do not change in length but slide past each other, which is why this process is known as the **sliding filament theory** of contraction. As the filaments contract and slide past each other, the muscle as a whole seems to become shorter. When the muscle is relaxed, the filaments slide apart and the muscle as a whole appears to become lengthened.

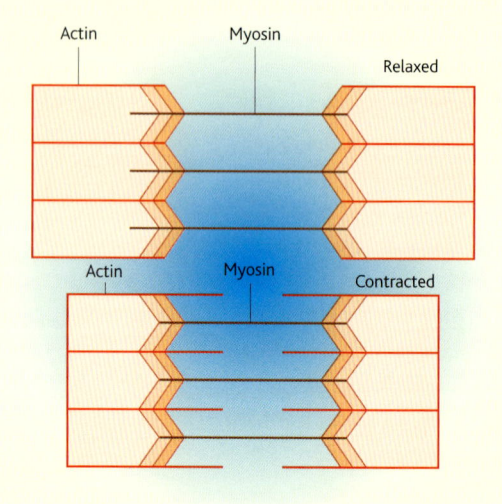

▲ The sliding filament theory of muscle contraction

Muscle fatigue

All cells and tissues require energy from food. Carbohydrates are broken down into simple sugars called **glucose** which supply the body with energy. If glucose is not immediately required it is stored in the muscles as glycogen. When glycogen mixes with oxygen it produces a compound called **adenosine** triphosphate (ATP), which is a rich energy source. ATP is released when needed to give muscles the energy required to contract.

Oxidation of glycogen also produces a by-product called pyruvic acid, which is broken down to produce more energy as well as waste products (carbon dioxide and water). During vigorous activity the body takes in more oxygen, which produces more ATP and more energy. If insufficient oxygen is available, pyurvic acid is converted to **lactic acid**, which builds up in the muscle and causes **muscle fatigue**. Fatigue is another term for tiredness and when muscles are fatigued they don't work efficiently. A fatigued muscle will feel sore and may become cramped due to a build-up of lactic acid. Over-exertion of fatigued muscles can lead to injury.

> **Link to learning**
>
> When you feel tired, you need to rest and recuperate. If you carry on working you might fall ill or have an accident. The same is true of fatigued muscles.

Variations in muscle performance

Muscles, like people, perform well in the right circumstances, but in the wrong circumstances things can go wrong. For example, if you have a busy day ahead the sensible thing to do is to make sure you precede it with a good night's sleep and then eat a healthy breakfast on waking. You will then have the energy required to perform well during the day. If, however, you stayed out until late and skipped breakfast, it is likely that you will be tired the following day, feel less prepared and perform less well. The same principles can be applied to muscles. Muscles require rest and energy in order to carry out their function. An absence of either of these can result in injury.

Muscle activity during exercise

Prior to any body workout it is important to warm up by beginning with slow, gentle movements and gradually increasing the pace. During the activity you will notice that you start to feel warmer, your cheeks might glow, and you might become short of breath. The reasons for these changes are due to contractions taking place in the muscles. Movement creates heat. Just as jumping up and down makes you feel hot, so repeated muscle contraction creates localised heat in the muscle.

As heat in the muscles is created with exercise, the skin turns red as blood is pumped faster around the body and to the surface of the skin in an effort to maintain body temperature. Similarly, heat in muscles causes increased blood circulation to the area. One of the main functions of blood is to transport oxygen and glucose to the cells to provide them with energy and to remove waste products such as carbon dioxide and water. So, increased blood supply to muscles provides them with the energy they require for contractions. During exercise it is also important to breathe deeply so as to increase the amount of oxygen being inhaled. This will ensure that enough oxygen is available for the muscles to produce ATP and the energy needed to maintain the activity (see muscle fatigue above).

Effect of treatments on muscle performance

> **Link to practice**
>
> Massage triples the blood flow to muscles which increases the supply of energy and removal of waste products. This, in turn, enhances performance.

All treatments have the effect of warming body tissues and increasing circulation of blood and lymph. As described above, these physiological changes have a positive effect on muscle performance. Massage manipulations can help to alleviate aches and pains in muscles caused by overexertion or muscular tension. This is achieved by warming the tissues, which encourages tight muscle fibres to relax and become more elastic.

It is useful to compare a manual or mechanical body treatment to an exercise routine. Just as you would not launch into a vigorous activity without a warm-up, neither should you over-stimulate muscles without proper preparation. It is important to warm the muscles with gentle manipulations, such as effleurage, before performing more stimulating techniques such as petrissage, or before administering deeply stimulating mechanical treatments such as gyratory massage.

> **Link to practice**
>
> A specialist area of treatment is sports massage. This is useful prior to activity to prepare muscles for action and improve performance. Post-event massage can reduce the effects of muscle fatigue. 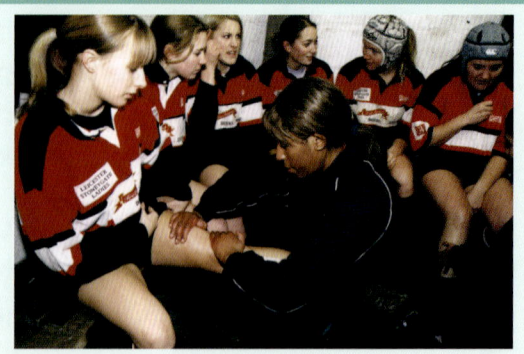
>
> ▶ Massaging the quadriceps in a crowded changing room

> **Case study**
>
> **Level 3**
>
> Samir is a teacher aged 30 years old. He keeps fit by running three times a week and plays football for his local team. Devise a treatment plan to improve Samir's performance and reduce the risk of injury.

Muscular diseases and disorders

Muscle disorders

Poorly trained muscles, wear and tear, over-exertion and injury can result in muscular disorders.

- One of the most common disorders is torn muscle, which is caused by sudden movement or over-exertion. Over-exertion of the thigh during a game of football can lead to a torn hamstring muscle, which can put a footballer out of action for some time. With sufficient rest, the muscle fibres will eventually heal themselves.
- **Sprains** are injuries to ligaments or muscles in the locality of a joint which occur when the joint is over-stretched. A sprain causes localised pain and swelling and should be rested. A good example again comes from football: the adductor muscles of the inner thigh can suffer a sprain if over-exerted. This is what is known as a groin strain.
- Excess muscular tension can lead to postural imbalances, usually resulting in pain and/or restricted movement.
- Muscular tension can also put pressure on nerves. Sciatica is the name of a common nervous disorder whereby the sciatic nerve is irritated causing pain in the lower back and leg. (Link to The Nervous System, page 133)

CHAPTER 4 Muscles and the Muscular System

> **Link to practice**
>
> Massage can be beneficial for the treatment of muscular disorders. However, it is important that the client seeks medical approval prior to treatment to rule out the risk of causing further harm. In some cases it may also be necessary to refer the client to a specialist, such as a physiotherapist or sports masseur.

Muscular diseases

- Multiple sclerosis (MS) is a **degenerative** disease of the nervous system which can affect mobility, speech or vision (Link to The Nervous System, page 133). It is the most common disabling **neurological** disease among young adults and affects around 85,000 people in the UK.
- Parkinson's disease is a degenerative disease less associated with age. (Link to The Nervous System, page 133) It is caused by a fault with the **neurotransmitters** which control movement. Individuals with this disorder suffer from muscular tremors or rigidity and a lack of facial expression.
- Motor neurone disease (MND) is a degenerative disease associated with middle age and the cause is unknown. It results in paralysis of nerves and muscles in the body and can be fatal.
- Cerebral palsy (CP) is a **congenital** disorder of the brain. Symptoms include a loss of muscle control and spasm.

Effects of ageing on the muscular system

Like all of the body's systems, the muscular system slows down with age. And without due care and attention, the body is more prone to disorders affecting the muscles.

Posture

Healthy people with a positive mental attitude tend to have good posture whatever their age. However, there are certain changes associated with age which can affect a person's posture, such as bone shrinkage and flattened cartilage in the vertebral column. Whilst this reduces height, slouching reduces height further and can make a person look older or less healthy than he or she really is. In other words, slouching can have an ageing affect on a person.

The chief muscles responsible for maintaining posture, and the effects of both good and poor muscle tone on posture, are described below.

> **Link to practice**
>
> It is possible to learn specialist remedial techniques to treat conditions such as sciatica and sports injuries. However, you must only perform such techniques if you are properly qualified to do so.

Postural muscle	Good muscle tone	Poor muscle tone
Erector spinae	Maintains upright position of the head; lengthens neck and spine	Slouching and decreases overall appearance of height
Trapezius	Pulls the head upright and the shoulders back	Rounded shoulders, humped back and drooping breasts
Rectus abdominus	Supports the trunk; acts as an antagonist to the muscles of the back	Protruding abdomen, lower back pain
Gluteals	Maintains upright posture of the trunk	Loss of firmness, lower back pain

Lifestyle factors

Lifestyle factors contribute to the maintenance of good muscle tone and the quality of a person's posture. These are often habits formed over a lifetime

> **Fascinating fact**
>
> All kinds of habits can affect posture, even the position you sleep in. Sleeping on your front on a soft bed can cause an exaggerated curve of the lower back, known as the **lumbar** curve.

PAGE 75

due to a person's occupation, weight or self-esteem, for example. They include how a person sits or stands at work, and how much exercise a person does; the quality of a person's diet.

> **Link to practice**
>
> - The best thing a person can do to look after their muscles is to use them regularly, which helps to maintain good muscle tone and keep them working effectively. Keeping fit and active maintains the strength and tonicity of the muscles responsible for good posture at any age, while long periods of inactivity cause them to become lazy and ineffective. It is important to advise clients to use their muscles in order to maintain good posture, which can take off or add years to a person's appearance.
> - It is also important to eat a healthy diet, to supply the muscles with the energy they need for contraction.
> - It is important to maintain a steady weight which is appropriate for your height, as any extra weight carried on the abdomen or buttocks puts a strain on the back muscles.

Case study

All levels

Donald is approaching 65 years and wants to make sure he stays fit and active during his retirement. What advice could you give to help him achieve this?

> **Knowledge check**
>
> 1. Describe briefly the structure and function of cardiac muscle tissue.
> 2. Describe briefly the structure and function of involuntary muscle tissue.
> 3. Describe briefly the structure and function of voluntary muscle tissue.
> 4. List the chief components of muscle tissue.
> 5. Name the two proteins in voluntary muscle.
> 6. Name the four main functions of skeletal muscle.
> 7. Explain what happens to the origin and insertion of a muscle during movement.
> 8. Describe muscle tone.
> 9. Name the two proteins in connective tissues.
> 10. Describe the sliding filament theory of muscle contraction.
> 11. Describe muscle fatigue.
> 12. Describe the physiological effects of manual massage treatment on muscles.
> 13. Explain how massage can reduce 'knots' and tension in muscles.
> 14. Name the chief postural muscles.
> 15. Describe the effects of ageing on the muscular system.
> 16. Name and describe three common disorders which can affect muscles.
> 17. Name the facial muscle responsible for each of the following:
>   a) crow's feet
>   b) lines on the forehead
>   c) double chin
>   d) frown lines.
> 18. Name the muscles likely to be responsible for shoulder tension.
> 19. Name the muscles responsible for the following postural complaints:
>   a) knock knees
>   b) bow legs
>   c) hollow back
>   d) hump back.
> 20. Name the muscles which form the following body parts:
>   a) the calf
>   b) the waist
>   c) a 'six pack'
>   d) the buttocks.

SECTION 2

CHAPTER 5 The Blood Circulatory System

Link to practice

The circulatory system is important to therapists for several reasons. Treatments and massage:

- Bring fresh blood containing oxygen and nutrients to the area being treated, helping with growth, maintenance and repair of body tissues. The extra oxygen and nutrients improve the look and texture of the skin, and improve the efficiency of muscles whilst helping to maintain them in the best possible state of nutrition.
- Assist with the removal of waste products from the area being treated (see page 86). This helps muscles to recover after exercise, reducing muscle fatigue and inducing relaxation.
- Cause blood vessels to **dilate**. **Erythema** occurs and warmth is produced, which helps to relax the client.

The blood vascular system consists of the **blood**, the blood vessels and the **heart**. This system is also known as the **blood circulatory system** because it circulates the blood around the body within vessels with the aid of a pump – the heart.

The circulatory system is responsible for transporting oxygen to the body's tissues and removing carbon dioxide to be excreted via the lungs. Thus the circulatory system is very closely related to the respiratory system (Link to The Respiratory System, page 111). Another system which is also closely related is the lymphatic system (Link to The Lymphatic System, page 99). A job of the lymphatic system is to return excess fluid in the tissues of the body back to the blood and with the blood defends the body against infection and disease.

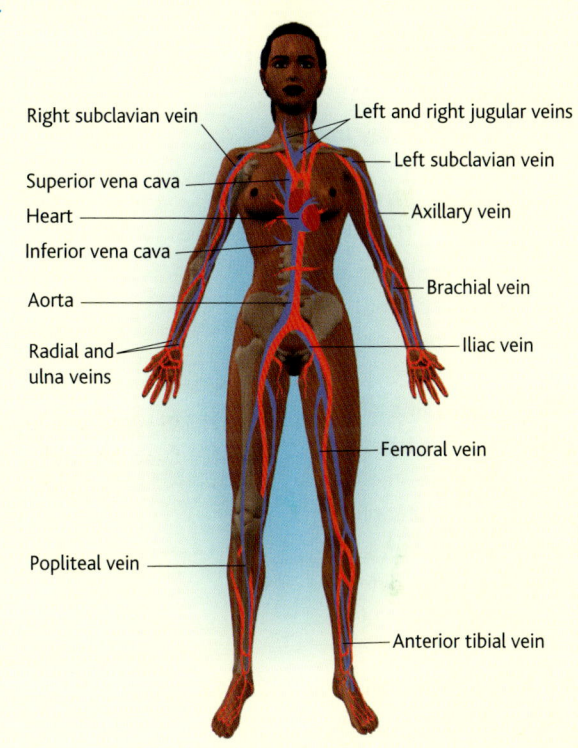

▲ The blood circulatory system and the major veins of the body

You will learn

In this chapter you will learn about:
- the functions of the circulatory system
- the composition of blood
- the types and functions of blood cells
- the structure and function of blood vessels
- the circulation
- the heart
- pulse rate and blood pressure
- diseases and disorders of the blood circulatory system
- ageing and the blood circulatory system.

SECTION 2

Link to learning
Remembering the functions of the blood can be made easier using the mnemonic, *Old Charlie Foster Hates Wild Women Having Double Chins.*
Use the first letter of each word to jog your memory and recall the functions of blood:

O – Oxygen transport (to the tissues)
C – Carbon dioxide transport (away from the tissues)
F – Food transport (to the tissues)
H – Heat regulation and transport
W – Water regulation and transport
W – Waste removal
H – Hormone transport
D – Defence of the body through white blood cells
C – Clotting to defend and prevent fluid loss.

Learn this mnemonic then try it out in pairs.

The functions of the circulatory system
Functions of blood
The three main functions of blood are regulation, transport and protection.

Regulation of:	Transport of:	Protection from:
• water (the amount circulating the body) • heat distribution around the body.	• nutrients • oxygen • water • hormones • heat • enzymes • waste products.	• infection and disease through white blood cells • blood and fluid loss through clotting.

Contents of plasma:
- Transports waste products from the cells to kidneys, lungs and sweat glands for excretion
- Transports hormones from the endocrine glands to the cells
- Transports enzymes to the appropriate cells
- Transports oxygen from the lungs to the cells of the body
- Transports carbon dioxide from the cells to the lungs
- Helps in the regulation of body temperature
- Regulates the water content of cells
- Transports white corpuscles to the source of infection, helping to protect the body against foreign substances
- Prevents fluid loss because of the clotting mechanism
- Transports nutrients from the digestive tract to the cells of the body

▲ The functions of blood

Regulation
Water regulation
The water content of the body has to be maintained within certain limits. This is achieved in two ways:
- The hypothalamus gland, situated in the brain, monitors the amount of fluid circulating in the blood and produces anti-diuretic hormone (ADH), which is secreted by the pituitary gland and sent to the kidneys. (Link to The Endocrine System, page 137) Blood passing through the kidneys is filtered and water levels in the blood are adjusted. Too much water and the kidneys pass the excess to the bladder for excretion. (Link to The Excretory and Urinary System, page 171) If fluid levels are normal or low, water is retained and passed back into the blood.

- If the hypothalamus detects that the fluid levels are too low, the thirst centre is stimulated in the brain, which gives rise to the feeling of thirst and the desire to drink.

Heat regulation

The blood is responsible for distributing heat around the body. The main organ which produces heat in the body is the liver, since many heat-producing metabolic processes are carried out there. As the blood circulates through the liver, it picks up the heat and then transports it around the rest of the body.

The blood vessels are also responsible for maintaining body temperature.
- When in a cool or cold climate, the blood vessels near the skin's surface **constrict** and divert blood away from the skin and extremities to the core of the body, to supply heat to the vital organs. (Link to The Skin, Hair and Nails, page 33) This explains why the fingers and toes are the first body parts to go cold – the body can survive without fingers and toes, but not without vital organs. In prolonged freezing conditions, fingers and toes can be lost to frostbite: this is when extreme cold causes damage to the skin and underlying tissues; it can result in amputation of the affected area.
- When the body is heated, as in a sauna or when in a hot climate, the blood vessels near to the skin's surface dilate so that more blood circulates to the outer areas of the body. This allows more heat from the body to escape through the skin into the air. This is why the skin goes red when you are hot.

Transport

The blood is responsible for transporting:
- substances that the body needs; oxygen, food, water, hormones and enzymes to the body's cells and tissues
- waste products from the cells and tissues to the lungs and kidneys to be excreted; these include carbon dioxide and toxins
- heat around the body.

Protection

Defence

The body has several defence mechanisms against invasion, and the blood assists with this.
- White blood cells attack, ingest and produce substances to kill invading bacteria, and this protects the body from disease. The body also builds up immunity (either naturally or through vaccination) by being subjected to small quantities of invading organisms.
- **Platelets** activate the clotting process when the skin is broken. The forming clots scab over and prevent bacteria from entering the body via the skin. Clotting also stops vital body fluids from being lost from the body.

Fascinating fact

The body contains around 5–6 litres (9–11 pints) of blood. The amount taken during blood donation is 300 ml (half a pint). Although the body can lose this amount and make up the missing red blood cells easily, it can leave the donor feeling light-headed and weak until the deficit is made up. About a litre (2 pints) of blood could be lost before the need for a blood transfusion (receiving another person's donated blood).

SECTION 2

> **Fascinating fact**
>
> The pH of blood is 7.4. It is vital for the blood to maintain this pH level. If the blood pH falls, it becomes too acidic (a condition known as acidosis); if the blood pH rises, it becomes too alkaline (a condition known as alkalosis). (Link to Cells and Tissues, page 27)

The composition and function of blood

Although blood appears as a fluid it is actually composed of solid parts held in a solution of fluid (**plasma**) and is classified as a connective tissue (Link to Cells and Tissues, page 23). Blood appears as a fluid because the solid parts are so tiny that they cannot be seen with the naked eye.

The solid elements in blood include:
- red blood cells (erythrocytes)
- white blood cells (leucocytes)
- platelets 'clotting particles'.

These elements make up about 45 per cent of blood. The other 55 per cent is blood plasma, a pale yellow fluid that is the liquid part of blood. Blood cells are also known as corpuscles.

55% Plasma

45% Blood cells

▲ The structure of blood

Blood corpuscles

Red blood cells (erythrocytes)	Carry oxygen and carbon dioxide
White blood cells (leucocytes)	Defend the body against invasion and infection. They include: • granulocytes (75%) eat or ingest invaders: • neutrophils • eosinophils • basophils • **lymphocytes** (20%) provide immunity: • B-cells • T-cells • monocytes (5%) eat or ingest invaders.
Platelets	Allow clotting and prevent blood loss

> **Fascinating fact**
>
> In childhood most bones are involved in the production of red blood cells. As we age, the areas which are no longer used to manufacture red blood cells are known as yellow marrow, and the actively producing areas are red bone marrow. The rates at which blood cells are formed and die are roughly equal. This means that you should have roughly the same amount of blood circulating in your body at any one time.

All blood cells originate and mature in the bone marrow (the sponge-like material in the cavities of bone). They begin in **stem cells** and then differentiate into the red cells, white cells and platelets.

Blood plasma

Plasma is a vital part of blood since it is the fluid in which all the important matter is transported. It is a pale yellow colour and consists mainly of water (90 per cent), but contains many other substances, crucial to health. These include:
- proteins, fats, glucose, vitamins and minerals
- salts
- waste products

> **Proving the point**
>
> Where else have you heard of stem cells?

CHAPTER 5 The Blood Circulatory System

> **Fascinating fact**
>
> Stem cells are primitive cells which have the ability to continuously divide and develop into other types of cells and tissues. The tissue or cell which each stem cell eventually becomes is dependant on the environment and chemicals it comes into contact with.

- gases
- hormones
- enzymes
- antibodies and antitoxins.

The types and functions of blood cells

Red blood cells

Red blood cells (Erythrocytes) are minute cells – there are more red blood cells than any other type of blood cell. Their job is to transport oxygen from the lungs to the tissues of the body and remove carbon dioxide from the tissues to be excreted by the lungs.

Red blood cells are biconcave discs, meaning they have a hollowed-out centre on each side of the disc. They are very flexible, can change shape and can squeeze through the tiniest of blood vessels. They contain a special substance called **haemoglobin**, which gives the cell its red colour. The job of haemoglobin is to carry large amounts of oxygen.

> **Fascinating fact**
>
> There are over 200 detectable components of human blood.

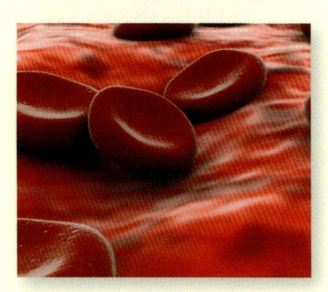

The life of a red blood cell

Red blood cells are made in the red bone marrow of the spongy bone of the sternum, the vertebrae, the pelvis, ribs, and parts of the humerus and femur (Link to The Skeletal System, page 50). During the production of a red blood cell, the cell nucleus is lost, so a red blood cell does not have the ability to reproduce. Erythrocytes live for about 120 days and are then ingested by the liver and spleen, where most of the iron in the haemoglobin is removed and reused. Other parts of the haemoglobin (the pigments) are converted into bile pigments and are excreted by the body.

▲ Red blood cells seen under an electron microscope

> **Link to practice**
>
> Research has shown that massage can improve the oxygen-carrying capacity of red blood cells. This means that more oxygen is available for all the body's tissues to use, which helps to improve the functioning of cells throughout the body.

> **Fascinating fact**
>
> Men have more red blood cells (5–6 million per cubic mm of blood) than women (4–5 million per cubic mm of blood). People who live in areas of high altitude, where there is less oxygen in the air, have about 8 million per cubic mm of blood.

White blood cells

White blood cells (leucocytes) are concerned with defending the body. There are several different types and they each have a specific role in protecting the body from invasion from micro-organisms and preventing disease.

Classification of leucocytes

Leucocytes are classified according to whether or not they have a granular appearance under the microscope.

- Those with granules are known as granulocytes, of which there are three types:

PAGE 81

SECTION 2

> **Fascinating fact**
> It takes approximately seven days to make a red blood cell, and approximately two million are formed every second.

- neutrophils
- basophils
- eosinophils.
- Those without a granular appearance are known as agranular (without granules), of which there are two types:
  - lymphocytes
  - monocytes.

Classification of granulocytes

Granulocytes		Function
Neutrophils	Neutrophill	Neutrophils in the blood squeeze through the capillary walls and move into infected tissue. They kill invaders such as bacteria; they then eat the remnants.
Basophils	Basophill	The number of basophils increases during times of infection in the body. Basophils leave the blood and accumulate at the site of infection or where they are needed. They release substances such as **histamine**, which increases the blood flow to the area.
Eosinophils	Eosinophill	The number of eosinophils in the blood is normally quite low. However, numbers increase sharply if certain diseases are present, such as asthma, eczema or parasitic infections. Eosinophils are toxic to cells (cytotoxic); they release substances to attack invader cells.

> **Fascinating fact**
> If red blood cells did not contain haemoglobin, they would still be able to carry oxygen but not nearly as much. Haemoglobin carries 100 times more oxygen! Reduced levels of haemoglobin results in the condition known as anaemia (see also page 94).

Classification of agranular leucocytes

Agranular leucocytes		Function
Lymphocytes	Lymphocyte	There are several kinds of lymphocytes, each with different functions to perform. The most common types of lymphocytes are: • *B-cells*: these are responsible for making antibodies • *T-cells*: these are concerned with defending the body from viruses and other types of infection.

> **Fascinating fact**
> For every 1 white blood cell there are 40 platelets and 600 red blood cells. This means that in 1 cubic mm of blood there are:
> - 4,000 to 11,000 leucocytes
> - 150,000 to 400,000 platelets
> - 5,000,000 erythrocytes.

> **Link to practice**
>
> Studies show that massage increases cytotoxic capacity (the activity level of the body's natural killer cells). This means that regular massage can help to strengthen a client's immunity.

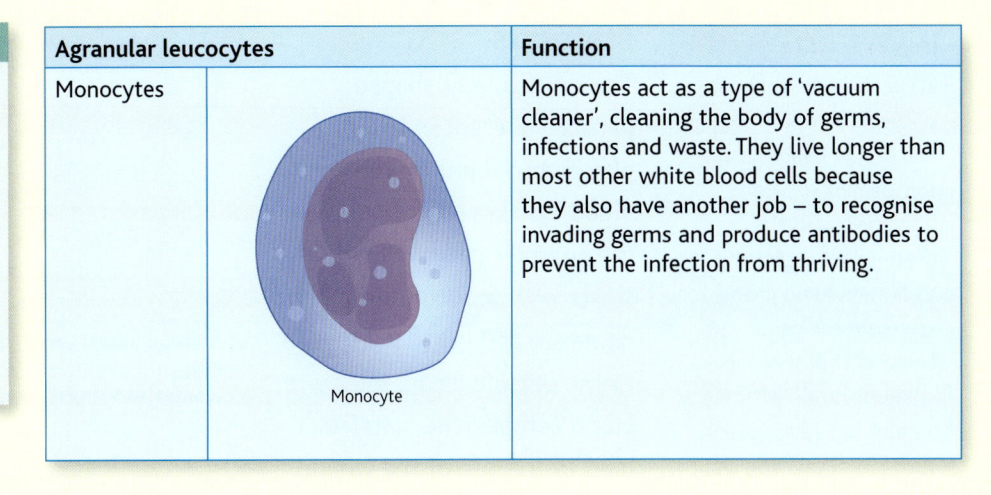

Agranular leucocytes		Function
Monocytes	Monocyte	Monocytes act as a type of 'vacuum cleaner', cleaning the body of germs, infections and waste. They live longer than most other white blood cells because they also have another job – to recognise invading germs and produce antibodies to prevent the infection from thriving.

Immunity

Some leucocytes produce **antibodies**. These are chemicals which attach to substances that do not belong in the body, such as toxins or disease-causing bacteria. **Antigens** are substances which cause the body to produce antibodies. Once a foreign substance has been in contact with the blood, white blood cells remember the antibody needed to defend against it. This means that the next time the body comes into contact with the substance, the necessary antibodies are produced quickly in large quantities. This is how the body develops **immunity** to disease and how vaccinations provide immunization. During a vaccination, a tiny amount of the disease-causing organism is injected into the blood. The amount is small enough that the person receiving it will not fall ill, but is sufficient to enable the body to develop resistance to it.

The life of a white blood cell

Most white blood cells are made in the bone marrow. T-cells then travel to the thymus gland to mature (which is why they are known as T-cells), whilst B-cells mature in the bone marrow.

When a granulocyte is released into the blood, it remains there for approximately four to eight hours. It will then migrate into the tissues of the body, where it remains for about four to five days. If there is an infection present, this process is speeded up.

Monocytes stay in the blood usually for 10 to 20 hours and then migrate into the tissues. Here they become tissue macrophages and will live for a few months to several years. Lymphocytes pass back and forward between lymphatic tissue, lymph fluid and blood. When they are in the blood, they stay for several hours. Lymphocytes can live for weeks, months or years.

SECTION 2

> **Link to practice**
>
> With some treatments, particularly reflexology and Indian head massage, self-healing is often discussed with the client when explaining treatments and giving aftercare advice.
> Some clients may feel uncomfortable with the idea of self-healing. In such situations you can use the example of a cut healing – from bleeding to clot to scab to raw scar to complete skin. This provides a good example of the body self-healing.

Platelets

These irregularly-shaped particles present in blood play a crucial part in the blood clotting process. This is a complex process which starts when a blood vessel is damaged and blood is exposed to the outside air. As the blood escapes, the platelets bind to the site of the wound and then to each other. At the same time, substances are released to form a network of fibres, and this forms a plug to prevent further blood loss. On the skin's surface, this process is seen as a scab.

▶ How a cut normally heals

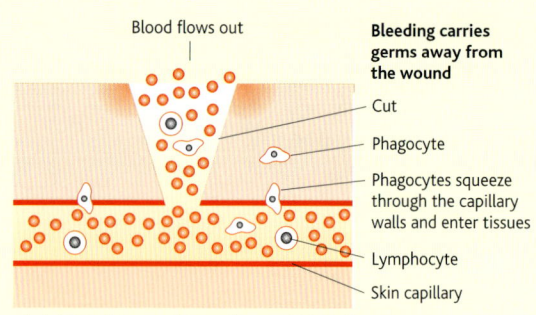

a) A blood vessel breaks and blood escapes. Platelets bind to the rough edges of the wound, forming a temporary plug.

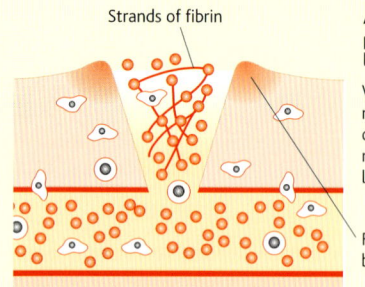

- Blood flows out
- Bleeding carries germs away from the wound
- Cut
- Phagocyte
- Phagocytes squeeze through the capillary walls and enter tissues
- Lymphocyte
- Skin capillary

b) Substances are released to form a network of fibres, and this forms a clot (plug) to prevent further blood loss.

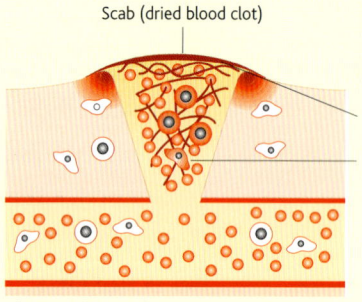

- Strands of fibrin
- A blood clot forms preventing further loss of blood
- White blood cells release histamine which causes vasodilation and makes the blood vessels leaky
- Fluid leaks out of the blood causing swelling

c) The blood clot dries and a scab forms. White blood cells clear away germs and dirt as the skin repairs itself. After several days, the scab falls off.

- Scab (dried blood clot)
- Pressure on the nerve endings causes pain and makes the area sensitive
- Blood clot
- Phagocytes engulf the germs and pus starts to collect
- Lymphocytes join in the defence

> **Fascinating fact**
>
> There are 100,000 km (60,000 miles) of blood vessels in an adult's body.

The structure and function of blood vessels

Blood is transported around the body in vessels. **Arteries** are the largest blood vessels. They connect to smaller **arterioles**, which connect to the tiniest of all the vessels – **capillaries**. Capillaries then connect to **venules**, which are smaller versions of **veins**. Arteries, arterioles, venules and veins all have the ability to dilate and constrict (open and close).

Arteries

Arteries take blood away from the heart to be delivered around the body. They have thick, muscular walls and lots of elastic tissue. They are constructed in this way because blood is under pressure leaving the heart, so the arterial walls

CHAPTER **5** The Blood Circulatory System

> **Fascinating fact**
> Macrophage literally means 'big eater' and is a monocyte that, true to its name, develops into a cell which ingests **pathogens** and cell debris.

have to be able to withstand this pressure. They must also expand to take the volume of blood, which pushes the walls of the artery outwards. The walls then constrict inwards to force the blood through the artery – it is this dilation and constriction process which creates the **pulse** of the blood in the arteries (see also page 89).

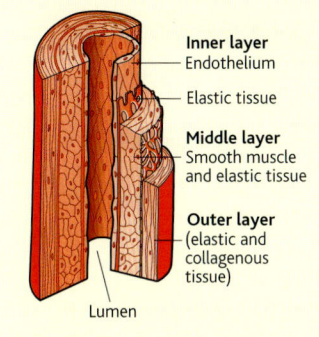

Arterioles

These are smaller versions of arteries and they connect arteries to capillaries. They have a special feature: they contain circular or sphincter muscles which allow the vessel to constrict and stop blood flow to certain areas of the body when it is not required (see also page 93).

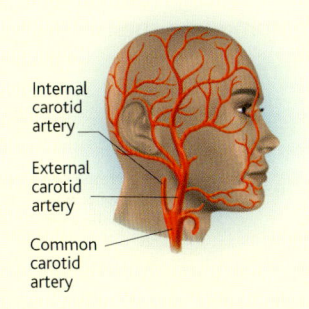

▲ The structure of an artery

Inner layer – Endothelium, Elastic tissue
Middle layer – Smooth muscle and elastic tissue
Outer layer – (elastic and collagenous tissue)
Lumen

▲ Arteries of the head and neck.

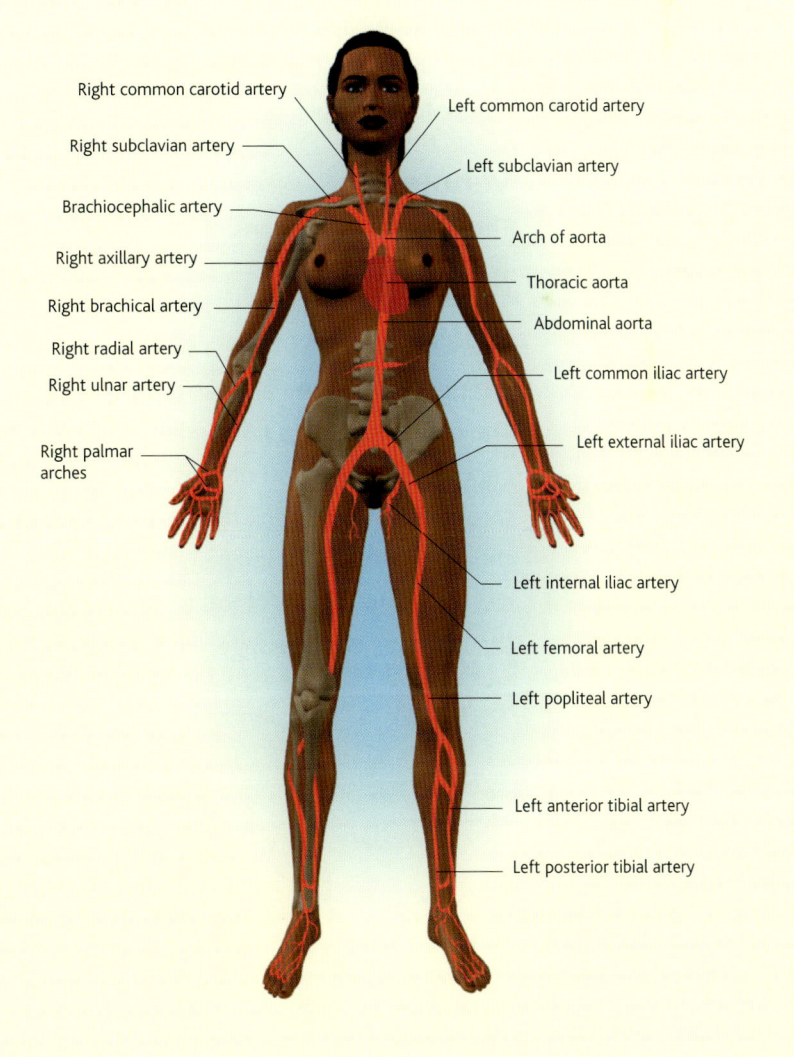

- Internal carotid artery
- External carotid artery
- Common carotid artery

▲ Veins of the head and neck.

- External jugular vein
- Internal jugular vein

▲ The major arteries of the body

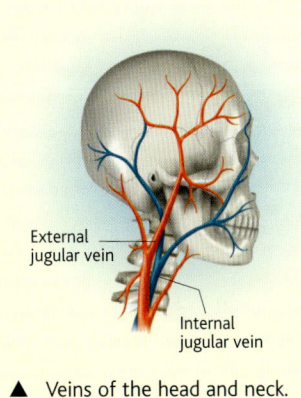

- Right common carotid artery
- Right subclavian artery
- Brachiocephalic artery
- Right axillary artery
- Right brachical artery
- Right radial artery
- Right ulnar artery
- Right palmar arches
- Left common carotid artery
- Left subclavian artery
- Arch of aorta
- Thoracic aorta
- Abdominal aorta
- Left common iliac artery
- Left external iliac artery
- Left internal iliac artery
- Left femoral artery
- Left popliteal artery
- Left anterior tibial artery
- Left posterior tibial artery

PAGE 85

SECTION 2

Link to practice

'Spider veins' are not actually veins, but are damaged capillaries.

Capillaries

These are the tiniest vessels within the blood circulatory system. They are microscopic – the walls are just one cell thick. The walls need to be this thin to allow for capillary exchange (see also page 87). This is when substances in the blood, such as nutrients and oxygen, pass through the capillary wall to reach the body's cells and tissues, and waste products in the cells and tissues, such as carbon dioxide, pass back to the blood for removal via the lungs or kidneys.

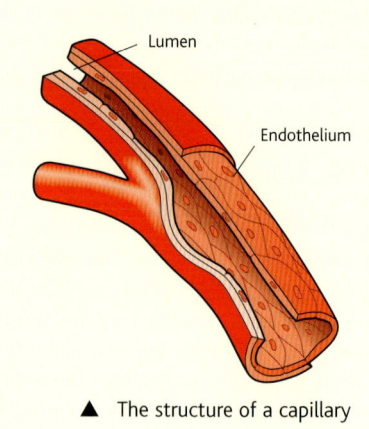

▲ The structure of a capillary

Fascinating fact

Capillaries are so small that you would need the width of ten of them to equal the thickness of one human hair. If you joined up all the capillaries in your body, they would reach round the world two and a half times.

Every capillary has an **arterial** end, which has come from an artery, and a **venous** end, which connects up to a vein. The pressure of the blood flowing through the capillary changes from higher at the arterial end to much lower at the venous end. Capillaries can dilate or constrict to accommodate the body's needs; for example, providing more oxygen to muscles during exercise.

Venules

These are small versions of veins, which connect capillaries to veins.

Veins

These blood vessels have a similar structure to arteries but they differ from arteries in that they are narrower, have less muscular tissue and contain valves. The blood in veins is not under pressure and valves prevent the blood flowing backwards. The action of muscles contracting and relaxing forces the blood up through the veins (Link to Muscles and the Muscular System, page 64). Gravity can also help venous blood to return to the heart, as can massage.

Link to practice

When performing skin analysis and other treatments, you might refer to 'split capillaries'. These are capillaries which have broken away from the main circulatory system, usually as a result of damage to the area. They can be caused by knocks to the area, tight clothing (particularly elasticated stocking tops), sun damage, and squeezing pustules and comedomes.

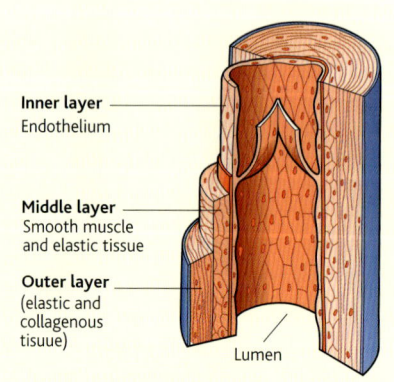

▲ The structure of a vein

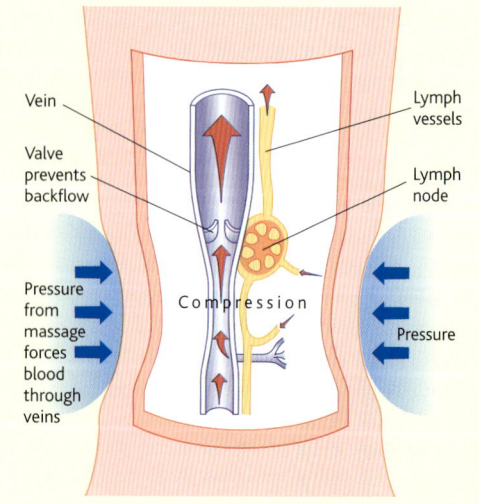

▲ Massage assists blood flow back to the heart (venous return), helping with removal of waste products from the body

Capillary exchange

As the blood flows through the arteries, they branch off into smaller arterioles, which eventually branch off into capillaries. The capillaries form a dense network around the tissues of the body. It is at this level that oxygen and substances such as nutrients, hormones and white blood cells, pass through the thin walls of the capillary into the fluid which bathes the tissues' cells. The cells use the oxygen and nutrients (metabolism) and produce waste products as a result. These waste products pass back through the cell wall and back into the blood stream. Some substances (fluid, white blood cells and waste) remain in the surrounding tissue fluid, where they are removed by the lymphatic capillaries and returned to the blood later on. (Link to The Lymphatic System, page 100)

▲ Capillary exchange

Water, food and oxygen can pass from the blood to get to the cell where it is needed because capillary and cell walls are **semi-permeable**; allowing the passage of certain substances through their walls. There are factors which affect how this occurs:

- **Hydrostatic pressure** is the pressure of the fluid (blood) in the capillary. It is greater at the arterial end of the capillary than at the venous end. This pressure allows fluid to 'force' its way out of the capillary wall.
- **Diffusion** is the movement of particles from a high solution on one side of the wall to a low solution on the other; this allows oxygen, glucose and nutrients, for example, to travel from the blood (where they are in high quantity) to the cells (where they are in low quantity).
- **Osmosis** is the diffusion of water from a high amount of water (low or dilute solution) on one side of a membrane to a lower amount of water (more concentrated solution) on the other side.

Link to practice

Massage is always carried out centripetally: this means towards the heart. This is for two reasons:
- to assist the flow of blood back to the heart – the **venous return**
- massage directed against the venous flow puts pressure on the valves, which can be very painful.

Proving the point

A helium balloon will gradually sink to the floor after a few days. Using the principle of diffusion, explain why this happens.

Link to learning

Capillary exchange also takes place in the alveoli in the lungs, where carbon dioxide is removed and replaced with oxygen. This is known as gaseous or gas exchange. (Link to The Respiratory System, page 115)

Fascinating fact

Apart from the pulmonary artery, which takes **deoxygenated** blood from the heart to the lungs, all other arteries in the body carry oxygenated blood.

The circulation

Humans have a double circulatory system consisting of:
- the **pulmonary circulation**, which takes deoxygenated blood to the lungs and returns oxygenated blood to the heart
- the **systemic circulation**, which transports blood around the rest of the body.

The heart is also divided into two, in effect providing two pumps, each with two chambers. This provides greater pressure than a single pump, giving the force necessary to supply the body with an adequate supply of oxygen.

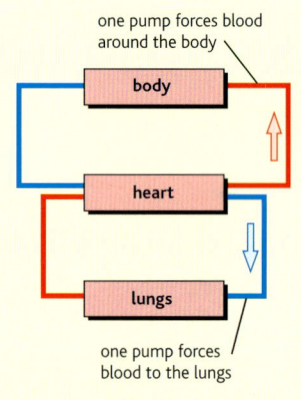

The heart

The structure of the heart

The heart is a hollow muscular organ which acts as a pump. It is situated in the middle of the chest, between the lungs. It is divided into two lengthways by a wall (**septum**); this creates two separate chambers and prevents oxygenated and deoxygenated blood passing from one side to the other.

Each chamber is divided into two further chambers, which form an upper **atria** and lower **ventricle** on either side. When the heart muscle contracts, the blood is forced through valves from the atria to the ventricles, then out of the heart via an artery.

▲ The double circulatory system

The cardiac cycle

A: The right side of the heart receives blood which is returning from the body and is low in oxygen (deoxygenated). It enters the right atria by the superior and inferior vena cavae veins. The blood passes into the right ventricle where it is pumped out through the pulmonary artery.

B: The pulmonary artery takes the deoxygenated blood to the lungs, where it is re-oxygenated. (Link to The Respiratory System, page 114)

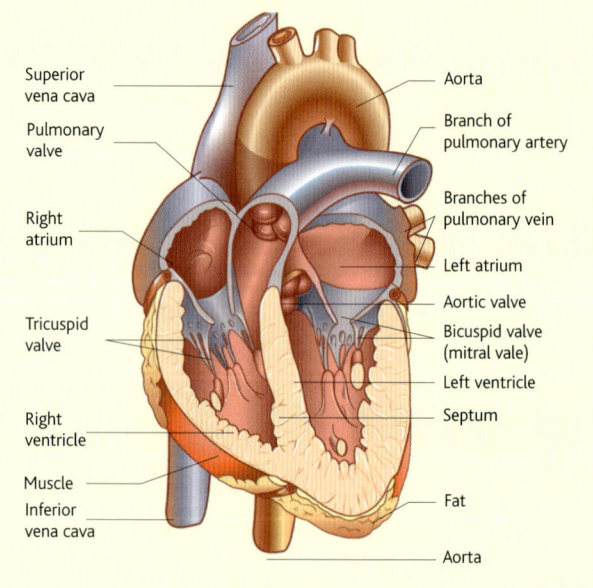

▲ The structure of the heart

Fascinating fact

Smoking causes the heart rate to increase because the red blood cells are carrying carbon monoxide instead of oxygen. This means that the heart has to beat more frequently to supply the body with the amount of oxygen it requires.

CHAPTER 5 The Blood Circulatory System

> **Proving the point**
>
> Pair up and take each other's radial pulse. To measure your pulse, the body should be at rest. The fingertips should be placed into the hollow at the base of the metacarpal of the thumb and pressed lightly over the artery. The number of beats in a minute should be counted, using a watch with a second hand count. The average pulse rate in an adult is 72 beats per minute but varies between 60 and 80 beats.

C: Oxygenated blood returns from the lungs to the left side of the heart via the pulmonary vein. It enters the heart at the left atria then passes through valves into the left ventricle, from where it is pumped out of the heart.

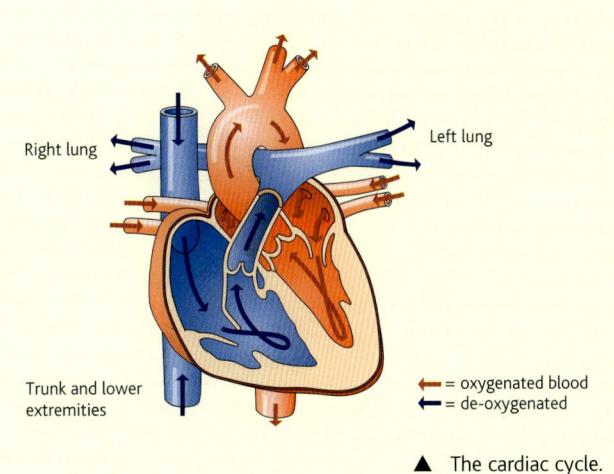

D: Oxygenated blood leaves the heart via the aorta, which is the largest artery in the body. The aorta then branches off to serve all areas of the body with oxygenated blood.

▲ The cardiac cycle.

Pulse rate and blood pressure

Pulse rate

The pulse is the rate at which the heart pumps blood out through the arteries and it is measured in beats per minute. It is the expansion and constriction of the artery as the blood passes through it, which can be felt as a wave of pressure at various points in the body.

Pulse rate is affected by many factors and will alter many times throughout a normal day.

Exercise and pulse rate

A low pulse rate is considered healthy as this means the heart is not working so hard. The way to lower pulse rate is to perform exercise which causes you to breathe harder and make the heart pump faster for a period of not less than 20 minutes, at least three times a week. Exercising the heart strengthens and develops the cardiac muscle, making it more efficient at pumping blood. This means that it can pump a higher volume of blood at each beat, and therefore does not have to work so hard.

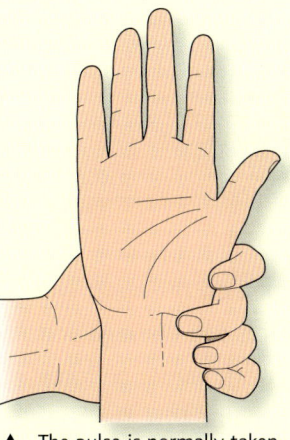

▲ The pulse is normally taken at the wrist just under the thumb on the palmar surface of the hand – this is called the radial pulse

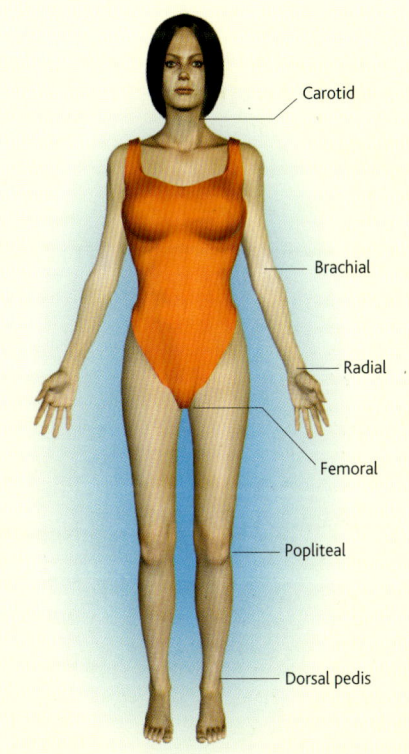

▲ Common pulse points

PAGE 89

Fascinating fact

Some athletes have a resting heart rate of around 32 beats per minute. This is a sign of being extremely fit!

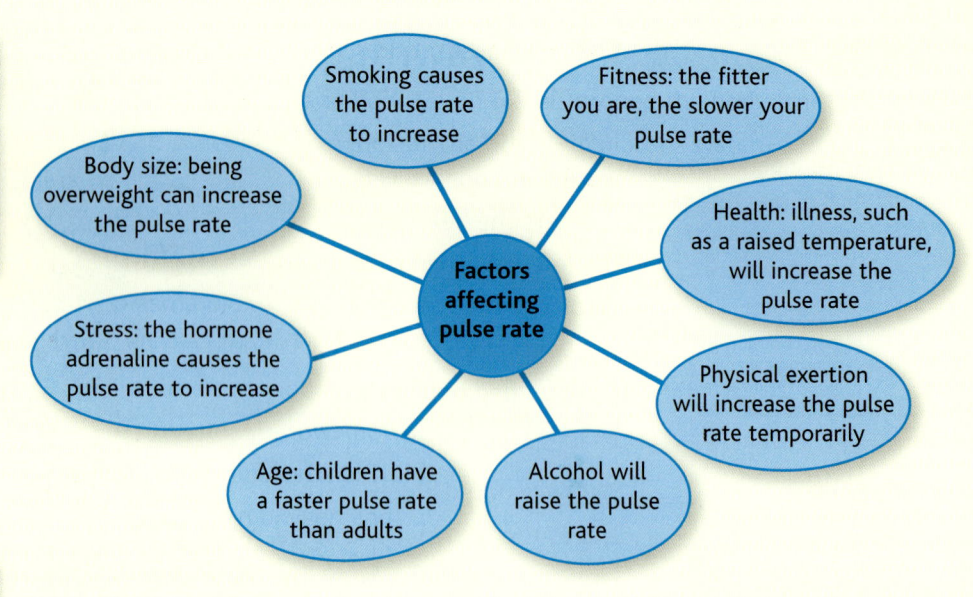

Factors affecting pulse rate
- Body size: being overweight can increase the pulse rate
- Smoking causes the pulse rate to increase
- Fitness: the fitter you are, the slower your pulse rate
- Health: illness, such as a raised temperature, will increase the pulse rate
- Stress: the hormone adrenaline causes the pulse rate to increase
- Physical exertion will increase the pulse rate temporarily
- Age: children have a faster pulse rate than adults
- Alcohol will raise the pulse rate

Proving the point

Take your pulse in the morning before you get out of bed. Then take your pulse at several intervals throughout the day after carrying out different activities. For example, take your pulse after drinking a strong cup of coffee, running for the bus, or when lying down. Make comparisons between these measurements.

Blood pressure

Every time the heart beats, it pumps out a volume of blood into the arteries. It is this force which is measured when taking blood pressure.

Blood pressure is measured at its highest and lowest, giving two figures.
- The highest pressure is when the heart contracts and the blood is pumped out. This is known as **systolic pressure**.
- The lower pressure is when the heart relaxes, which is known as **diastolic pressure**.

These two numbers are usually written with the systolic measurement over the diastolic measurement. For example, the average healthy blood pressure is written as $\frac{120}{80}$ and is said as '120 over 80'.

The range of blood pressure	Measurement
Low	90/60 or less
Normal	120/80 or less
Mild	140/90 or less
Moderate	160/100 or higher up to
Severe	180/110 or higher up to
Crisis	210/120 or higher

High blood pressure

High blood pressure (HBP) relates to the force of the blood on the heart walls and the walls of the arteries. If the force is very strong, this can damage and weaken the artery walls, meaning that the heart has to work harder to force the blood around the body to reach all the vital parts. In doing this, the heart enlarges but also grows weaker and is more prone to injury. HBP increases the risk of a heart attack and stroke. Stress causes the heart to work even harder as adrenaline will make the heart rate rise, thereby increasing those risks.

Factors affecting blood pressure

Blood pressure is maintained within normal limits by minor adjustments within the body. There are several factors which affect blood pressure, as shown in the diagram below.

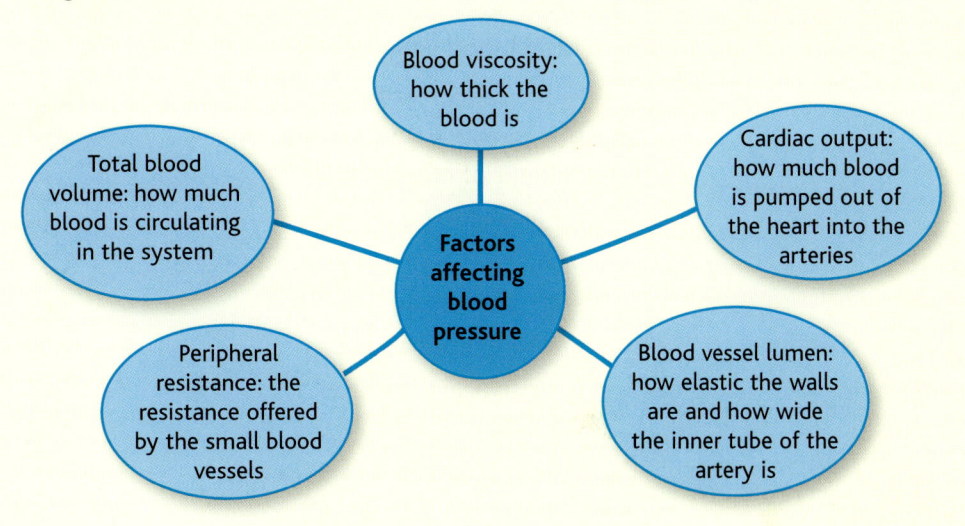

Factors affecting blood pressure:
- Blood viscosity: how thick the blood is
- Cardiac output: how much blood is pumped out of the heart into the arteries
- Total blood volume: how much blood is circulating in the system
- Peripheral resistance: the resistance offered by the small blood vessels
- Blood vessel lumen: how elastic the walls are and how wide the inner tube of the artery is

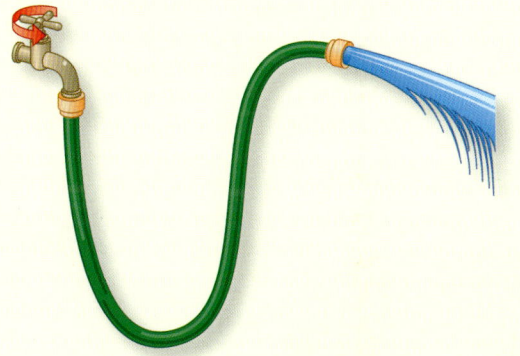

▲ Cardiac output: as the tap is turned and water flows, the pressure inside the hose rises. The more the tap is turned, the higher the pressure becomes.

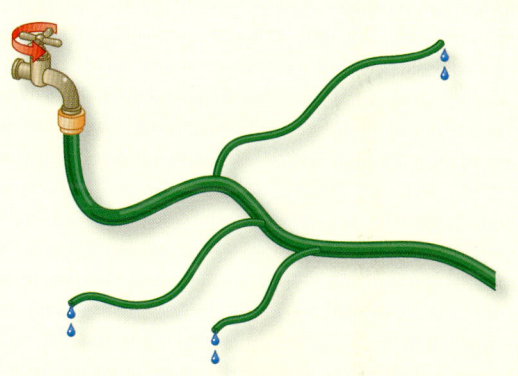

▲ Peripheral resistance: imagine that the hose is punctured many times for tiny tubes to be inserted into it (to feed plants all over the garden as in an irrigation system). Because the tubes are narrow, the flow of water in the tiny tubes slows down; this helps to maintain the water pressure inside the main hose. If the tubes were much wider, the flow of water would speed up and greater pressure would be lost.

In order to understand blood pressure it is useful to imagine a garden hose attached to a tap. The tap is the 'heart' and the hose is the aorta and other arteries.

- **Cardiac output**: how much blood is pumped out of the heart into the arteries. The cardiac output rises, for example, during exercise, when a greater amount of oxygenated blood is required around the body.
- **Peripheral resistance**: the resistance offered by the small blood vessels. The flow of blood in the capillaries slows down because they are so narrow; if the capillaries were wider, blood flow would speed up and greater pressure would be lost. It is the fact that the blood capillaries are so tiny which helps to maintain blood

pressure when blood flows to the peripheral areas, for example, as erythema during a massage.
- **Total blood volume**: how much blood is circulating in the system. If a significant amount of blood is lost, for example, from severe bleeding (haemorrhage) after an accident, the blood pressure drops and does not rise again until the lost blood is replaced.
- **Blood viscosity**: how thick the blood is. Blood is about three times thicker than water, and this thickness is known as **viscosity**. Thick blood does not flow freely and causes pressure to build up.
- **Blood vessel lumen**:
  - How wide the inner tube of the artery is: if blood vessels become narrow, for example, because of cholesterol build-up, the blood pressure will increase.
  - How elastic the walls are: in the aorta, the arterial walls expand and then recoil again; this pushes the blood through the body and helps to maintain blood pressure. If the arterial walls could not change shape in this way, the blood would not be forced onwards and the blood pressure would drop.

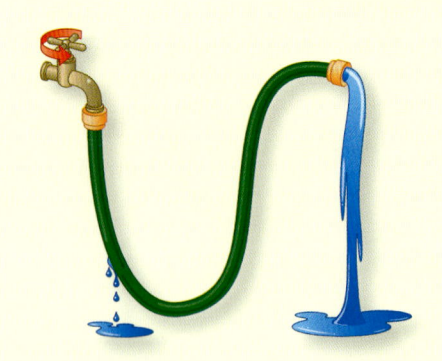

▲ Total blood volume: if the hose was split and water escaped, the water pressure would drop dramatically. It would not rise again until the tear was repaired and the lost water replaced.

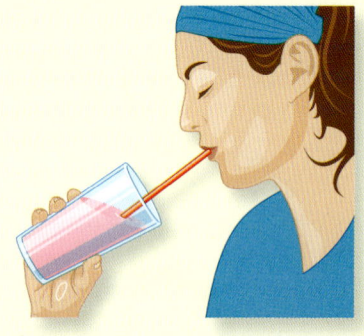

▲ Blood viscosity: imagine water in the hose being replaced with a thick syrup. The syrup would flow more slowly but causes pressure to build up.

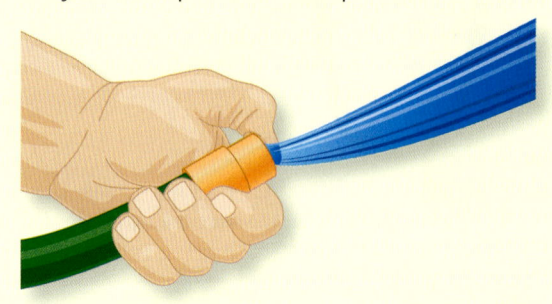

▲ The lumen of the vessels: if you want to increase the water pressure to reach the far end of the garden, partially close the end of the hose with your thumb.

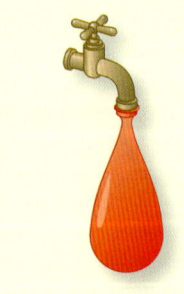

▲ Elasticity of the arterial walls: if the hose is made of a more pliable rubber, like a balloon, the tube would expand to contain the water and then recoil again, pushing the water along the hose. This would not be possible if the hose was a rigid, metal tube with no elasticity in the walls.

Link to practice

Blood pressure can fall during a treatment as vasodilation occurs when capillary activity rises. Research has shown that regular massage can reduce blood pressure, heart rate and stress.

> **Case study**
> **Level 3**
> Mrs Hamilton books in for an Indian Head Massage. Halfway through the treatment, she tells you that she is feeling really dizzy. What action should you take and why? How might the treatment have caused the client to feel dizzy?.

Other factors affecting blood pressure

Blood pressure can rise or fall at different times during the day. It is usually lowest first thing in the morning, when you are fully rested after sleep. It may fall slightly after eating, as the blood flows to the digestive system. Smoking and alcohol also cause an increase in blood pressure.

Stress can increase blood pressure, whether psychological (such as a stressful day at work) or physiological (such as in extreme heat, when blood pressure rises to create heat loss). In some cases, the thought of going to the doctor's for a blood pressure check can cause it to rise (known as 'white coat syndrome').

It is also thought that excess salt in the diet may cause the blood pressure to rise. Salt (sodium chloride) is vital for the body to function normally, but an excess in the blood will attract extra fluid from the body's cells and tissues, raising the total blood volume. If the total blood volume is increased, the blood pressure rises too.

> **Link to practice**
> Heat treatments are contra-indicated if a client has been drinking alcohol or after consuming a heavy meal. This is because alcohol causes the blood vessels to dilate close to the skin's surface and digestion diverts blood to the stomach and intestines. Both of these can make the client light-headed and prone to fainting.

> **Case study**
> **Level 3**
> A new client has booked in for an aromatherapy massage (at the suggestion of her doctor) to de-stress because she has high blood pressure. Mrs Cheng says that she knows having high blood pressure is a bad thing but she doesn't understand why. What advice would you give Mrs Cheng?

Blood shunting

Blood shunting is the ability of the circulatory system to shut down and open up arterioles, thereby restricting or increasing blood flow to an area as required. To enable this, arterioles contain tiny sphincter muscles which allow them to be constricted; this diverts blood flow away from one area to be rerouted to another. For example:

- During exercise, to provide oxygen and nutrients for energy, the muscles are given priority over other areas of the body, such as the stomach.
- After eating, the body begins the process of digestion and blood is shunted towards the stomach and intestines, away from the muscles and skin.

> **Link to learning**
>
> **Blood glucose**
>
> Sugar is required by the body and is utilised in its simplest form: **glucose**. It is important that the levels of glucose are maintained correctly and there is a mechanism in the body which ensures that they do not rise or drop beyond safe levels. This mechanism involves the **secretion** of the **hormones insulin** and **glucagon**, which are both released by the pancreas. (Link to The Endocrine System, page 141)
> - If there is too much sugar in the blood, insulin is released. This converts the sugar to **glycogen**, which can then be stored in the liver.
> - If there is too little sugar in the blood, glucagon is released. This ensures that glycogen is taken from the liver and converted to glucose for use within the body.
>
> This mechanism is known as **negative feedback**.

> **Fascinating fact**
>
> If you were to exercise after eating a heavy meal, the blood that is needed by the stomach and intestines to digest and absorb nutrients would be diverted towards the muscles. This would stop or slow the digestive process and potentially give you abdominal or muscle cramps. This is why you should wait for at least two hours before exercising after a meal.

> **Link to learning**
>
> The blood circulatory system and the lymphatic system are very closely linked; they could not work efficiently without each other. (Link to The Lymphatic System, page 99)

Diseases and disorders of the blood circulatory system

Anaemia

A condition where the blood lacks the ability to provide the body with an adequate supply of oxygen – anaemia literally translates as 'without blood'. It is caused by several different factors, such as loss of blood or lack of iron, and there are several different types.

- Pernicious anaemia is where the body is unable to absorb or utilise vitamin B12, which is essential for the production of red blood cells.
- Sickle cell anaemia is a disorder affecting the red blood cells, making them inflexible and unable to pass through the capillaries. This results in a lack of oxygen to areas of the body and is extremely painful for the sufferer; there is no cure for this disorder.

Aneurysm

A weak point in a blood vessel wall which creates a bulge; this increases in size until it eventually bursts, usually resulting in instant death. Aneurysm can be treated surgically.

Angina

Angina occurs when the heart muscle does not receive enough oxygen due to a narrowing of one of the arteries that supply blood to the heart muscle, causing pain. It is an indication of heart disease. It is usually brought on by an extra need for oxygen, i.e. during physical exertion or emotional stress. The symptoms are pain, burning or squeezing in the chest spreading to the arms, face, back or stomach.

Anti-coagulants

Anti-coagulants are types of medication which help to keep the blood thin and allow it to flow freely. They are commonly given to people who have narrowed arteries, or those who have suffered strokes or heart attacks.

Arteriosclerosis

Hardening of the arteries which occurs when plaque (cells, cholesterol and other substances) builds up in the arterial walls. This narrows the arteries, makes the walls inelastic and eventually blocks the passage of blood to vital organs, such as the heart and the brain.

It may be caused by:

- high cholesterol (and other fat levels) in the blood
- high blood pressure
- smoking.

Bruising

Leakage from a blood vessel under the skin. Some people bruise more easily than others. A possible cause of bruising more easily maybe a deficiency in certain nutrients, chiefly vitamins C, E, K, bioflavonoids and zinc.

Chilblains

A condition which occurs when fingers (usually) and toes are subjected to very cold temperatures and then warmed; the skin becomes irritated, red and itchy.

Chronic heart failure

This occurs when, because of heart disease, the heart does not pump enough blood around the body to meet its needs. It is caused by:
- blocked arteries
- a previous heart attack which has caused damage to the heart muscle
- a heart defect which may have been present since birth
- high blood pressure
- infection of the heart or valves
- heart muscle or heart valve disease.

It results in blood backing up in the veins around the body, causing swelling (oedema) in the feet, ankles and legs. (Link to The Lymphatic System, page 105) Fluid may also build up in the lungs.

Signs of heart failure are shortness of breath, even when lying down, feeling tired and run-down, oedema in the feet, ankles and legs, weight gain from fluid build-up, and confusion or the inability to think clearly.

Haemophilia

A disorder where the sufferer lacks a factor in the blood which prevents it from clotting normally; the factor is administered as a drug, but haemophiliacs are susceptible to haemorrhage (bleeding resulting in severe blood loss).

> **Fascinating fact**
> Around 1 in 5 adults in the UK are obese. This means that a person's weight gain is such that his or her health has been put at risk.

Heart attack

This is where the blood supply to the heart muscle is cut off. It accounts for half of all coronary heart disease deaths. The main symptoms of a heart attack are:

- pressure or pain in the centre of the chest lasting minutes or is intermittent
- pain in the shoulders, neck or arms
- discomfort in the chest, feeling light-headed, fainting, sweating, nausea or being out of breath.

Other warning signs of a heart attack include:

- chest, stomach or lower abdominal pain
- nausea or dizziness
- shortness of breath or difficulty in breathing
- unexplained anxiety, weakness or fatigue
- palpitations or paleness.

Heart disease

In the UK, heart disease is responsible for the death of more men and women than any other disease. The term 'heart disease' is in fact a number of conditions that affect the health of the heart and its performance. The commonest form of heart disease is where the blood vessels which feed the heart tissue are blocked, usually due to a build-up of deposits in the blood vessel. This can result in a variety of symptoms, including:

- *angina* – pain in the chest caused by a lack of blood to the cardiac muscle
- *heart attack* – when a coronary artery (supplying the heart muscle) becomes completely blocked, so parts of the heart muscle receive no oxygen; permanent damage can occur
- *arrhythmia* – an irregular heartbeat, which can increase the chances of suffering a stroke or heart attack.

Hypertension

High blood pressure.

Hypotension

Low blood pressure.

> **Fascinating fact**
> Research carried out in the 1960s on a group of seven countries showed that people from the Greek island of Crete had the lowest incidence of heart disease. This was attributed to their Mediterranean diet. The Mediterranean diet is one which is high in olive oil, fresh vegetables, salads, fruit, beans, herbs, fish and red wine. More recent studies have concluded that having a diet of this type significantly reduces the chances of heart disease.

Leukaemia

Cancer of the white blood cells, caused by the tissue which manufactures white blood cells, to make an excessive amount; these extra cells overpower the red blood cells. It is a malignant disease and can be fatal.

Pacemaker

A device fitted internally which regulates an irregular heart beat.

Peripheral arterial disease
Narrowing of the arteries in the legs, abdomen and pelvis. Pain is the first sign, usually in the muscles of the thighs, buttocks or calves, especially when exercising or walking.

Raynaud's Disease
This is when the blood vessels of the fingers and thumbs constrict, causing them to go white/blue and cold.

Septicaemia
Blood poisoning. May be caused by bacteria entering the bloodstream; it can be life-threatening.

Shock
This describes a lack of blood flow to the body and may be mild or severe. It is usually treated with intravenous fluids (fed directly into the vein) and oxygen.

Thrombosis
A clot of blood inside a blood vessel. It can block the flow of blood, cutting off the supply of oxygen. If this happens in an artery to the brain, a stroke occurs and may cause brain damage, paralysis, loss of sensory functions, or even death.

Varicose veins
Veins whose valves have collapsed, causing circulation pools in the veins. Varicose veins are painful and swollen and should not be massaged. Being overweight, pregnant, standing for long periods, crossing legs, wearing tight jeans and socks can cause varicose veins and make existing ones worse.

> **Link to practice**
> Because of the risk of brain damage, paralysis or death, it is very important not to perform treatments on anyone with thrombosis or a history of thrombosis.

> **Link to practice**
> Varicose veins are a contra-indication to many treatments where blood flow is increased, as this places extra strain on the veins. They are also painful if massaged or pressure/exertion (as in waxing) is applied.

Ageing and the blood circulatory system
The heart muscle deteriorates with age: it reduces in size and ability to contract, the heart valves become less efficient and the muscle may produce irregular rhythms. Older people may have a reduced tolerance to physical exercise and may be unable to withstand stress.

- There is also an increased likelihood of bruising. Ageing and sun damage weaken tiny vessels in the skin, which break and cause bruises to develop and they take longer to heal.
- Varicose veins are more likely to occur with age, since valves in the veins become less effective. Reduced activity and a lack of exercise may create complications where varicose veins already exist; for example, ulceration (open sores on the skin's surface).
- Diabetes (a disorder of the endocrine system) is more likely to occur with age; it damages the small blood vessels, which causes bruising and poor circulation. The reduced circulation has a particularly negative effect on the feet.

Link to practice

Some older clients will be on types of medication (for example, anti-coagulants such as aspirin or warfarin), which can cause the skin to bruise more easily.

Link to practice

Diabetes is considered to be a contra-indication to most treatments. This is because the circulation to the lower limbs is poor, the walls of the blood vessels are weakened and bruising is likely. However, with approval from a doctor, superficial massage to the lower limbs and feet can improve the circulation and assist with mobility.

Link to practice
Looking after your heart

Looking after your heart will keep it healthy and allow it to last a lifetime. Your lifestyle, including your diet, the amount of exercise you do, your mental attitude and drinking and smoking habits, will all have an effect on the health of your heart and, maybe, how long you live. Here are some top tips for a healthy heart:

- Increase the amount of exercise you do: just 30 minutes of fairly intensive activity (anything which gets you slightly out of breath) several times a week can halve the chance of developing heart disease than if no activity is done at all.
- Stop smoking: giving up will significantly reduce your risk of developing heart disease. Five years after stopping smoking, the risk of developing heart disease falls to the same level as someone who has never smoked.
- Reduce high blood pressure by:
  - maintaining a healthy weight and losing weight if you are overweight
  - limiting salt intake to no more than six grams a day
  - stopping smoking
  - reducing stress levels
  - exercising for at least 30 minutes every day.
- Moderate drinking (limiting alcohol consumption to no more than one to two units a day).
- Healthy eating – eating five portions of fruit and vegetables each day has been shown to decrease the risks of heart disease. Reducing saturated fat intake, using healthy methods of cooking (not frying) and increasing starchy foods will also all have a positive effect.

Knowledge check

1. State the functions of the blood.
2. Define erythema.
3. List the causes of erythema.
4. What is high blood pressure?
5. State 3 factors which can affect blood pressure.
6. State 4 reasons why the pulse rate may increase.
7. Why should you not massage over a varicose vein?
8. Define capillary exchange and state where this takes place.
9. Describe blood flow through the heart.
10. Name the 4 vessels entering and leaving the heart.
11. Name the arteries supplying the leg.
12. Describe the structure of arteries.
13. How do veins differ from arteries?
14. What is the job of platelets?
15. How does massage affect the circulation?
16. What causes broken capillaries?
17. What is the job of white blood cells?
18. Where are blood cells manufactured?
19. What is thrombosis and why is it a contra-indication?
20. Briefly explain how blood sugar levels are maintained in the body.

SECTION 2

CHAPTER 6 The Lymphatic System

The **lymphatic system** can be thought of as the body's waste disposal and recycling system. It collects up all the unwanted material in the body which has come from the blood and the tissues, then filters it by taking out the rubbish and returning all the good bits back to the blood. The lymphatic system is also a drainage system: it removes excess fluid and proteins from around the tissues, then deposits them back into the blood once they have been filtered.

The lymphatic system is thus very closely connected to the blood circulatory system (Link to The Blood Circulatory System, page 77); so much so that it is sometimes called the 'second circulatory system'. However, the lymphatic system differs from the blood circulatory system in three fundamental ways:
- it does not have a pump like the heart
- unlike blood vessels, **lymph vessels** are not connected up in a circular pathway
- it does not contain blood – instead, it contains a fluid called **lymph**.

Because the lymphatic system does not have a pump, it relies on pressure within the body (breathing and blood pressure help to maintain this), muscular action and gravity to force the fluid up towards the heart.

The lymphatic system also acts with the blood circulatory system to help defend the body and keep it free from disease. It is therefore part of the **immune system**.

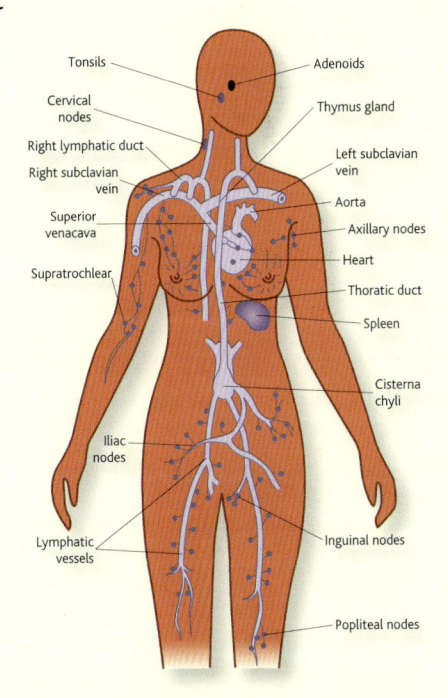

> **Link to practice**
>
> Massage can play a big part in assisting the passage of lymph around the body. Applying pressure on the muscles and therefore the lymphatic vessels, pushes the fluid upwards and onwards on its journey. (See also page 102.)

▲ The lymphatic system of the body

> **You will learn**
>
> In this chapter you will learn about:
> - components of the lymphatic system
> - functions of the lymphatic system
> - the lymphatic pathway
> - the major lymph nodes in the body
> - the spleen
> - the tonsils and adenoids
> - the thymus gland
> - disorders and diseases of the lymphatic system
> - ageing and the lymphatic system.

PAGE 99

Proving the point

Although lymph fluid is normally clear, after leaving the digestive system it contains digested fat molecules, which makes it go a milky colour (lymph is then called chyle). To reproduce this effect, place some oil in a jar of water and shake it. The water will become cloudy when the fat droplets mix with the water.

The components of the lymphatic system

The lymphatic system is composed of:
- lymphatic fluid
- lymphatic capillaries
- lymphatic vessels
- lymphatic tissue
- lymphatic nodes
- lymphatic ducts.

Lymphatic fluid

Lymphatic fluid, or lymph, is the liquid which flows in the lymphatic system. It is normally clear or pale yellow in colour. It is very similar to blood plasma and tissue fluid because this is where it comes from. The actual composition of lymph varies considerably according to where it is in the body, and may include any of the following:

- water
- large protein molecules
- foreign bodies
- **white blood cells**
- waste products from **cellular metabolism**
- **lymphocytes**
- large fat molecules
- bacteria and viruses.

Functions of lymph

The main functions of lymph are transport and defence. It acts as a means of transport for various substances in the body, both beneficial and harmful. By taking up any harmful substances, lymph keeps unwanted substances out of the blood. It also provides an abundance of white blood cells to destroy bacteria and viruses, and **antibodies** to protect against disease.

Lymph passes from **lymph capillaries** into lymph vessels and then through **lymph nodes** and into **lymph ducts**.

Lymph capillaries

Lymph capillaries are minute vessels which are similar to blood capillaries, but they do not join one vessel to another as blood capillaries do (Link to The Blood Circulatory System, page 86). They begin as round-ended tubes, like a tiny test tube, that join up to lymphatic vessels. Lymph capillaries have a larger and more irregular **lumen** (inner space) than blood capillaries and are more **permeable**. This allows the lymphatic system to pick up larger molecules, such as protein which has escaped from the blood but cannot easily return there.

Fascinating fact

If you have ever sobbed your heart out, you will be aware that the delicate skin around the eyes swells up and remains swollen for some time afterwards. This is because the body recognises that the eye area has suffered a trauma and sends extra blood (and thus tissue fluid) to the area. Your eyes remain swollen for some time because the lymphatic system takes a while to remove all the excess fluid!

CHAPTER 6 The Lymphatic System

> **Fascinating fact**
> The tonsils are the body's first line of defence at the back of the mouth, and 'Peyer's patches' help with prevention of infection in the intestines.

> **Fascinating fact**
> When you get a throat infection or the start of a cold or flu, which nodes swell up first? Why do you think this is?

The wall of a lymph capillary is constructed of endothelial cells that overlap one another. When fluid outside the capillary pushes against the overlapping cells, they swing slightly inward, like a swinging door that moves in only one direction. Fluid inside the capillary cannot flow out through these openings; they are one-way doors only.

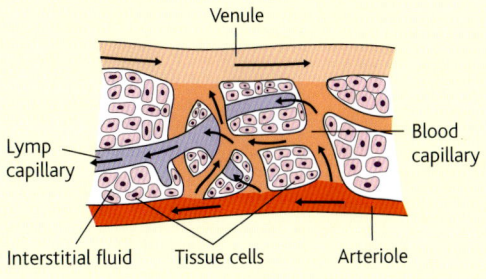

▲ Lymph capillaries in relation to blood capillaries.

Lymph vessels

Lymphatic capillaries join lymph vessels. These are similar to veins but they have wider lumens and far more **valves**, to assist the flow of lymph away from the tissues.

Lymphatic tissue

Lymphatic tissue, also known as lymphoid tissue, consists mainly of a mass of lymphocytes. It is found all over the body but typically at sites where infection may enter the body, such as the mouth or ears, or where infection is more likely to occur. Certain organs within the lymphatic system consist of lymphatic tissue; these include the spleen, the thymus gland and the lymphatic nodes.

The structure and function of lymph nodes

There are hundreds of lymph nodes all over the body. These filter the lymph fluid that passes through the lymph vessels (each vessel passes through at least one node). Lymph nodes tend to be clustered in groups around the body; for example, many hundreds are found in the abdomen and intestinal tract.

▲ The structure of a lymph node.

▲ The flow of lymph fluid through lymph vessels. a) When pressure is exerted on the vessel walls, valves are forced open to allow lymph to pass through. b) The valves close to prevent the backflow of lymph in the vessels.

PAGE 101

Lymph nodes vary in diameter from 1 mm to 20 mm. They contain lymphatic tissue and numerous white blood cells. It is the job of the white blood cells to filter **cell debris** and ingest bacteria and micro-organisms from the incoming lymphatic fluid. Lymphocytes multiply in the lymph nodes and are added to the lymph as it flows through the node. Thus the lymph leaving the node is cleaner and richer in lymphocytes.

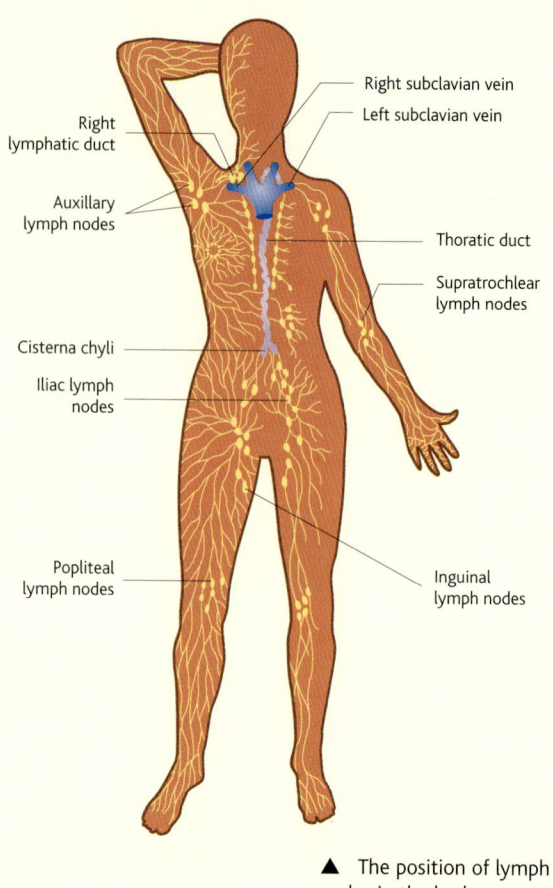

▲ The position of lymph nodes in the body.

> **Link to learning**
> Debris is another word for rubbish.

> **Link to practice**
> The removal of cell debris via the lymphatic system is speeded up by massage, which assists the flow of lymph through the body.

Cell debris
Cell debris is the unwanted waste which accumulates all over the body as a result of the many different processes which are constantly taking place.
- Some debris is from the processes of metabolism – the breaking down of nutrients into useable units. For example, protein metabolism produces a waste product known as **urea**. This has to be moved to the kidneys for **excretion**. (Link to The Excretory and Urinary Systems, page 174)
- Other debris is the result of white blood cells (**macrophages**) eating invaders, which produces pus-like material.
- Carbon dioxide is a waste product produced when oxygen is used for **respiration**. (Link to The Respiratory System, page 115)

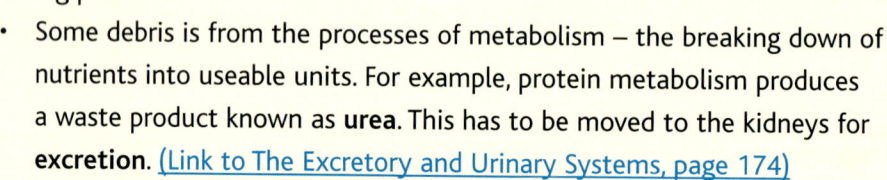

The lymphatic ducts
After lymph fluid has passed through at least one lymph node, it travels to one of two lymph ducts. These are basically collecting tubes for lymph fluid from around the body. They are:
- the thoracic duct
- the right lymphatic duct.

The thoracic duct
The thoracic duct is the larger of the two lymph ducts. It collects lymph mainly

▲ The position of lymph nodes in the head and neck.

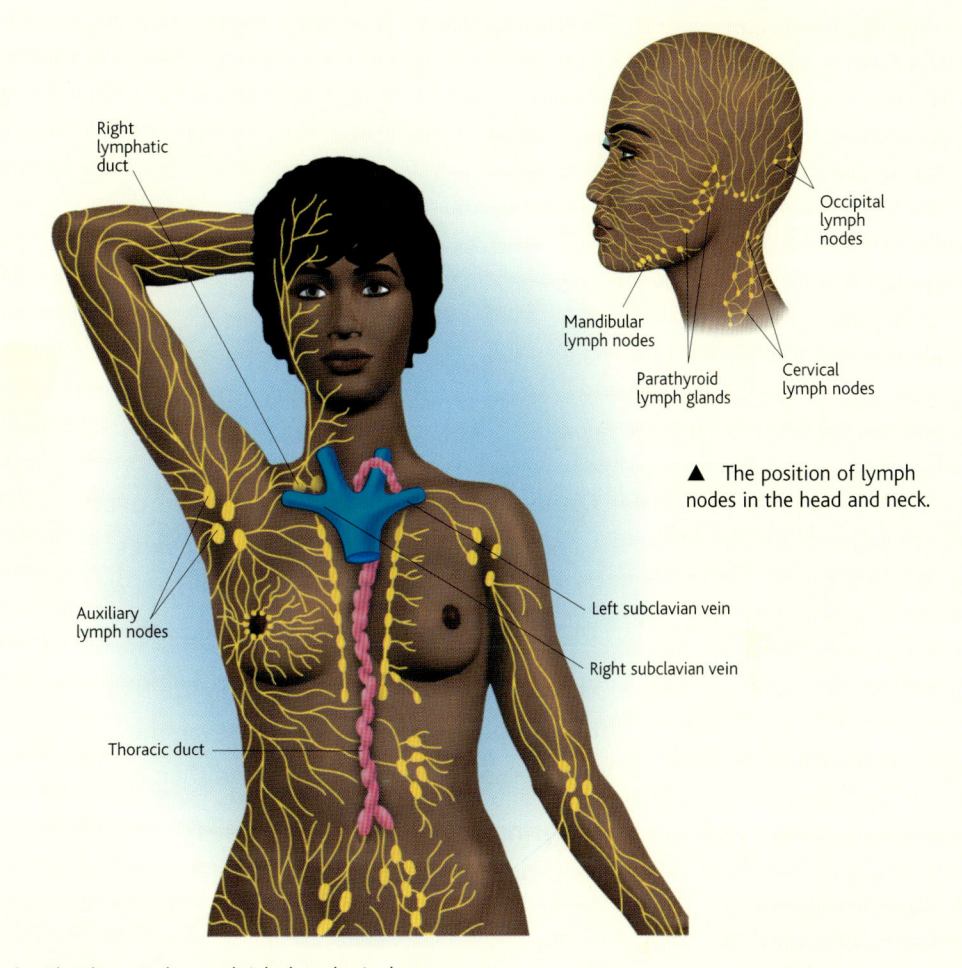

▲ The thoracic duct and right lymphatic duct.

from the lower portion of the body. The lower vessels of the body unite to form a widened lymph vessel known as the cisterna chyli (pronounced sis-ter-na kylie). This is a pouch about 6 cm (2¼ inches) long and is situated in the lumbar region of the abdominal cavity (just above the waist). At the level of the twelfth thoracic vertebra, the cisterna chyli narrows and becomes the thoracic duct. It is about 30 cm (12 inches) in length.

The right lymphatic duct

The right lymphatic duct is much smaller – only 1 cm (⅓ inch) long. It collects lymph fluid from the right side of the head and neck, the right arm and the shoulder.

Both ducts take the lymph fluid to the left and right subclavian veins in the upper chest (Link to The Blood Circulatory System, page 85). From here, lymph rejoins the blood circulation: the subclavian veins join up to the superior vena cava, which takes blood directly to the heart.

Link to practice

Aromatherapy massage in particular uses lots of long, stroking movements to assist lymphatic drainage.

Functions of the lymphatic system

Proving the point
Think of an occasion in a woman's life when she may be affected by swollen ankles. As a therapist, what advice could you give to help female clients with this problem? How would you explain what has caused this condition?

Functions of the lymphatic system:
- Absorption of fat from the intestines
- Drainage of tissue spaces and removal of excess fluid
- Production of lymphocytes and antibodies
- Filtering of waste in the nodes

Link to practice
It is very important that therapists understand the functioning of the lymphatic system and the influence treatments have upon it. For a sluggish lymphatic system, massage is very effective in assisting the passage of lymph upwards.

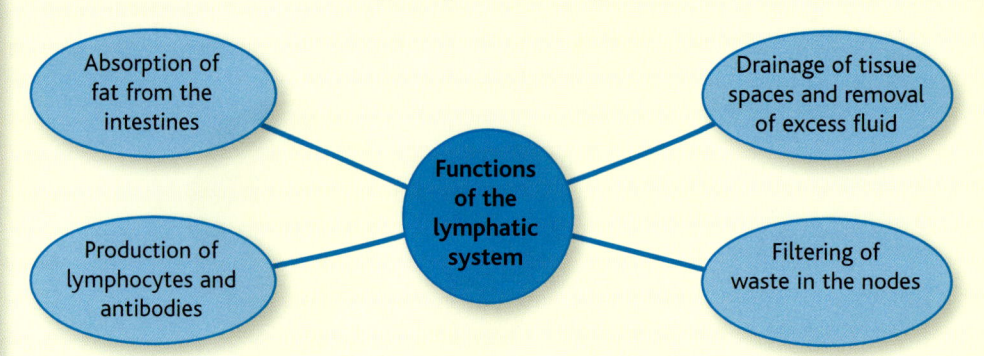

Drainage of tissue spaces and removal of excess fluids
Lymphatic capillaries collect up any excess fluid from around the tissue cells. This allows fresh fluid to flow into the area to bathe the tissue cells. The lymphatic system returns the fluid to the blood via the subclavian veins.

Excess proteins may be present in the tissue fluid which are too large to pass back into a blood capillary. However, they can pass into the more permeable lymph capillaries; the system can then return the proteins to the blood.

Filtering of waste in the nodes
As lymph passes through the nodes, it is filtered of unwanted particles, such as debris from cell metabolism and bacteria. The white blood cells in the nodes engulf and destroy the waste matter and harmful substances. This prevents any poisonous substances and germs which may be present in the tissues from entering the bloodstream. As the nodes deal with infection, they often become inflamed, swell up and may be painful.

Link to practice
If a client has an accumulation of excess tissue fluid, there may be serious reasons for this. It is therefore important that clients check with their doctor if oedema is present before commencing treatment.

Production of lymphocytes and antibodies
The nodes provide extra white blood cells; the fluid leaving the node has a higher concentration of white blood cells. Lymphocytes are able to produce antibodies which are important in fighting infection. (Link to The Blood Circulatory System, page 83)

Absorption of fat from the intestines
There are special lymphatic vessels in the intestines which absorb digested fat and transport it to the areas where it is needed, for example, the liver, or to be further metabolised. The vessels are called lacteals.

The effects of poor lymphatic drainage on the body
A sluggish lymphatic system has an effect on other body systems, such as the blood circulatory and respiratory systems. If fluid is not removed efficiently from around the tissues, fresh fluid, which is high in oxygen and nutrients,

CHAPTER 6 The Lymphatic System

> **Proving the point**
>
> Go for a walk on a hot day and swing your arms fairly vigorously as if marching. What happens to your hands and fingers? Why do you think this has happened? What can you do to reverse this effect? What is happening physiologically when you counteract the effects of walking in this way?

cannot move from the blood to the tissue spaces. This means that the tissues become low in oxygen and high in carbon dioxide. As a result, the heart and lungs work harder in an attempt to get oxygen to the tissues. This puts a strain on the heart and, in extreme cases, breathing can become more difficult.

Excess tissue fluid

The term for excess tissue fluid is **oedema** (o-deema). Oedema is a sign that the lymphatic system is not functioning efficiently and is caused by several factors. For example, it may be due to the body carrying excess weight, which makes it more difficult for the fluid to return up the body to the blood. Oedema is often seen around the ankle area and can occur during pregnancy. Medical conditions such as varicose veins, thrombosis, heart failure, liver disease, kidney disease, malnutrition and certain allergic conditions can all lead to oedema.

> **Link to practice**
>
> Vacuum suction is a piece of equipment which is designed to redistribute lymph in the body, so it is useful where there is a build-up of excess fluid. It also speeds up the interchange of tissue fluid, thus removing waste products and bringing oxygen and nutrients to the tissues.

> **Link to practice**
>
> Body wraps are a popular salon treatment for clients wishing to slim on a temporary basis. The wraps are firmly applied from the lower legs up the body and the client is then left to relax for up to an hour. The pressures of the wraps force the tissue fluid into the lymphatic system and speed up removal of toxins and waste products. It is effective in reducing inches for up to 2–3 days, so is an excellent treatment before a big night out or special occasion.

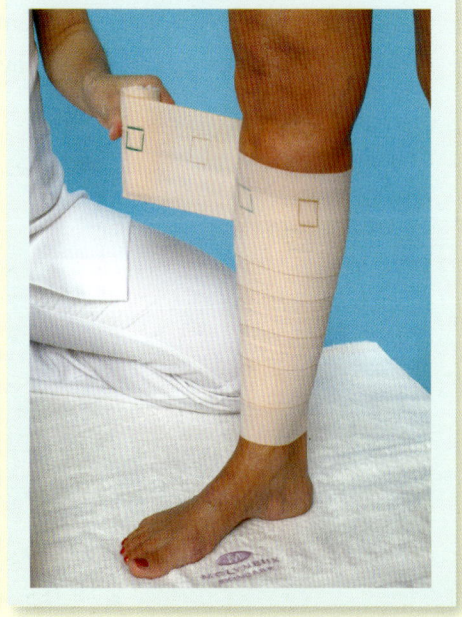

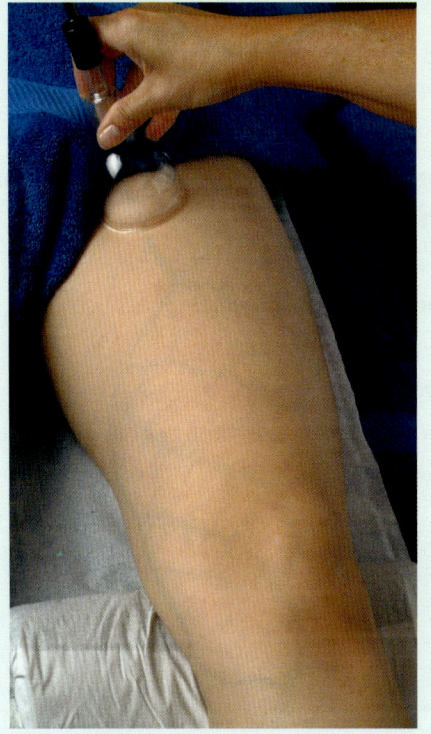

The lymphatic pathway

In order to fully understand how lymph travels around the body (the lymphatic pathway), it is necessary to look at the blood circulatory system at the same time. (Link to The Blood Circulatory System, page 87)

From plasma to tissue fluid to lymph

- The **plasma** in blood passes out through the blood capillary wall and into the surrounding tissue spaces. The fluid is now known as **tissue fluid** or **interstitial fluid**.
- This fluid, rich in oxygen and nutrients, surrounds the cells so that the cells may take up the oxygen and nutrients. The cells use the oxygen and nutrients to metabolise, grow or repair, depending upon the type of cell.
- The waste products of metabolism pass out of the cell membrane and back into the tissue fluid.
- Most of the tissue fluid, along with the waste products, is taken back up by the blood capillary. However, because the **blood pressure** in the capillary is greatly reduced, not all the fluid passes back.
- The remaining fluid is drawn into the lymphatic capillary. It is now known as lymph.

> **Link to practice**
> When you perform massage, you must direct massage strokes towards the main groups of lymphatic nodes. However, you must never apply pressure directly over the major groups of nodes (the inguinals and popliteals, for example) as pressure over these areas would be painful.

> **Fascinating fact**
> If the spleen is damaged or ruptured, which can happen during contact sports such as rugby, it must be removed. This does not have a major negative effect on the health of the body as other organs and mechanisms within the body take over the spleen's functions. However, resistance to certain types of infections may be reduced in someone who has had a splenectomy (surgical removal of the spleen).

The plasma in the blood passes out through the blood capillary wall and into the surrounding tissue spaces, where the cells are bathed in tissue fluid

The blood capillary cannot take all the fluid containing waste products back, so the excess passes into the blind-ended lymph capillary

The cells use the oxygen and food, and then pass the waste products back into the tissue fluid. Most of this fluid returns to the blood capillary.

▲ From plasma to tissue fluid to lymph

▲ The lymph nodes of the face and neck
- Pre-auricular
- Post-auricular
- Occipital
- Sub-mandibular
- Buccal
- Superficial and deep cervical
- Sub-mental
- Supraclavicular

The flow of lymph through the lymphatic system

Lymphatic capillaries join up to larger lymphatic vessels. These pass through lymphatic nodes, where the lymph is filtered and white blood cells (lymphocytes) are added. The lymphatic vessels generally follow the same course as arteries and veins.

Lymphatic vessels from the lower body join to form the cisterna chyli, which becomes the thoracic duct (see page 102).

CHAPTER 6 The Lymphatic System

Proving the point

Holding a mirror in front of you, open your mouth as wide as you can and look at the back of the throat. The tonsils are visible to the left and right as lumps of fleshy tissue. The next time you have a sore throat, have another look at your tonsils and make a comparison.

Fascinating fact

Both the adenoids and tonsils can be removed if persistent infections occur, although because of the role of the tonsils in **immunity** when growing up, removal is not carried out unless it is considered to be absolutely necessary and the person suffers from infected tonsils on a very regular basis.

Link to learning

The thymus gland is also an organ of the **endocrine system** (Link to The Endocrine System, page 139).

The right lymphatic duct collects lymph fluid from the right side of the head and neck, the right arm and shoulder (see page 103).

Lymph returns to the blood circulatory system

Both lymphatic ducts empty into the left and right subclavian veins (see page 103). The lymphatic fluid has now been returned to the blood circulatory system, where it is taken up and becomes part of the plasma again in the blood.

The major lymph nodes in the body

Link to practice

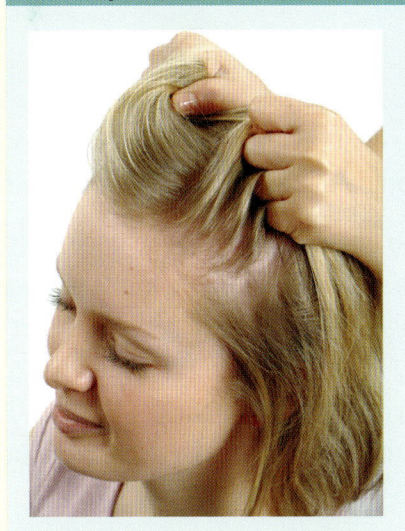

Indian head massage concentrates on lymphatic drainage of the face. This is very useful in helping to remove waste products and bring fresh oxygen and nutrients to the skin. It also assists in draining excess fluid from under the eyes, thereby reducing puffiness, and from around the cheek bones (zygomatic) when the sinuses are inflamed.

The spleen

The spleen is the largest organ associated with the lymphatic system. It acts very much like a lymphatic node in that it filters the blood (not lymph) which flows through it.

The spleen lies in the abdominal cavity below the diaphragm, behind and slightly to the left of the stomach. It does not have a specific shape but is malleable, meaning that its shape changes according to the other organs surrounding and pressing against it (namely the stomach, kidney and colon). The spleen varies in size but is approximately 12 cm by 7 cm (5 x 3 inches).

Function

The spleen has two main functions:
- the destruction of worn-out red blood cells (erythrocytes)
- the production of lymphocytes.

It is thought that the spleen is involved in fighting infection in the body, particularly when the blood becomes infected, as in diseases such as malaria.

PAGE 107

> **Fascinating fact**
>
> The thymus gland of young animals such as lamb or veal is considered to be quite a delicacy. The thymus (and also the pancreas) are known as sweetbreads in culinary terms and are highly prized by chefs and connoisseurs for their mild flavour, tenderness and velvety texture. They can be prepared by sautéing, poaching, grilling, frying and roasting.

> **Link to practice**
>
> **Massage and cancer**
> It was initially thought that massage spread cancer cells so was contra-indicated. However, today's thinking is that massage will not spread the cancer to other parts of the body and is extremely beneficial to cancer sufferers in the majority of cases. It is essential to have the approval of the person's doctor before going ahead. Attending training on '**oncology massage**', as it is sometimes known, is also advisable in order to best adapt your massage techniques.

Structure

The spleen's internal structure is similar to that of a lymph node, with fibres or trabecula supporting splenic pulp. There are two types of splenic pulp: red and white.

- The white pulp is circular in structure and is made up mainly of lymphocytes.
- The red pulp surrounds the white pulp and contains mainly red blood cells and macrophages. The main function of the red pulp is to destroy old red blood cells (erythrocytes).

The tonsils and adenoids

The tonsils

The tonsils are masses of lymphatic tissue which are concerned with the filtration of tissue fluid (not lymph). The tonsils are actually named the **palatine tonsils** and are located either side at the back of the mouth.

The tonsils are the body's first line of defence when infection strikes, which is why it is common to have a sore throat at the start of any illness (in particular colds, flu and coughs). They work to prevent the infection from passing further down the body. When an infection is present, the tonsils swell up and feel sore. If there is a considerable amount of bacteria present, they will develop pustular blisters on their surface. The condition when the tonsils are inflamed is tonsillitis.

Adenoids

The adenoids are masses of lymphatic tissue situated on the wall behind the nose. They are known as the **pharyngeal tonsils** because they are in the upper part of the **pharynx**. (Link to The Respiratory System, page 113)

The thymus gland

The thymus **gland** lies in the chest cavity under the sternum. It is concerned with the development of **T-lymphocytes** (Link to The Blood Circulatory System, page 83) and immunity. It is really only active up until **puberty**, after which time the organ atrophies (wastes away and reduces in size).

Disorders and diseases of the lymphatic system

Hodgkin's disease

This occurs when a lymphocyte in the lymph node multiplies at an abnormal rate, causing swelling. The abnormal lymphocytes then spread to other nodes. Hodgkin's disease begins in the same way as lymphoma (see below) but the cells in Hodgkin's are less malignant and the disease is more curable.

> **Fascinating fact**
>
> The old-fashioned word for oedema is 'dropsy'. This word is derived from the Greek word 'hydrops' (*hydro* means water). It is no longer a scientific term.

> **Proving the point**
>
> If you have flown on an aircraft, you may have experienced swollen feet and ankles. This is mainly due to the lack of movement and activity whilst flying, but the reduced air pressure in the cabin also has an effect. What advice do airlines give to reduce the effects of oedema whilst flying?

> **Link to learning**
>
> The word 'gland' is often used when referring to a lymph node. For example, saying 'my glands are up' actually means that the lymph nodes are swollen and fighting an infection. Remember: lymph nodes are not glands as they do not produce secretions. (Link to The Endocrine System, page 135)

Immunodeficiency

This is where the body's ability to defend itself is reduced or non-existent, usually as a result of other diseases such as leukaemia or lymphoma.

Leukaemia

This is a type of cancer which affects white blood cells. It starts when a white blood cell divides at an abnormal rate and produces other abnormal cells. This leads to a large amount of abnormal white blood cells, which then impair functioning of the body's systems. There are two main types of leukaemia:

- lymphatic leukaemia affects the white blood cells manufactured in the lymph nodes (lymphocytes)
- myeloid leukaemia affects the white blood cells manufactured in the bone marrow (neutrophils).

Both types of leukaemia can be **chronic** (long-term) or **acute** (short-term). Sufferers of chronic leukaemia may live for as long as 15 years; for those with acute leukaemia, death can occur within weeks if the disease is not treated.

Lymphadenitis

Inflammation of the lymph nodes, which indicates that the body is fighting infection.

Lymphandenopathy

Disease of the lymph nodes. It is a common symptom in many cancerous diseases. Swollen nodes throughout the body are also an early sign of AIDS (Acquired Immune Deficiency Syndrome), arising from HIV (Human Immunodeficiency Virus) infection.

Lymphangitis

Swelling and inflammation of the lymphatic vessels, appearing as deep pink or red lines on the skin. Lymphangitis may start where an infection is already present in the body. If the lymph nodes fail to fight and control the infection, it may pass to the blood causing septicaemia (blood poisoning).

Lymphoma

Lymphoma occurs when a white blood cell (lymphocyte) in the lymph node multiplies at an abnormal rate and produces other abnormal lymphocytes. These cause the node to swell. Lymphomas or tumours can be malignant (cancer-causing) or benign (non-cancerous).

Non-Hodgkin's lymphoma

This is more common than Hodgkin's disease and includes a wide range of cancerous disorders which affect lymphoid tissue. It generally affects older people.

Oedema
Excess fluid in the tissues.

Tonsillitis
Inflammation of the tonsils

Ageing and the lymphatic system

Recent research has suggested that the body's ability to develop immunity from a vaccine diminishes from about 65 years of age. Also, the likelihood of contracting Non-Hodgkin's lymphoma increases with age.

Because the lymphatic system is closely related to the blood circulatory system, if the heart loses strength in old age, the ability to pump blood is reduced; this means that the lymph fluid will have less suction to help it on its return journey. If there is the added complication of obesity, lymph fluid is more likely to remain in the tissues, preventing fresh fluid from reaching the area. The body will then struggle to provide sufficient oxygen and nutrients to the cells, putting excessive strain on the heart.

Knowledge check
1. What is lymph?
2. Explain how lymph is formed.
3. Describe what a lymph node does.
4. What is oedema?
5. Name the two lymphatic ducts in the body.
6. Which body parts do each of the lymphatic ducts drain?
7. Name two other types of lymphatic tissue in the body.
8. What is the function of the spleen?
9. What role does the thymus gland play in the lymphatic system?
10. Name the group of lymph nodes in the underarm area.
11. What does it mean if your tonsils are swollen?
12. Name four groups of nodes in the head and neck.
13. Name the nodes in the groin.
14. Where does lymph rejoin the blood circulation?
15. State the basic constituents of lymphatic fluid.
16. How does lymph move around the body?
17. How does a lymphatic capillary differ from a blood capillary?
18. List the functions of the lymphatic system.
19. How do lymph vessels prevent the backward flow of lymph?
20. When and why does lymph fluid appear milky?

CHAPTER 7 The Respiratory System

SECTION 2

Fascinating fact

People breathe on average approximately sixteen times per minute, but this rate is slower during sleep and rises during exercise.

Breathing is something that you do every moment of your life, whether waking or sleeping, and yet you probably rarely notice this **automatic** process. However, if breathing stops for more than three minutes, the body's cells will stop working properly and will quickly begin to die. The respiratory system is thus crucial to the body's functioning.

The respiratory system is a network of tubes and passages ending in tiny air sacs, connecting the outside air with blood. The movement of air in and out of the lungs is called breathing, and the breakdown of **oxygen** and glucose to form heat energy in the cells is called respiration.

Cells need a continuous supply of oxygen in order to produce energy for the body. This process of **metabolism** gives rise to a gas called **carbon dioxide**. It is the **respiratory system** that allows oxygen and carbon dioxide to enter and leave the body during breathing.

The **blood circulatory system** transports oxygen to the cells and takes carbon dioxide from the cells back to the lungs. [(Link to The Blood Circulatory System, page 77)](#) In order to maintain **homeostasis**, carbon dioxide must be removed quickly or the cells will not function effectively. When you breathe harder, for example, during exercise or stress, the cells demand more oxygen and will therefore produce more carbon dioxide. The rate of breathing must change to allow for these changes; this rate is controlled by a specialised part of the brain.

It is important to have a thorough understanding of the respiratory system because treatments such as Indian head massage, aromatherapy and reflexology have an effect on it.

> **You will learn**
>
> In this chapter you will learn about:
> - the organs of respiration
> - gaseous exchange (the process of respiration)
> - the process of breathing
> - different types of breathing
> - the effects of pollution on the respiratory system
> - common disorders of the respiratory system
> - ageing and the respiratory system.

SECTION 2

Proving the point

The mucous membranes of the nose secrete up to 1 litre (2 pints) of mucus per day. Can you suggest a function for this mucus?

The organs of respiration
The nose and nasal cavities

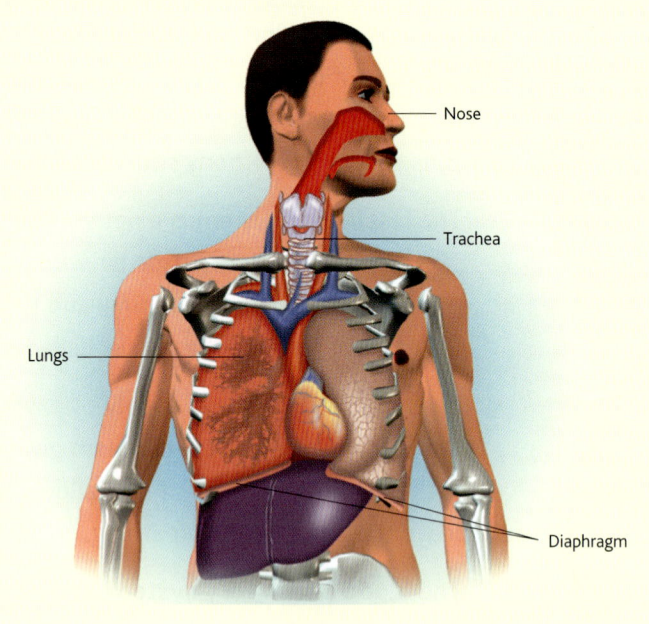

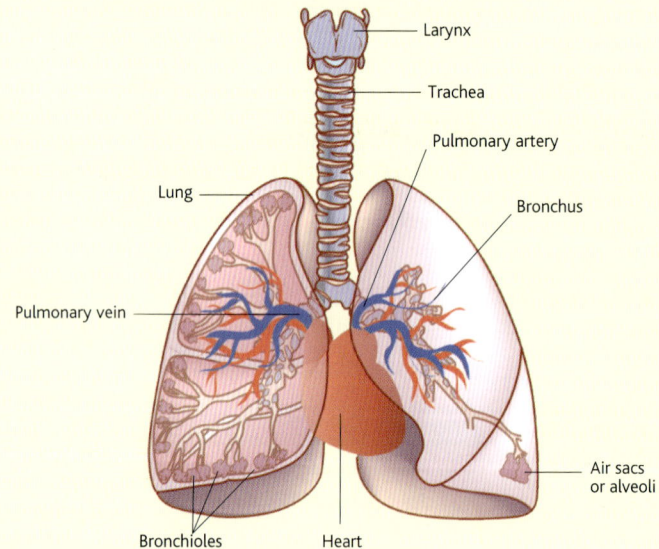

▲ The respiratory system

Fascinating fact

The vocal cords in men are longer than in women, which accounts for the deeper voice in men.

Fascinating fact

Laryngitis is an inflammation of the voice box resulting in soreness and hoarseness in the voice. It can be caused by irritants such as cigarette smoke or by overuse, for example, performers who sing for hours a day. Cancer of the larynx is also linked to smoking.

Air enters the respiratory system through the nose, and the mouth. The main function of the nose is to warm and moisten the air before it enters the lungs. The nose is divided into two cavities by the nasal septum. These cavities are situated between the roof of the mouth and the cranium, and are lined with **mucous membrane**, which contains many blood vessels to deliver heat and moisture. As the air passes over the mucous membranes it is warmed and moistened by the blood vessels and filtered by the tiny hairs found there. The protective nature of the nasal cavities can only be realised by breathing through the nose rather than the mouth.

The pharynx
The pharynx or throat is a funnel-shaped tube that links the back of the mouth with the larynx or voice box. It serves as a passage way for food as well as air.

The larynx
Commonly called the voice box, the larynx is located between the pharynx and the trachea, or windpipe. The larynx is composed of cartilage and has a protruding section commonly known as the Adam's Apple. The larynx houses the vocal cords, which vibrate forming a sound as air passes out of the lungs.

At the top of the larynx is a leaf-shaped flap of **cartilage** called the epiglottis. This closes over the top of the larynx (or glottis) during swallowing and prevents any food or liquid passing into the lungs.

The trachea
The trachea, or windpipe, is a tube, approximately 12 cm (4.5 inches) long, which carries air into the lungs. It extends from the larynx to the point of bifurcation (splitting) and is situated in front of the oesophagus. The trachea is formed from C-shaped hoops of cartilage to ensure that it is kept open at all times. The base of the trachea bifurcates or splits to form two bronchi.

The bronchi
The structure of the bronchi is similar to the trachea but they are narrower. The bronchi carry air into the lungs. On entering the lungs they divide into smaller airways called bronchioles.

Lining of the air passageways
The respiratory tract is lined with **ciliated epithelial tissue** interspersed with mucus-producing goblet cells. (Link to Cells and Tissues, page 20)

The cilia are hair-like projections that sweep dust and dirt out of the lungs. This is rolled into a ball with the mucus and swept towards the pharynx so that it can be coughed or sneezed out or swallowed and destroyed by stomach acid.

The lungs
The lungs are large, spongy, elastic, cone-shaped structures that almost fill the thoracic cavity, extending right down to the diaphragm. They are the centre of the respiratory system. They are divided into sections called lobes. The left lung is slightly smaller than the right lung because of the position of the **heart**; it only contains two lobes whereas the right lung has three.

The lungs' function is to bring oxygen-rich air into the body and to expel the carbon dioxide made by the cells during respiration. As each bronchus

---

Fascinating fact

The lungs are designed to fit neatly into the thoracic cavity but they have an extremely large surface area. It is calculated that if all the alveoli were opened up they would cover an area of about 60 square metres (646 square feet) – that's roughly the size of a tennis court!

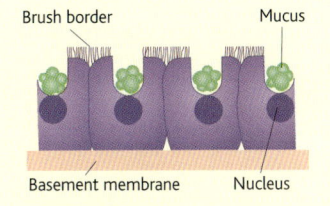

▲ Goblet cells line the respiratory tract

Fascinating fact

The harmful effects of smoking
The tar in cigarette smoke will damage and finally destroy the cilia, leaving them flattened and ineffective. This means that there is no defensive barrier to keep unwanted substances out of the lung. Mucus is still produced, but to prevent it entering the lung the smoker must cough it out. This is unpleasant and, ultimately, weakens the muscles around the air passages causing permanent damage.

SECTION 2

Fascinating fact
The lungs contain so many air spaces that if dropped in water they float. No surprise then that the word lung means 'light'.

enters the lung, it branches and divides into many smaller branches resembling the branches on a tree – hence it is often referred to as the 'bronchial tree'. The smallest branches are called bronchioles. Unlike the bronchi these tiny tubes are not held open by cartilage but contain tiny muscles controlled by the **autonomic nervous system.** (Link to The Nervous System, page 129) The bronchioles end in air sacs called **alveoli**.

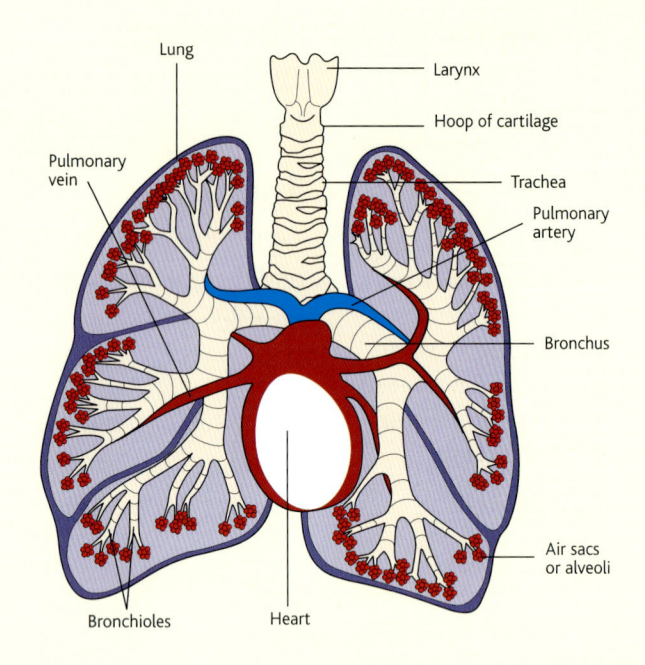

▲ The lungs

The alveoli
The alveoli are microscopic air sacs located at the end of the bronchioles. Each lung contains 300 million alveoli. It is here that oxygen and carbon dioxide are exchanged in a process called **gaseous exchange**.

The walls of the alveoli are made from a single layer of epithelium covered by a layer of moisture. Each alveolus is covered with a network of **capillaries** to allow for the easy exchange of gases. Deoxygenated blood, rich in carbon dioxide, is brought to the lung from the heart in the pulmonary artery. When the blood has been oxygenated it returns to the heart in the pulmonary vein.

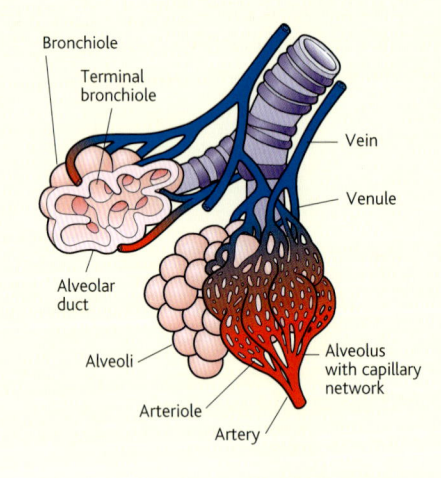

▲ Gaseous exchange takes place in the alveoli

The pleura
The lungs are covered by a tough double-layered sac or membrane called the pleura. Between the two layers is a space filled with pleural fluid to lubricate the membranes. These membranes allow the lungs to increase in capacity during breathing.

CHAPTER 7 The Respiratory System

Overview of the respiratory system

> **Link to learning**
>
> The pulmonary artery brings blood low in oxygen but high in carbon dioxide to the lungs from the right ventricle of the heart. The pulmonary vein takes blood rich in oxygen from the lungs to the left atrium of the heart so that it can be pumped through the left ventricle into the aorta and on to all the tissues of the body. (Link to The Blood Circulatory System, page 88)

Organ	Structure	Function
The nose	Linked to the outside world; lined with ciliated mucus membrane.	To warm and filter air that is breathed in.
The pharynx	A muscular tube forming the throat.	To act as a passageway for food and air.
The larynx	A box-shaped structure formed from cartilage.	Contains the vocal cords which enable speech.
The trachea	A tubular passageway for air; kept open by semi-circular hoops of cartilage.	To carry air to and from the lungs during breathing.
The bronchi	Two tubes formed when the trachea bifurcates. When the trachea divide, the right bronchi is wider.	To carry air to the lungs.
The lungs	Large spongy organs that almost fill the thoracic cavity.	To allow the exchange of gases.
The bronchioles	Tiny branches of the bronchi containing muscles.	To carry air to the alveoli.
The alveoli	Tiny air sacs with walls that are one-cell thick.	To allow oxygen to enter the bloodstream and carbon dioxide to be breathed out.

> **Link to learning**
>
> The breathing rate is regulated by the hypothalamus gland and the respiratory centre in the brain. (Link to The Endocrine System, page 137) They respond to increased levels of carbon dioxide by stimulating the muscles of respiration.

Gaseous exchange

Gaseous exchange takes place in the alveoli of the lungs. Because the walls of the alveoli and the walls of the surrounding blood capillary are only one cell thick, it is relatively easy for gases such as oxygen and carbon dioxide to pass through.

- When you breathe in, oxygen from the air accumulates in the alveolus and diffuses through into the blood capillary and then into the bloodstream.
- At the same time, carbon dioxide is released from the blood through the wall of the alveolus to be breathed out.

Thus, the purpose of breathing is to keep the oxygen concentration high and the carbon dioxide concentration low in the alveoli so that gaseous exchange can occur. (Link to Cells and Tissues, page 13)

> **Proving the point**
>
> During exercise, the levels of carbon dioxide in the air leaving the lung will be higher. Can you account for this?

> **Summary of gaseous exchange**
> - Oxygen enters the lung as you breathe in.
> - Oxygen diffuses through the wall of the alveolus.
> - Oxygen binds to the haemoglobin in the blood.
> - Blood carries oxygen to the cells as required.
> - Cells make energy in the form of heat, creating the waste product carbon dioxide.
> - Carbon dioxide is carried in the blood back to the lungs.
> - Carbon dioxide diffuses out of the blood into the lungs.
> - Carbon dioxide is breathed out.

> **Proving the point**
>
> Why does mouth-to-mouth resuscitation work in first aid?

PAGE 115

> **Link to practice**
>
> Because it is slower, nose breathing has a more calming effect than mouth breathing and is often recommended to aid relaxation. It also helps maintain elasticity of the lungs and improves posture. Try sitting with your client and doing a few slow, deep breaths in through the nose and out through the mouth. This is an ideal way to start a treatment like Indian head massage or aromatherapy.

The process of breathing

There are two distinct phases of breathing:
- inhalation or breathing in
- exhalation or breathing out.

The internal and external intercostal muscles, located at an angle between the ribs, and the dome-like diaphragm muscle move the chest up and down during breathing to allow air into and out of the lungs. (Link to Muscles and the Muscular System, page 70)

Inhalation

When breathing in, the lungs are inflated. The first step involves the diaphragm becoming flatter and the external intercostals muscles contracting. This means that the ribs are pulled upwards and outwards, increasing the capacity of the lungs and reducing the air pressure inside the lungs.

As the pressure inside the lungs falls, air from outside rushes in to equalise the pressure.

Exhalation

At a signal from the respiratory centre, located in the medulla oblongata in the brain (Link to The Nervous System, page 124), the process of exhalation or breathing out begins. The diaphragm returns to its dome shape, the internal intercostal muscles contract and the ribs are forced downwards and inwards. This action squeezes that air out of the lungs.

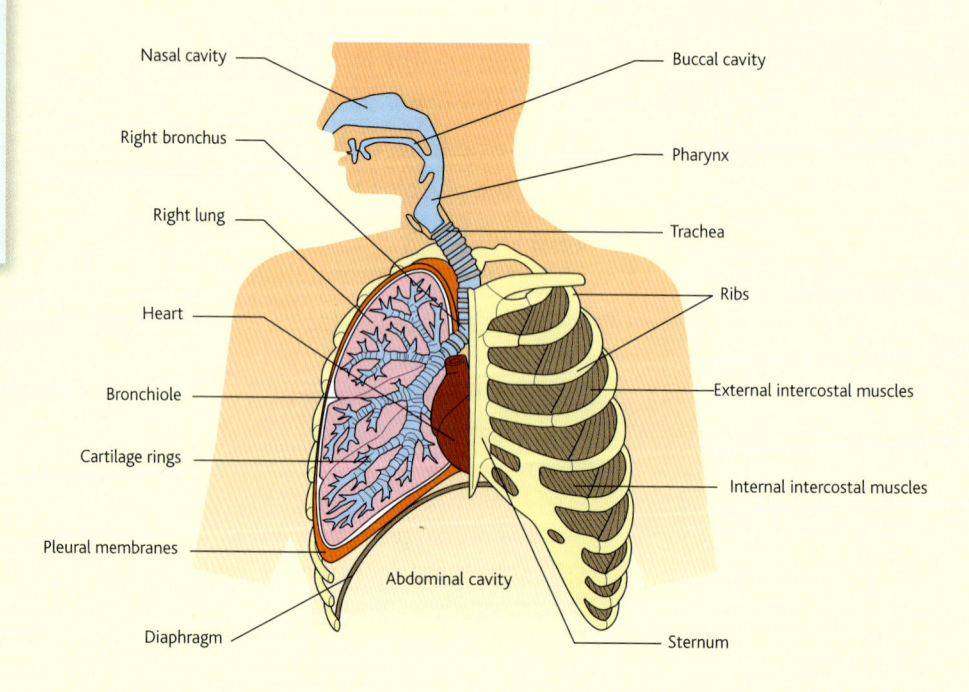

> **Link to practice**
>
> If you are about to start a reflexology treatment, apply gentle thumb pressure on the reflex point for the solar plexus as your client breathes in. Then release the pressure as your client exhales. As you do this, breathe with your client so that you become attuned with each other.

▲ The process of inhalation and exhalation

Gases entering and leaving the lungs

Gas	Entering the lung	Leaving the lung
Oxygen	21%	16%
Nitrogen	79%	79%
Carbon dioxide	0.04%	4.5%
Other gases	Trace	Trace
Water vapour	Variable	Saturated

The effects of pollution on the respiratory system

Air pollution

People are becoming more and more concerned about air pollution and its effect on health. Car exhaust fumes and industrial smoke pollute the air in cities and built-up areas. In the countryside, wind carries pollen and agricultural chemicals into homes.

- There has been a worrying rise in asthma in children, and this may be related to air pollution.
- Pollution can trigger bouts of coughing in people who are more susceptible to respiratory problems, such as young children and the elderly; recent studies show that even low levels of pollutants reduce lung function.
- The majority of smoke in cities comes from vehicle exhausts; larger smoke particles are trapped in the upper air passages causing an increase in nasal secretions, but smaller particles travel deeper into the lungs where they can cause breathing difficulties.

Most researchers now agree that air pollution is a major public health problem, second only to smoking in the damage that it can do to the lungs. Giving up smoking will make the lungs less vulnerable to the effects of pollutants as well as bestowing other health benefits. You can help to reduce air pollution by leaving your car at home as often as possible and, when you do drive, using a car with a catalytic converter. Some modern buildings are fitted with filters to prevent pollutants from entering offices and workplaces.

The effects of smoking

Cigarette smoking causes permanent, irreversible damage to the lungs. Cigarette smoke contains over 4,000 chemicals, many of which are harmful. The government has become so concerned about the effects of passive smoking that it has imposed a ban on smoking in all enclosed public spaces (due to come into effect in mid-2007).

Proving the point

When you breathe very quickly or very deeply, you use the accessory muscles of respiration such as the abdominals, pectoralis major and latissimus dorsi. (Link to Muscles and the Muscular System, page 70) Try taking a few deep breaths yourself and feel the muscles involved in this process. Then list the actions of these muscles. Why are they so useful in rapid breathing?

Proving the point

What advice would you give to a client who was worried about the effects of pollutants?

Fascinating fact

One out of every two lifetime smokers will die early because they smoke.

> **Link to practice**
>
> Clients with chronic bronchitis may not be comfortable lying flat for a treatment as it can be hard for them to breathe – always ask if your client would prefer to sit.

The main effects of smoking are:
- the tar in cigarette smoke coats the lungs like soot in a chimney
- carbon monoxide replaces oxygen in gaseous exchange meaning that the muscles and the heart have to work harder
- fat deposits build up on the walls of the blood vessels, causing them to narrow and thus increasing the likelihood of strokes and heart attacks
- blood vessels to the limbs may also become narrow; smokers sometimes have their hands and feet amputated
- babies born to smoking mothers are more likely to have a low birth weight
- **chronic bronchitis** and emphysema are caused by smoking
- it can exacerbate the symptoms of asthma
- it is highly addictive so people find it terribly difficult to stop
- it increases the risk of lung cancer.

Disease and disorders of the respiratory system

Acute laryngitis
During this illness, the throat becomes sore and the voice is hoarse (reduced to a whisper). It usually clears up within a few days.

Asthma
Asthma attacks occur when the muscles of the bronchioles go into spasm (known as bronchospasm). This makes it difficult to get oxygen into the body and to remove carbon dioxide, so air becomes 'trapped' in the lungs. This can be a very serious condition and sufferers usually carry an inhaler in case of a sudden attack.

Bronchitis
Inflammation of the bronchi is called bronchitis. This may be **acute**, which is usually caused by an infection, or chronic, which does not clear up. Chronic bronchitis is common in middle-aged smokers and tends to be worse in the winter.

Common cold
The common cold is a disorder of the upper respiratory tract but can lead to bronchitis or other more serious respiratory conditions. It is a highly infectious and very common disorder. It is caused by a virus and is spread by droplet infection. On average, an individual will suffer two to three colds per year but this lessens with age, possibly as a result of accumulating immunity.

Emphysema
The air spaces in the lungs become enlarged making exhalation difficult. The exchange of gases becomes impaired and any movement will leave the sufferer short of breath. Emphysema is a very serious condition often seen in smokers

and can follow chronic bronchitis.

Lung cancer
When cells in the lung reproduce abnormally, they can produce useless tissue that is malignant. The early signs of lung cancer include a cough that does not clear up. The main cause of lung cancer is cigarette smoking.

Pleurisy
Inflammation of the pleural membrane is called pleurisy. This is an extremely painful condition, particularly when coughing. Pleurisy can be caused by a number of factors, including viral infection.

Pneumonia
Pneumonia is an acute infection of the alveoli of the lungs, which can be viral or bacterial. Oxygen cannot diffuse properly and breathing is difficult. It is more common in people with a low resistance to infection, for example, the elderly and the young, and is potentially fatal.

Pulmonary embolism
This refers to the presence of a blood clot in a pulmonary blood vessel, thus obstructing the flow of blood to the lungs with very serious consequences. The blood clot originates in another blood vessel, often a vein in the leg (deep vein thrombosis, or DVT). Pulmonary embolism can occur following a long airline flight. Smokers and those with other risk factors are particularly vulnerable.

Tuberculosis
Tuberculosis (TB) is caused by the presence of a microbe called the tubercule bacillus and is spread by droplet infection. Small lesions or tubercles destroy the lung tissue, restricting their function. Tuberculosis can be prevented by a vaccine called the BCG now given routinely. However, TB is on the increase in the UK and remains the world's leading cause of death.

Ageing and the respiratory system
With age the respiratory system becomes more rigid and loses its elasticity. The muscles of respiration become weaker, resulting in loss of lung capacity. The cilia lining the air passages are reduced and because the immune system is less efficient, there is a vulnerability to infections such as pneumonia. Smokers are more likely to develop bronchitis and emphysema as they get older. Because the cardiovascular system and the respiratory system are so closely linked, damage to one system usually affects the other. People who take regular aerobic exercise throughout life are less susceptible to the effects of ageing.

Case study

Level 3/Holistic

Manjeet is a 45-year-old woman who is booked in for a complementary therapy. She is married with two children, one at university and one about to leave school. She is a non-smoker who has a good diet and a moderate consumption of alcohol, and she enjoys good physical health. She works part-time as a legal secretary.

During the consultation she reveals that she is occasionally overwhelmed by frightening physical symptoms when driving. These take the form of rising feelings of terror accompanied by nausea, sweating and difficulty in breathing. The last time this happened she had to stop the car and call her husband to come and collect her, despite having been driving for many years. She is confused and frightened by these episodes. What do you sugest?

Knowledge check

1. Distinguish between respiration and breathing.
2. State three structures found in the respiratory system.
3. What happens to air as it passes over the nasal mucosa?
4. Explain why it is better to breathe through the nose than the mouth.
5. Name the part of the respiratory system that contains the Adam's Apple.
6. Explain how food particles are prevented from entering the lungs.
7. Give the correct names for throat, voice box and windpipe.
8. Explain how dirt and dust are prevented from entering the lungs.
9. Explain why the right lung is larger that the left.
10. State why the bronchi are sometimes referred to as a tree.
11. Describe the function of the alveoli.
12. How does the pulmonary artery differ from the other arteries in the body?
13. Name the respiratory muscles.
14. Name two accessory muscles of respiration.
15. Identify the two phases of breathing.
16. Which part of the brain controls the breathing rate?
17. Where does gaseous exchange take place?
18. Respiration occurs as the same rate as breathing. True or false?
19. Where in the body is carbon dioxide produced?
20. Describe the functions of the respiratory system.

CHAPTER 8 The Nervous System

SECTION 2

Fascinating fact

The brain never sleeps and it uses 20 per cent of the body's total energy supply.

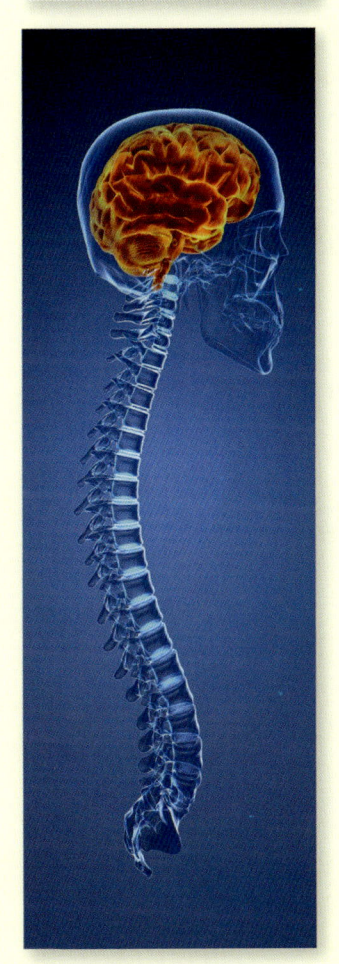

How do you know what a flower looks like, how a song sounds, how cotton wool feels, how chocolate tastes, how freshly baked bread smells? You might answer that you know these things because of your sense organs, which is correct but only partly so. The sense organs pick up information from the external and internal environment, but what happens next is an extraordinary journey along many miles of tiny fibres, to the brain and back again. This journey takes place within the **nervous system**, a major system of the human body whose role is communication and co-ordination.

The nervous system also controls those things which happen automatically in your body – things that you might be less aware of. It makes sure that the heart continues to beat, that food is digested, that air passes in and out of the lungs, and that wounds heal. In fact, the nervous system controls everything that the body does, whether you are aware of it or not.

The nervous system is a collection of billions of specialist cells and **connective tissue** and it consists of two main parts. The central part consists of the brain and spinal cord and is called the **central nervous system** (CNS). The part around the outside is called the **peripheral nervous system** (PNS).

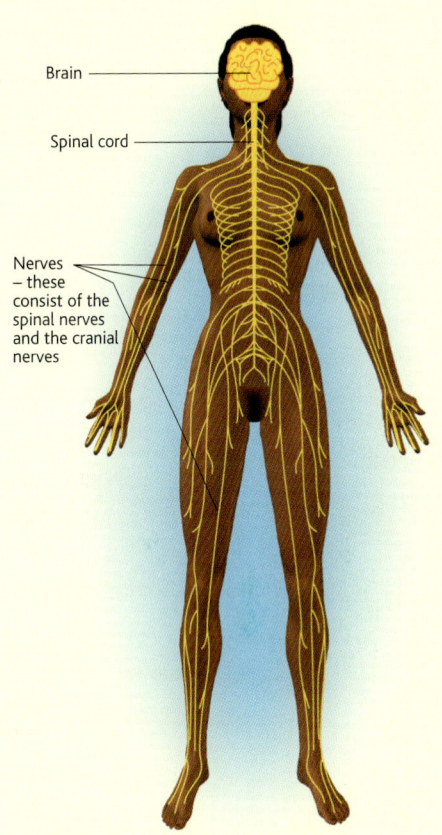

▲ The brain and spinal cord form the central nervous system

▲ The nervous system (Brain, Spinal cord, Nerves – these consist of the spinal nerves and the cranial nerves)

Link to learning

The nervous system behaves like a telephone system. It can send internal messages to the brain as well as transmitting messages to and from the world outside.

You will learn

In this chapter you will learn about:
- the structure and function of a nerve cell
- the structure and function of the central nervous system (CNS)
- the structure and function of the peripheral nervous system (PNS)
- the sensory system
- the structure and function of the **autonomic nervous system** (ANS)
- the nature of a reflex action
- disorders and diseases of the nervous system
- the effects of ageing on the nervous system.

PAGE 121

SECTION 2

> **Fascinating fact**
>
> The brain produces more electrical impulses than all the telephones in the world!

The nervous system provides a network of communication between different areas of the body so that all the systems remain in contact with each other and the body maintains co-ordination. The nervous system also acts as a receiver for information from the external environment so that the body knows what is happening in its surroundings and can respond in the appropriate way. These external stimuli are transmitted by sense organs in the form of sensations.

It is necessary to have knowledge of the nervous system because it plays such a central part in co-ordinating the functions of the body. An understanding of the functions and structures within this system will enable you to explain why the body behaves as it does in certain situations. For example, the nervous system plays an important role in defining the body's reaction to stress. There are also a number of disorders and diseases associated with the nervous system which may have implications for treatment.

> **Link to practice**
>
> There are millions of nerve endings in the skin. (Link to The Skin, Hair and Nails, page 31) This means that every time you touch a client, your nervous system is interacting with the nervous system of your client.

The structure and function of a nerve cell

What is commonly known as a 'nerve' is actually a bundle of many smaller cells called **neurones**. The shape and size of neurones varies according to their position and function in the body. They have a fairly large cell body which contains the **nucleus** of the cell, and this is what makes up the grey matter of the brain and spinal cord.

Information coming into the cell travels along short, branched processes called **dendrites**. Information going away from the cell is carried along longer nerve fibres called **axons**. Axons and dendrites make up the white matter of the brain and spinal cord.

> **Link to learning**
>
> It is worth remembering that the nervous system is closely related to the endocrine system in that they are both systems of communication and co-ordination. (Link to The Endocrine System, page 135)

Axons, and some dendrites, are protected by a fatty sheath of myelin between the cell and the connective tissue. The **myelin sheath** insulates the nerve fibres so that impulses are contained and not transmitted to neighbouring nerves. The sheath also protects the fibres from pressure and injury. It is grooved, which enables contact with surrounding tissue fluid; this is necessary for the exchange of nutrients and waste matter.

▲ A neurone

CHAPTER 8 The Nervous System

Fascinating fact

The human nervous system comprises around twelve thousand-million (12,000,000,000) neurones. I wonder who counted them...

Axons have tiny expanded ends which are a bit like frayed wire. They lie very close to but do not touch the cell body or dendrites of adjacent neurones. The minute space between neurones is called a **synapse** or reflex arc. Nervous impulses travel across a synapse in one direction only and it is here that communication between neurones takes place.

Nerves

A collection of neurones is called a nerve. Nerves carry information in one direction only – either towards the Central Nervous System (CNS) or away from it.

- Nerves which carry information towards the CNS from the sensory organs are called **afferent** or **sensory nerves**. Their job is to pick up sensory impulses.
- Nerves which carry information away from the CNS towards other parts of the body are called **efferent** or **motor nerves**. Their role is to initiate movement.

Link to learning

To recall the difference between axons and dendrites, remember:
- *AAA:* Axons carry information A-long (they are longer fibres) and A-way from the nerve cell.
- Dendrites are shorter fibres that carry information towards the nerve cell.

The structure and function of the central nervous system (CNS)

As the name suggests, the central nervous system (CNS) is the central part of the nervous system. It is both centrally located and has central importance. The CNS is made up of two main structures: the brain and spinal cord. These have overall control of the millions of nerve cells and fibres in the body.

The CNS is surrounded by a liquid component called cerebrospinal fluid. This fluid, along with the brain and spinal cord, is enclosed in a membrane called the meninges.

Link to learning

The neurones which make up a nerve are all the same length and lie alongside each other, protected by a myelin sheath. They are a bit like individual electrical wires within an insulated plastic cable.

The CNS is like the control station of the body, receiving and sending out millions of messages each day. It receives messages about external temperature, the sound of a conversation, pain or the taste of your favourite food. The CNS then sorts out all this information and instructs the body to act, either consciously or unconsciously. Thanks to the nervous function of the CNS you can walk, talk, see and hear. The CNS also controls involuntary actions such as heartbeat, digestion of food and blinking of the eyelids.

The brain

The brain receives and analyses all information internal and external to the body. This information is translated into sensations and reactions and is stored as memories.

The brain has three main components, which are named according to their location. These are the forebrain, the midbrain and the hindbrain.

SECTION 2

Fascinating fact

The human brain is 85 per cent water. You may have noticed that one of the early signs of dehydration (not drinking enough water) is that you get a headache.

Fascinating fact

As human intelligence has evolved, so has the size of the human brain. The size of your brain is three times that of your early human ancestors.

Link to learning

The area known as the brain stem is made up of the midbrain, the pons and the medulla oblongata.

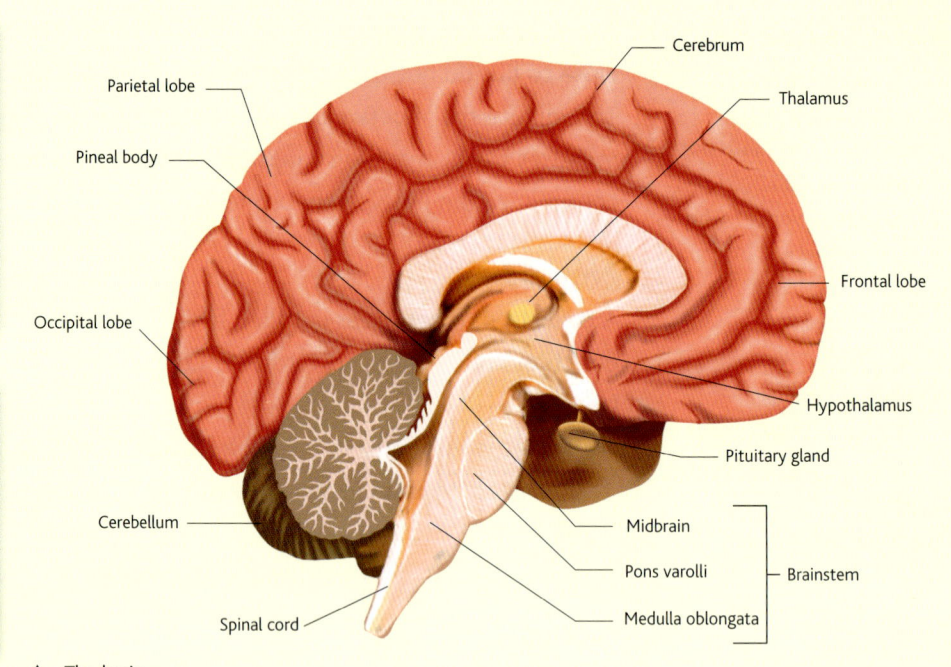

▲ The brain

The forebrain

The largest part of the brain is the forebrain or **cerebrum**. This is the upper part of the brain and its main function is to co-ordinate movement.

The forebrain is divided into two halves called the right and left **cerebral hemispheres**. Each hemisphere is further subdivided into four lobes. These are named according to their location and are the frontal lobe, parietal lobe, occipital lobe and temporal lobe.

The midbrain

The midbrain is located between the forebrain and the hindbrain. Its function is to transmit messages to and from the CNS and it is also responsible for co-ordinating sight and sound.

The hindbrain

The hindbrain has three parts called the pons, cerebellum and medulla oblongata.

- The pons is located between the midbrain and the medulla oblongata and it transmits impulses between these two areas.
- The medulla oblongata is located between the pons and the spinal cord. It controls the vital centres which are the blood circulatory and

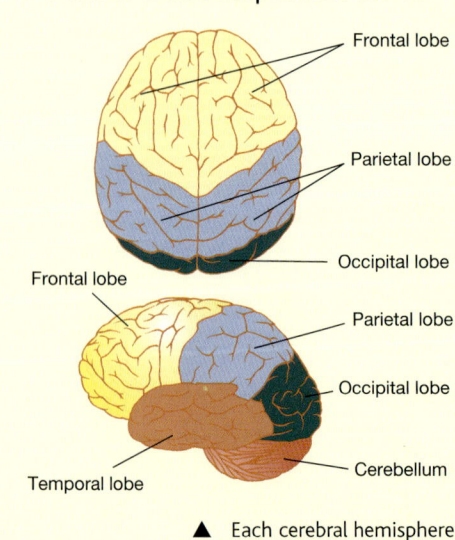

▲ Each cerebral hemisphere is divided into four lobes

PAGE 124

CHAPTER 8 The Nervous System

> **Fascinating fact**
> Sensations picked up from the left side of the body are interpreted by the right side of the brain because the nerve fibres cross over.

> **Link to practice**
> There are a number of disorders of the brain which may require medical approval prior to treatment, such as Parkinson's disease (see also page 133).

respiratory systems. (Links to The Blood Circulatory System, page 77 and The Respiratory System, page 114)

- The cerebellum is underneath the occipital lobe of the forebrain. Its function is to control muscular activity. (Link to Muscles and the Muscular System, page 62)

The spinal cord

The spinal cord is about 45 cm (18 inches) in length, running from the midbrain to the level of the first lumbar vertebra. (Link to The Skeletal System, page 48) The cord is ridged down the centre and so appears to have a left and right side, like the forebrain. It is thicker at the top than at the bottom and swells in the cervical and lumbar regions due to the location of a large nerve supply to the arms and legs. The spinal cord consists of motor fibres which run downwards from the brain, and sensory fibres which run upwards towards the brain.

The spinal nerves

There are 31 pairs of spinal nerves on each side of the spinal cord. These are sub-divided into:

- 8 pairs of cervical nerves
- 12 pairs of thoracic nerves
- 5 pairs of lumbar nerves
- 5 pairs of sacral nerves
- 1 pair of coccygeal nerves.

Each nerve is divided into an anterior motor root and a posterior sensory root. The anterior motor root transmits information from the CNS to the body. The posterior sensory root transmits information from the body to the CNS.

Nerve plexus

The network of nerves which surrounds the spinal column is called the **nerve plexuses**. ('Plexus' simply means a network of structures.) The nerve plexuses are named according to their location along the vertebral column and are found in all areas except the thoracic region (where individual thoracic nerves supply the chest and abdomen). The main nerve plexuses are:

- the cervical plexus in the neck
- the brachial network in the region of the arms

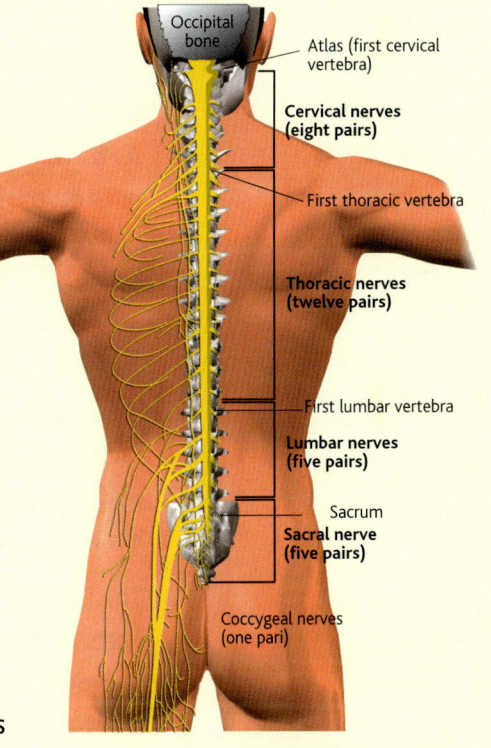

▲ The spinal cord and spinal nerves

PAGE 125

SECTION 2

> **Link to practice**
>
> The sciatic nerve branches from the sacral plexus. It can become trapped due to muscular or joint injury, causing pain in the hip and leg known as sciatica. Sciatica can be relieved by massage but only with prior medical consent.

- the lumbar and sacral networks in the lower part of the trunk.

Nerve plexus	Part of the body supplied
Cervical plexus	Neck, shoulder and **diaphragm**
Brachial plexus	Outer arm, inner arm and hand
Lumbar plexus	Lower back and legs
Sacral plexus	Pelvis, front of leg, back of leg and foot

> **Link to practice**
>
> The solar plexus is located just below the sternum in the centre of the body. Its name derives from the fact that the nerve fibres were thought to radiate outwards to other areas of the body, rather like the rays of the sun. This area has central importance in holistic philosophies and therapies. It is a concentrated area of sympathetic nerve endings and it is believed that light pressure here can have a calming effect on the body. Many therapies start and end with the practitioner placing their hands over the area of the solar plexus as it is thought that this, quite literally, calms the body.

The structure and function of the peripheral nervous system (PNS)

As the name suggests, the peripheral nervous system is on the periphery, or outside, of the central nervous system. In other words, it is the part of the nervous system which supplies the arms, legs, back, abdomen and internal organs – in fact, every part of the body other than the brain and spinal cord.

The PNS has two parts: the **somatic nervous system** and the autonomic nervous system, because not all nervous functions are the same. For example, if you want to get up and walk across the room, you are able to do

▲ The peripheral nervous system and its actions

> **Link to practice**
>
> Motor nerves enter a muscle at the motor point and cause a contraction. Treatments such as EMS stimulate the motor point artificially via an electrical current.

PAGE 126

Link to learning

A sensory nerve fibre which terminates in a muscle, gland or organ and stimulates a particular action is called an effector nerve because it effects an action.

Fascinating fact

Medical or dental treatment might require a local anaesthetic to numb an area. Anaesthetics work by preventing sensory impulses from travelling to the CNS. An epidural, which is often administered during childbirth, prevents all sensations below the point of the spinal cord at which it is administered.

so because your conscious mind sends a message to your brain informing it of your intentions; the brain then sends a message back to your muscles instructing them to move. These conscious movements are controlled by the somatic nervous system. Movements which are not under conscious control are effected by the autonomic nervous system.

Cranial nerves

There are twelve pairs of cranial nerves which originate in the brain stem. Some of these are sensory nerves which transmit information from the body to the CNS. These include the olfactory nerve which originates in the nose, the optic nerve which originates in the eye and the vestibulocochlear nerve which originates in the ear. Other cranial nerves are motor nerves which transmit information from the CNS to the body. These include the oculomotor nerve which controls the eye and the hypoglossal nerve which controls the tongue. Some cranial nerves transmit both sensory and motor information.

The sensory system

The sensory system transmits information from the skin, sense organs and internal structures of the body to the CNS where it is translated. Sometimes this translation occurs immediately and without conscious effort, as in breathing or heartbeat. Other sensations, which you may be more aware of, are caused by information received from the external environment.

All sensory impulses are sent to the thalamus in the brain, which is like the main sorting office of the internal communication system. The thalamus then distributes the information, to the particular part of the brain which deals with that particular kind of information. For example, one part of the brain deals with visual information, so sensory impulses received from the eyes are sent there. Another area of the brain deals with auditory information, so sensory impulses received from the ears are sent there. Some impulses are dealt with by the CNS automatically such as heartbeat or the contraction of muscles in the internal organs.

Summary of the functional areas of the brain

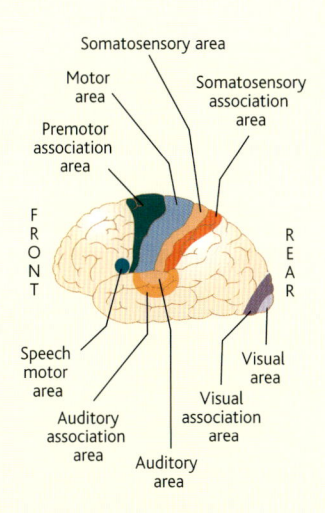

▲ The functional area of the left cerebral hemisphere

Area of the brain	Function
Left hemisphere	Language, rational, logical, analytical
Right hemisphere	Visuo-spatial, artistic, emotional, intuition, creativity
Motor cortex in frontal lobe	Fine movement
Pre-frontal cortex	Planning, working memory, goal-oriented behaviour
Limbic system	Emotions
Hypothalamus	Regulates ANS and endocrine system

Fascinating fact

The sense of smell and the sense of taste are so closely linked that only a few tastes can be interpreted without the corresponding sense of smell.

Proving the point

In pairs, try tasting different foods while you pinch your nose so that you can taste but not smell them. Which flavours are hardest to taste when you remove the sense of smell? Are the answers the same for each person?

The sense organs

The sense organs are the eyes, ears, nose, mouth and skin, (See Skin, Hair and Nails, page 39) and their function is to communicate information from outside of the body to the brain. The sense organs receive information from the external environment in the form of sensory impulses, which they transmit to the CNS via nerves. The CNS then instructs the body to provoke a physical or physiological reaction.

Information is transferred from the sense organs to the CNS and then interpreted in the following ways:

Sensory impulse	Path from sense organ to CNS	Point of interpretation
Sight	Optic (sensory) nerve (2nd cranial nerve)	Interpreted in the visual areas of the occipital lobes
Hearing	Vestibulocochlear (sensory) nerve (8th cranial nerve)	Interpreted in auditory areas of temporal lobes
Smell	Olfactory (sensory) nerve (1st cranial nerve)	Interpreted in the temporal lobe
Taste	Facial nerve (7th cranial) and glossopharyngeal nerve (9th cranial) (Sensory and motor)	Interpreted in the temporal lobe with the corresponding smell
Pain, heat and cold	Nerve endings that transmit pain and temperature changes	Sensory nerve fibres
Light touch	Nerve endings that transmit light touch	Sensory nerve fibres in spinal nerves
Firm pressure	Nerve endings that transmit firm pressure	Posterior nerve roots in the spinal cord

The olfactory system

Smell is one of the most primitive responses although it is less acute in modern humans than it was in our ancient predecessors. The sense of smell is also the sense most directly connected to the subconscious mind and memory function. A particular smell can summon vivid memories of a person or an event. Have you ever entered a school and been reminded of your own school days by the smells around you – perhaps by the smells of school dinners or disinfectant? Perhaps you have visited a relative in hospital and the smells have conjured up memories of a time when you were ill.

The sense of smell works in a similar way to the other senses. External stimuli are carried as gases in the air to the nose. **Olfactory** cells at the back of the nose transmit this sensory information along the first cranial or olfactory nerve to the olfactory bulb in the frontal lobe of the forebrain. Different smells are then translated in the temporal lobe and information about them is transmitted along motor nerves to the nose.

CHAPTER 8 The Nervous System

> **Link to practice**
>
> A client with no sense of smell would not benefit from treatments in the same way as other clients. Imagine not being able to smell a peppermint foot lotion, a strawberry face mask or a lavender and geranium massage oil.

The structure and function of the autonomic nervous system (ANS)

As the name suggests, the actions of the autonomic nervous system (ANS) are automatic. This part of the nervous system supplies the internal organs. The autonomic nervous system is mostly made up of efferent or motor nerve fibres, which run outwards from the organs, including the stomach, bladder, heart and blood vessels.

There are relatively few afferent or sensory nerve fibres running towards the organs. This is because the ANS is mostly responsible for causing an action (effect/efferent/motor) in an organ rather than picking up a message (sensation/sensory/afferent).

There are two branches to the ANS, which work together to co-ordinate the body. These are the **sympathetic** branch and the **parasympathetic** branch, and as their names suggest, they have opposing actions. Each organ has a double nerve supply, one from each branch of the ANS.

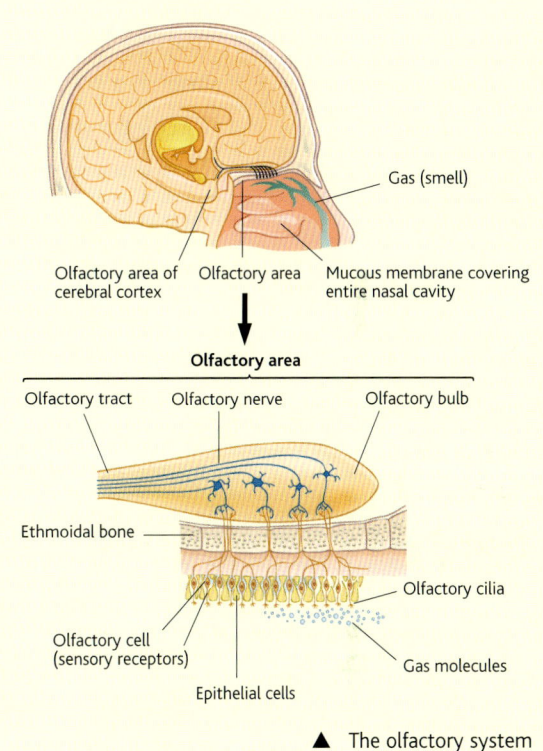

▲ The olfactory system

The sympathetic branch

The sympathetic branch of the ANS is stimulated by strong positive or negative emotions such as fear, anger and excitement. Its role is to prepare the body to respond in these situations. The sympathetic nervous system works closely with the adrenal glands, which it stimulates. The adrenals secrete the hormone adrenaline, which is known as the 'fight or flight hormone' and similarly, the sympathetic branch of the ANS prepares the body for fight or flight. It does this by stimulating the blood circulatory and respiratory systems and in doing so, the muscles are provided with a better supply of oxygen-rich blood which enables them to function more effectively. (Links to The Blood Circulatory System, page 90 and The Respiratory System, page 114) The sympathetic branch of the ANS also slows down the activity of the digestive system, which may result in a dry mouth, vomiting or bowel movements – these are all

> **Link to learning**
>
> Use mnemonic SS/PP to remember the two branches to the ANS.
> - **S**ympathetic branch of the ANS reacts to **S**trong emotions.
> - **P**arasympathetic branch of the ANS responds to **P**leasant emotions.

fairly common reactions to highly emotional situations. (Link to The Digestive System, page 164)

The parasympathetic branch

The parasympathetic branch of the ANS is stimulated by pleasant emotions and its reactions are the opposite of those of the sympathetic branch. The parasympathetic branch stimulates the digestive system to produce more **gastric** secretions and increase **peristaltic** action. The sensations you feel might be a watering mouth or a rumbling tummy (often described as 'butterflies'). (Link to The Digestive System, page 152) The parasympathetic branch also slows down blood circulation and respiration. (Links to The Blood Circulatory System, page 90 and The Respiratory System, page 114) Its role is to restore calm and preserve energy.

The normal functioning of the ANS is a bit like co-ordinating the pedals when driving a car. The accelerator and brake pedals have opposite actions and so, as you press the accelerator to speed up, you release the brake. To slow down, on the other hand, you would release the accelerator and press down on the brake. The sympathetic and parasympathetic branches of the ANS work in a similar way. However, during times of extreme anxiety or stress the two branches can work **antagonistically**, causing a state of flux and leading to the physical symptoms felt at such times.

The nature of a reflex action

A reflex action is one which occurs involuntarily without conscious control. It occurs when afferent or sensory nerves react to a stimulus causing stimulation of motor nerves and subsequent action. A good example of a reflex action is when you accidentally touch something hot. The temperature sensors in the skin transmit information to the brain very quickly, which causes you to immediately withdraw from the stimulus. The purpose of reflex actions of this kind is to protect the body from harm. Reflex actions also describe involuntary movements such as swallowing and sneezing which occur without effort. These actions enable the body to function effectively without conscious control.

Control of the urinary bladder is an example of a reflex action controlled by the autonomic nervous system. (Link to The Excretory and Urinary Systems, page 175) As urine enters the bladder, muscle in the bladder wall relaxes to accommodate the increasing volume of urine. Normally, urine does not leak out of the bladder because of two rings of muscle known as the internal sphincter and external **sphincter**, which form a tight grip on the opening of the bladder. These muscles are supplied by sympathetic and parasympathetic nerves. Once the bladder is full, the reflex contraction of muscle in the bladder

> **Fascinating fact**
> A reflex action depends on the co-ordinated activities of around 100,000 nerve cells in less than one second.

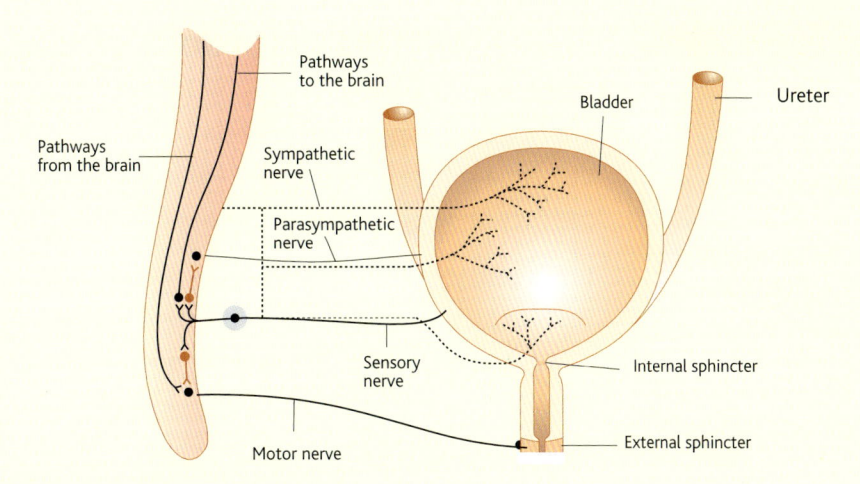

▲ Control of the urinary bladder is a reflex action controlled by the autonomic nervous system

is strong enough to open the internal sphincter. Nervous impulses are sent to the brain to give the sensation of the bladder being full. The brain then sends a message back to the bladder, via a motor nerve, which causes the external sphincter to relax resulting in voluntary urination.

> **Case study**
>
> **Level 3 and holistic**
> Francesca is a young mother of two small boys. She has been feeling short of breath and nauseous on and off for several months. Her GP has recently diagnosed panic attacks and high blood pressure and has prescribed beta blockers. Design a treatment plan for Francesca with aftercare advice.

Summary of the nervous system

Structure	Function	Illustration
Sense organs	Initiates the process of communication between internal and external environments	Stimulation of the nerve endings as a response to sound, sight, smell, taste or touch
Afferent or sensory impulses	Impulses travel from sense organs to the CNS; transmission of the nerve impulse	Temperature communicated by afferent or sensory neurones in the skin. The nerve impulse travels from the axon of one neurone to the dendrite or cell body of another
Efferent or motor impulses	Impulses which travel from the CNS to a gland or organ	Command sent via efferent or motor neurones
Autonomic nervous system	Controls voluntary functions	Heartbeat and secretions from glands
Sympathetic nervous system	Prepares body for 'fight or flight' in response to strong emotional situations	Stimulates blood circulatory and respiratory systems; slows digestive system
Parasympathetic nervous system	Restores balance in response to pleasant emotions	Stimulates digestive system; slows blood circulatory and respiratory systems

> **Link to practice**
>
> Therapists should be aware of basic first-aid procedures for dealing with a client or colleague who suffers an epileptic fit. Epileptic episodes can be prompted by flashing lights, intermittent noises or pulsing sensations, and certain treatments, such as EMS, are therefore contra-indicated to clients with epilepsy.

Diseases and disorders of the nervous system

Alzheimer's disease
This is a severe form of **dementia** which affects about 50 per cent of senile dementia sufferers. This disorder affects **cognitive** (brain) functions such as memory, thought, language and personality.

Bell's palsy
Bell's palsy is characterised by paralysis in one side of the face and is caused by a swollen facial nerve. The swelling occurs suddenly and may be the result of a virus.

Cerebral palsy
Cerebral palsy (CP) is a congenital disorder of the brain. Symptoms include a loss of muscle control and spasm.

Case study

Holistic

Tamir is 38 years old and suffers from cerebral palsy. Her posture is distorted and she suffers constant pain in the lower back, hips and legs. You find it difficult to understand Tamir's speech and she is often tearful. Design a treatment plan with aftercare advice to help Tamir feel mentally and physically better.

Epilepsy
Epilepsy is the name of a disorder caused by abnormal brain function. It results in seizures, fits or spasms in the face and body.

Case study

Level 3

Jenna comes to the salon because she has heard about body toning treatments using EMS and gyratory massage. During the consultation you discover she has epilepsy. Design a suitable treatment plan for Jenna with aftercare advice.

Meningitis
Meningitis is an inflammation of the membrane of the CNS. It can be caused by a head injury but is more commonly the result of a viral infection, such as mumps or measles. Symptoms include headache, backache, stiffness in the neck and vomiting. Bacterial meningitis is accompanied by flu-like symptoms as well as a rash.

Motor neurone disease
Motor neurone disease is associated with age. It commonly effects men over 50 years, and sufferers usually survive only five years or less from diagnosis. It is caused by degeneration of the motor nerves, and symptoms include clumsiness, cramp in the limbs and difficulty with swallowing and breathing.

CHAPTER 8 The Nervous System

> **Link to practice**
> With the recent increase in disorders such as mumps and meningitis, it is vital that you can recognise symptoms and refer individuals whom you suspect to be affected by these diseases to a GP prior to treatment.

Multiple sclerosis
Multiple sclerosis (MS) is a **degenerative** disease which effects nervous tissue in the CNS. (Link to Muscles and the Muscular System, page 75) Symptoms may vary according to the section of tissue which is damaged but can affect mobility, speech or vision.

Parkinson's disease
Parkinson's disease is a degenerative disease less associated with age. (Link to Muscles and the Muscular System, page 75) It is caused by a fault with the **neurotransmitters** which control movement. Individuals with this disorder suffer from muscular tremors or rigidity and a lack of facial expression.

> **Link to practice**
> Holistic therapies can be physically and mentally beneficial to clients suffering from multiple sclerosis or cerebral palsy. Be led by your client with regards to pressure and manipulations.

Sciatica
Sciatica is the name of a common disorder whereby the sciatic nerve is irritated, causing pain in the lower back and leg. (Link to Muscles and the Muscular System, page 74) Manipulation of the affected area can be beneficial but should only be carried out with medical approval.

Senile dementia
This is an age-associated disorder which affects people over the age over 65 years ('senile' literally means old age). The main symptom is confused memory and thought processes. As well as age, a further risk factor for senile dementia is atherosclerosis, which decreases blood flow to the brain.

> **Link to practice**
> If you suspect that a client may be suffering from motor neurone or Parkinson's disease, you should refer them to a GP prior to treatment.

The effect of drugs on the nervous system
The nervous system is affected by all kinds of drugs which have the effect of altering nervous transmission. This can have immediate and/or long-term effects.

	Prescription drugs	Common drugs	Illegal drugs
Examples	Painkillers, sedatives, sleeping pills	Alcohol, tobacco, caffeine	Cocaine, heroin, cannabis, ecstasy
Effects	Interact directly with the CNS by altering the body's reactions	Can slow reactions and alter physical and emotional state	Instant mental alteration; deterioration of cerebral cells
Complications	Can be addictive and have unpleasant side-effects	Can be addictive and can cause physical deterioration	Can cause tolerance so a higher dose is required to achieve the same effect

> **Link to practice**
> Senile dementia and Alzheimer's disease are distressing conditions for the sufferer as well as for family, friends and acquaintances. As with all clients, treat sufferers with respect and in a non-judgemental way.

The effects of ageing on the nervous system
Like all of the body's systems, the nervous system slows down and performs less effectively with age. From about the age of 40 years, the brain starts to shrink at an average rate of 9 grams each year. As with other systems, it is important to take care of the brain and exercise it regularly, just as you would

your muscles or bones. Maintaining an active mind, eating a balanced diet and living a healthy lifestyle will help to keep the nervous system in good shape and can help to prevent the onset of certain age-associated disorders.

Case study

Level 3 and holistic

Mary is a regular client. She and her husband enjoyed an active retirement until he passed away 12 months ago. Since that time you have noticed that Mary seems confused and forgetful. She also seems less vivacious and you are growing concerned about her physical and mental well-being. Mary's family live oversees. Design a treatment plan with aftercare advice for this client.

Link to practice

It is important that a client discloses information about drug use as it may affect treatment, particularly holistic therapies such as aromatherapy, Indian head massage and reflexology.

Knowledge check

1. Name and describe the main parts of a neurone.
2. What is a synapse?
3. What is a nerve?
4. State the alternative names for afferent and efferent.
5. Name the main parts of the central nervous system.
6. Name the three main sections of the brain.
7. What is the main function of the three main sections of the brain?
8. In what direction do motor and sensory fibres run in the spinal cord?
9. How many spinal nerves are there in the human body?
10. What are nerve plexuses?
11. Name the main nerve plexuses.
12. State the location of the sciatic nerve.
13. Name the two parts of the peripheral nervous system.
14. How many cranial nerves are there in the human body?
15. Describe the process involved in the sense of smell.
16. Describe what happens in a reflex action.
17. What are the two branches of the autonomic nervous system?
18. Name and describe two disorders of the nervous system which affect mobility.
19. Name and describe two disorders of the nervous system which affect mental functioning.
20. What are the effects of ageing on the nervous system?

CHAPTER 9 The Endocrine System

SECTION 2

> **Link to learning**
>
> The prefix *endo-* means within and the suffix *-crino* means to secrete.

> **Link to learning**
>
> A gland is a group of cells that produce, secrete or give off substances such as chemicals. These chemicals are sent to other parts of the body where they become active.

The **endocrine system** comprises a number of ductless **glands** that release powerful chemicals called **hormones** directly into the bloodstream. These endocrine glands and their hormones are vital to our health and well-being. They help to regulate metabolism, growth and reproduction, and can also influence behaviour and mood.

Hormones (literally meaning 'to set in motion') are released by the endocrine, or ductless glands, in response to the body's requirements. There are over twenty different hormones which enter the bloodstream directly and are carried to the point of need in the **plasma** by binding to a protein. The recipient cells are called **target cells**. Some hormones, such as thyroid hormone which regulates **metabolism**, will affect almost every cell in the body, whereas other hormones only affect specific cells. For example, gonadotrophin which only acts on the gonads. When their action is complete, hormones are de-activated by the liver.

An abnormally high or low hormone output will soon show itself as a disorder in the body. Because hormones play such an important role in **homeostasis,** it is essential that you understand how the endocrine system can affect clients and their treatments. For example, an imbalance in some hormones may cause male pattern hair growth in women; these clients may seek advice about epilation. In reflexology you will find that an imbalance in one gland may have consequences in another gland or another part of the body. For example, an obvious reflex over the pituitary gland may be linked to the thyroid gland or may be an indication of stress.

> **Link to learning**
>
> The endocrine system works closely with the nervous system. (Link to The Nervous System, page 122)

> **Proving the point**
>
> Pre-menstrual tension (PMT) occurs in women when levels of the hormone oestrogen are low. To give you an idea of the powerful effect of hormones on the body, make a list of the possible symptoms of PMT.

> **You will learn**
>
> In this chapter you will learn about:
> - the names and positions of the main endocrine glands
> - the names and functions of the major hormones
> - how the pituitary or 'master gland' regulates the other glands
> - diseases and disorders of the endocrine system
> - the effects of ageing on the endocrine system.

The endocrine glands and their hormones

The pituitary gland

The pituitary gland is located at the base of the brain behind the sphenoid bone. It is about the size of a small pea and is attached to the brain by a stalk. The pituitary gland is often referred to as the master gland because it plays an important role in regulating the other glands in the endocrine system, such as the thyroid gland. It does this by producing trophic or stimulating hormones

PAGE 135

SECTION 2

Proving the point

Endocrine glands are ductless glands. Exocrine glands differ from endocrine glands because they have ducts. Can you name three exocrine glands?

Fascinating fact

The pituitary gland produces hormones called **endorphins** which act on the nervous system and reduce feelings of pain. (Link to The Nervous System, page 124)

Fascinating fact

The production of pituitary hormones is influenced by mood, emotions and changes in the seasons.

Proving the point

What do you think will be the effect of over- and under-production of growth hormone during childhood?

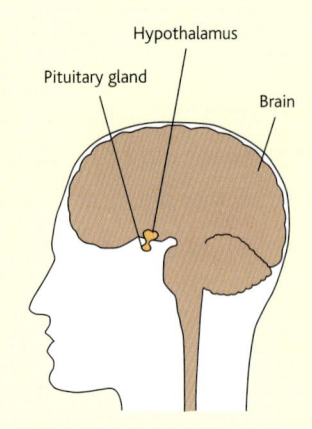

▲ The location of the hypothalamus and pituitary gland

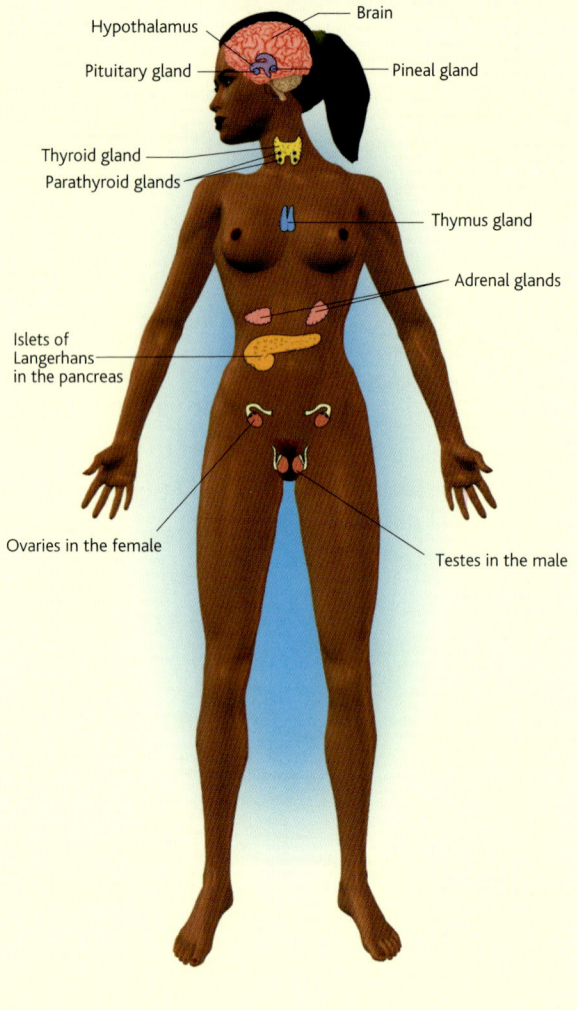

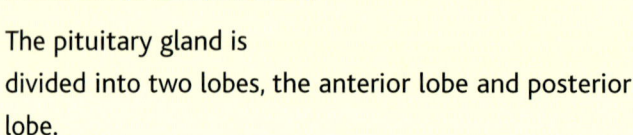

▲ The endocrine system

that are sent to the other glands to increase their output. The pituitary gland is itself controlled by a part of the brain called the hypothalamus (see also page 137). (Link to The Nervous System, page 124)

The pituitary gland is divided into two lobes, the anterior lobe and posterior lobe.

Hormones of the anterior pituitary lobe

Hormone	Function
Growth hormone (GH)	Responsible for promoting the growth of long bones during childhood. Its secretion is increased during sleep
Thyroid Stimulating hormone (TSH)	Essential for the production of thyroxin from the thyroid gland
Adrenocorticotrophic hormone (ACTH)	Needed for the release of steroids from the adrenal cortex
Prolactin	Produced during lactation or breastfeeding
Follicle stimulating hormone (FSH)	Needed to regulate the menstrual cycle in women
Lutenising hormone (LH)	Needed to regulate the menstrual cycle in women

Fascinating fact

Adults who secrete too much growth hormone develop a condition called acromegaly. Because the long bones in adults are fused, they cannot get longer, so they become wider. The hands and feet become larger and the cheeks and jaw thicken.

Proving the point

Diuretics are chemicals that cause an increase in urine production. Therefore a diuretic drink will produce a greater volume of urine than is found in the drink itself. In the 19th century children were told not to eat dandelion leaves since these would cause them to 'wet the bed'. Can you name two popular modern-day drinks that have a diuretic effect? What advice would you give to a client partial to this type of drink?

Hormones of the posterior pituitary lobe

The hormones of the posterior lobe are produced in the hypothalamus and stored, until needed, in the pituitary. They are:

Hormone	Function
Anti-diuretic hormone (ADH) or vasopressin	Regulates the levels of fluid in the body (hydration) by promoting the amount of water absorbed by the kidneys and therefore the amount of urine produced
Oxytocin	Produced during labour and makes the uterus contract. It is also produced during breastfeeding when it causes the milk to enter the breasts

The hypothalamus

The hypothalamus is the main link between the endocrine and nervous systems. (Link to The Nervous System, page 127) It is formed from nervous tissue and plays a crucial role in controlling the **parasympathetic** part of the **autonomic nervous system**. It also has a very important part to play in the regulation of the endocrine system, and one of its main functions is to control the pituitary gland and to produce certain hormones. It plays a vital role in homeostasis and regulates, amongst other things, body temperature, breathing rate and appetite.

The hypothalamus is situated at the base of the brain just above the pituitary gland. It is connected to the pituitary gland by a stalk; this carries nerve impulses and hormones from the hypothalamus to the pituitary.

The pituitary will not release its trophic (stimulating) hormones until **releasing hormones** arrive from the hypothalamus.

Regulation of the endocrine system by the pituitary and hypothalamus

It is very important that levels of hormone are maintained within normal limits. If the levels become too high or too low, problems will occur that result in physical symptoms.

The hormonal control mechanism is complex. It involves the pituitary gland which works with the

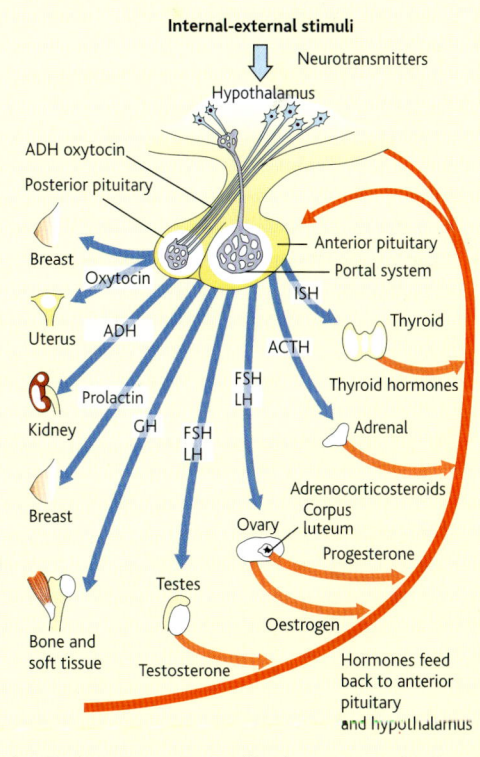

▲ The hormones secreted by the pituitary gland

> **Proving the point**
>
> 'Hooking' is a pressure technique used in reflexology to pinpoint a reflex. Instead of walking the thumb, firm pressure is applied by dragging the thumb over a reflex point until the thumb is flexed and then pressing or hooking over the reflex until the thumb is extended. The pituitary 'hook' is a very effective movement – can you explain why?

hypothalamus to play a very important role in the regulation of many of the hormones. This regulation is called **negative feedback** because very low levels of hormone will be picked up by the hypothalamus, which in turn stimulates the pituitary gland to produce trophic (stimulating) hormones. By producing varying levels of these trophic hormones, the pituitary gland regulates the amount of hormones in the blood.

> **Link to learning**
>
> Try to imagine that the hypothalamus is like a thermostat on a heater. If the temperature starts to rise, the thermostat will switch off the heater; as the temperature starts to fall, the heater will come back on again. Thus a constant temperature is maintained.

The thyroid gland

The thyroid gland is the largest endocrine gland. It is situated in the neck on either side of the trachea or windpipe and consists of two lobes joined together by a band of tissue called an isthmus. Its shape resembles a bow tie or butterfly.

Thyroxin

The main hormone produced here is thyroxin but only in the presence of the mineral iodine. The main function of thyroxin is to regulate metabolism in all the cells. This means that thyroxin controls the speed at which the body converts food into energy or heat. The more thyroxin is produced, the faster these changes relating to growth and development occur. A person with higher levels of thyroxin is said to have a quick metabolism. Slow metabolism usually results in weight gain.

> **Fascinating fact**
>
> Because of its crucial role as the master gland, the pituitary gland is often called the 'conductor of the orchestra'. When the importance of the hypothalamus began to emerge in the 20th century, physiologists said that 'the hypothalamus writes the music'.

Thyroxin is particularly important in tissue growth in children and during pregnancy, but it remains important throughout life as it affects blood flow, heartbeat, blood pressure and blood chemistry. (Link to The Blood Circulatory System, page 77)

Calcitonin

The thyroid gland produces a second hormone – calcitonin. This regulates the levels of calcium in the blood by promoting the absorption of calcium into the bones for storage. Calcium in the bloodstream is essential for normal muscle contraction and relaxation.

The parathyroid glands

> **Proving the point**
>
> In the endocrine system, homeostasis refers to maintaining the correct balance of hormones in the blood. List other organs that play a vital role in homeostasis elsewhere in the body.

The parathyroids are tiny glands embedded in the thyroid gland. There are usually two pairs, but three pairs or one pair is not uncommon. These glands secrete a hormone called parathormone or parathyroid hormone. Working closely with calcitonin, its function is to regulate the amount of calcium in

> **Fascinating fact**
>
> Because alcohol is a diuretic, drinking too much alcohol will speed up the loss of water from the body – you will lose more water in urine than you take in through drink. The resulting dehydration causes headache, dizziness and nausea (a hangover!). The alteration in fluid balance and the excessive production of urine is a result of the affect of alcohol on the production of ADH.

the blood. Most of the calcium entering the body is stored in the bones, but it is essential that some calcium (about 5 per cent of the total) remains in the blood as it plays a vital role in the mechanism of muscle contraction and relaxation.

The thymus gland

The thymus gland is located behind the sternum in front of the heart. It is composed of **lymphatic tissue** and plays a very important role in **immunity** by producing specialist **white blood cells** called T-lymphocytes to help fight infection. It produces a hormone, thymosin, which helps these specialised cells to reach maturity. (Link to The Lymphatic System, page 108)

The pineal gland

This is a small pine-cone shaped structure (hence its name) about 1 cm long found at the base of the brain. It produces the hormone melatonin during the night. Melatonin communicates information about environmental lighting to the brain and thus regulates the wake/sleep cycle. Because of its links to light and dark it is sometimes referred to as the 'third eye'.

The pineal gland's other function is to delay the development of the **secondary sexual characteristics** until **puberty**. (Link to The Reproductive System, page 181)

> **Fascinating fact**
>
> Iodine deficiency is now very rare as iodine is routinely added to salt.

> **Proving the point**
>
> Find three foods that are good sources of iodine.

The adrenal glands

There are two adrenal glands, each situated above a kidney (hence their name – *ad* meaning of, and *renis* meaning kidneys). These triangular glands are divided into two sections that have no direct relationship to each other. The outer part is called the cortex, which makes up the bulk of the gland, and the inner part is called the medulla.

The adrenal medulla and the hormone adrenaline

The adrenal medulla produces a hormone known as adrenaline or the 'fight or flight' hormone. Adrenaline is linked to the autonomic nervous system and is produced all the time in low levels. Output is increased in times of stress, excitement or in an emergency, when adrenaline has a powerful effect.

The effects of adrenaline include:
- increased blood pressure
- increased heart rate
- increase in metabolic rate
- dilation of the bronchioles
- release of **glucose** into the bloodstream.

> **Proving the point**
>
> Regular aerobic exercise is a good way of increasing metabolism and preventing weight gain. Measure your pulse rate when you are at rest, then do five minutes of brisk exercise (running on the spot or skipping) and measure your pulse rate again. If your pulse has increased, you have raised your metabolic rates.

Fascinating fact
Parathyroid deficiency is very rare and causes low levels of blood calcium. This can result in abnormal muscle contractions, a condition known as tetany.

Fascinating fact
Lack of melatonin is linked to the unpleasant symptoms of jet lag, although recent studies involving melatonin supplements for travellers on long haul flights have been inconclusive.

Link to practice
Techniques such as meditation or yoga help to control stress, whilst other symptoms may be relieved by a change in diet. Soothing body treatments or a relaxing facial will also help but they do not treat the underlying causes of stress – or 'stressors'.

Link to learning
Secondary sexual characteristics include an increase in body hair and the development of pubic hair. In females, the breasts develop and the hips broaden, and **menstruation** starts. In males, the voice breaks and facial hair develops.

Link to practice
Stress and the effects of adrenaline on the body
Stress is an everyday part of modern life, and during a client consultation, many of your clients may complain of feeling 'stressed out'. However, research shows that unmanaged stress may lead to distress, which has unpleasant psychological and physical consequences. Why is this?

When you experience a stressful or traumatic event, the nervous system signals the adrenal medulla to produce adrenaline so that you can react in an emergency. If you encounter excessive stress over the long-term, adrenaline will build up in the bloodstream causing adverse physical symptoms such as restlessness, tiredness, insomnia, feeling jittery and an inability to concentrate. Some diseases are referred to as being 'stress-related'. These include irritable bowel syndrome, headaches, migraine, stomach ulcers and asthma.

The adrenal cortex and its associated hormones

The adrenal cortex has a separate function from the adrenal medulla, despite their close proximity. It produces a group of hormones known collectively as steroids.

There are three main steroid hormones:

- *Glucocorticiods* – these help to release energy from carbohydrates by converting them into **glycogen** for storage. The production of these hormones is increased in times of stress to help the body cope with unfavourable conditions. Cortisone or cortisol are the best examples of these hormones.
- *Mineralocorticoids* – as the name suggests, these hormones work to maintain the balance of minerals such as potassium and sodium in the body. They do this by controlling the reabsorption of minerals in the kidneys. (Link to The Excretory and Urinary Systems, page 174)
- *Sex hormones* – namely **testosterone** (or androgens) and **oestrogen**. These are secreted in small amounts by both sexes. Their influence is slight because larger amounts of the male and female hormones are secreted by the **testes** and **ovaries**. (Link to The Reproductive System, page 182)

Link to practice
After the menopause, levels of oestrogen start to fall and women can develop some male pattern hair growth or **hirsutism** because of the natural production of testosterone which stimulates hair growth. Doctors often refer women with facial hair for electrolysis.

The pancreas

The pancreas is a sausage-shaped structure situated in the abdomen, just below the stomach. It is sometimes described as a dual organ because it also has a role in the digestive system. (Link to The Digestive System, page 157)

CHAPTER 9 The Endocrine System

> **Proving the point**
>
> Can you remember the last time you felt very nervous – perhaps before an exam or an interview? Make a list of the physical symptoms you experienced. This will give you an idea of the effects of adrenaline on the body.

The pancreas contains clusters of specialised cells known as pancreatic islet cells or the Islets of Langerhans. The main hormones produced by these cells are **insulin** and **glucagon**. These important hormones are responsible for regulating blood sugar or blood glucose.

The role of insulin and glycogen in maintaining blood sugar levels

The body tries to keep a constant supply of glucose for the cells by maintaining a constant glucose concentration in the blood; otherwise the cells would have too much glucose after a meal and not enough at night during sleep.

After eating, carbohydrate is broken down into glucose, which is absorbed into the bloodstream and distributed to all the cells. This causes blood glucose levels to rise. When the levels of glucose exceed normal, insulin is produced by the Islets of Langerhans. Insulin converts the blood glucose into a substance called **glycogen** that can be stored in the liver and muscles, or as subcutaneous fat, until needed. (Links to Muscles and the Muscular System, page 64 and The Blood Circulatory System, page 94)

Later, when blood glucose levels begin to fall and hunger is felt, the second pancreatic hormone, glucagon, converts the stores of glycogen back into glucose so that the blood glucose remains within normal limits.

▲ Target areas for androgen-stimulated hair growth in women.

Labels: Lip, Chin, Neck, Underarm, Chest centre, Back and shoulders, Chest/breast, Pubic, Thigh, Lower leg

> **Fascinating fact**
>
> Vitamin D is a steroid. It helps to regulate calcium and phosphorus levels in the body and is present in foods such as dairy products and oily fish. It can only be converted into an active form in the skin by UV rays from the sun.

Hormone	Action
Insulin	Brings blood sugar levels down by storing glucose as glycogen after meals. The major target cells for insulin are the liver, muscles and fat.
Glucagon	Converts stores of glycogen back into glucose to prevent blood sugar levels falling below normal limits.

Insulin and glycogen are said to be antagonistic in action – they have opposite functions but they work together to maintain homeostasis. The diagram on the next page shows the changes that occur in blood glucose levels during the morning of a typical day.

PAGE 141

Fascinating fact

Very low levels of blood glucose will seriously affect the way the brain functions and may lead to unconsciousness and ultimately death.

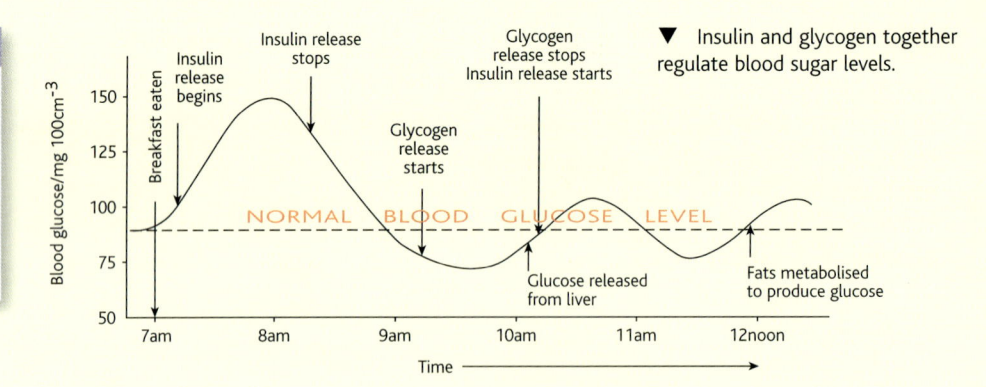

▼ Insulin and glycogen together regulate blood sugar levels.

The ovaries

The ovaries play an important part in reproductive life. They are situated in the female pelvic cavity on either side of the uterus and produce oestrogen and progesterone from puberty to the menopause. (Link to The Reproductive System, page 183)

The testes

The testes are situated in the scrotum. They produce hormones called androgens. The main androgen is testosterone; this contributes towards the male secondary sexual characteristics which occur at puberty. Testosterone is produced from puberty until the end of life. High levels of testosterone are associated with competitiveness and risk taking; low levels are associated with depression, loss of strength and libido, and reduced concentration. (Link to The Reproductive System, page 191)

Summary of the endocrine glands and their functions

Gland	Hormones	Function	Disorders
Anterior lobe of pituitary	Growth hormone (GH)	To regulate growth of all body tissues	Giantism; dwarfism; acromegaly
	Adrenocorticotrophic hormone (ACTH)	To regulate the production of steroids. To regulate the ovarian follicle and the production of progesterone. To stimulate milk production in the breast	
	Gonadtrophins	To regulate the function of the ovaries and testes.	

CHAPTER 9 The Endocrine System

Link to learning

The maintenance of blood sugar levels in the body is a good example of homeostasis. The key is to keep a constant blood glucose level.

Fascinating fact

Diabetes mellitus is a medical condition caused by a lack of insulin. This means that, although the levels of blood glucose are high after a meal, glucose cannot be stored in the cells as glycogen. It is a potentially fatal condition. To counter the effects of this disease, diabetics have to inject themselves with insulin every day. (For more information see the diseases and disorders section on pages 144–146.)

Fascinating fact

Chemicals similar to hormones known as prostaglandins can accumulate in the muscles that form the wall of the uterus, causing cramp-like pains and discomfort before a period (known as dysmenorrhoea). The best way to break down these hormones is to stretch and take some gentle exercise. Ironically, most women tend to curl up and move as little as possible – which makes the situation worse!

Gland	Hormones	Function	Disorders
Posterior lobe of pituitary (These hormones are merely stored in the pituitary gland until needed. They are secreted by the hypothalamus.)	Anti-diuretic hormone (ADH)	To regulate the absorption of water in the kidney, thus regulating urine output	Diabetes insipidus
	Oxytocin	To control milk production during breastfeeding and to promote the contraction of the smooth muscles of the uterus during childbirth	
Thyroid	Thyroxin	To regulate the metabolic rate; influences mental and physical activities	Hypothyroidism; hyperthyroidism
	Calcitonin	To regulate calcium levels in the bloodstream	
Parathyroid	Parathyroid hormone	Promotes the absorption of calcium which is needed for muscle contraction	Tetany
Pineal gland	Melatonin	To regulate the sleep–wake cycle; it is produced at night	Affected by flying from west to east (jet lag)
Thymus	Thymosin	To assist the production of T-lymphocytes	
Adrenal medulla	Adrenaline	To raise blood pressure and pulse as part of the 'fight or flight' response	Stress-related symptoms
Adrenal cortex	Steroids	To assist in the metabolism of carbohydrates, fats and proteins; to regulate the water balance in the body	Cushing's syndrome; Addison's disease
Pancreas	Insulin and glucagon	To regulate blood glucose	Diabetes mellitus (Types 1 and 2)
Ovaries	Oestrogen and progesterone	To regulate menstruation and secondary sexual characteristics in women; to prepare for and maintain pregnancy	Hirsutism; precocious puberty (early onset)
Testes	Testosterone	To regulate sperm production and secondary sexual characteristics in men	Low levels may cause delayed puberty

SECTION 2

Fascinating fact

If the ovaries do not respond to the trophic (stimulating) hormones from the pituitary gland, oestrogen levels will fall. One result of this is that the hair follicles will be influenced by the testosterone from the adrenal cortex. This can result in male pattern hair growth known as hirsutism (see also page 140).

Summary of the function of hormones

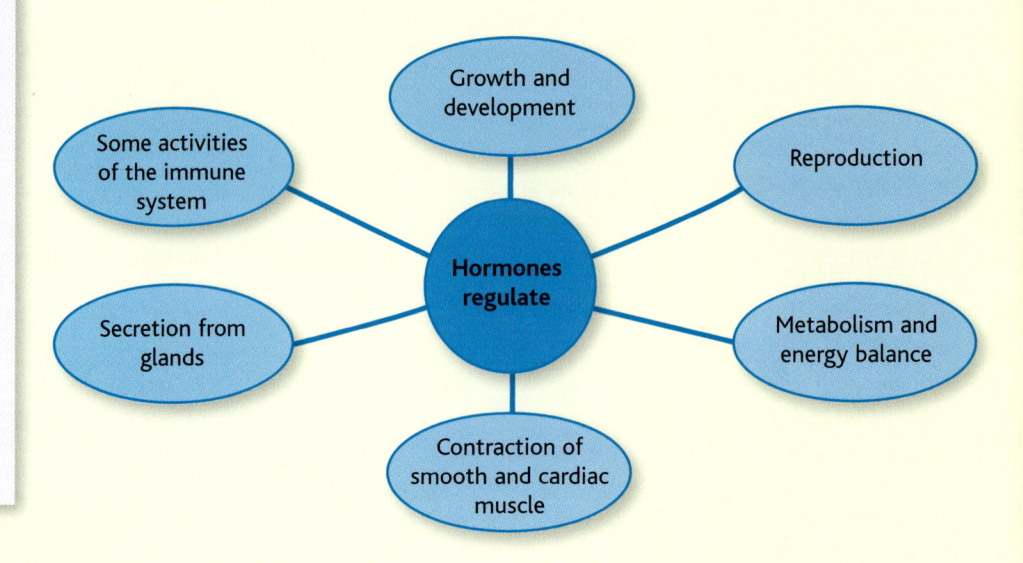

Hormones regulate:
- Growth and development
- Reproduction
- Metabolism and energy balance
- Contraction of smooth and cardiac muscle
- Secretion from glands
- Some activities of the immune system

Fascinating fact

Although it's considered a male hormone, women need testosterone too. Although they produce only a small amount (in the ovaries and adrenal glands), testosterone helps women to maintain the strength of muscle and bone.

Diseases and disorders of the endocrine system

Disorders of the pituitary gland

Diabetes insipidus

Insufficient ADH, or vasopressin, causes a very rare disorder called diabetes insipidus in which the kidneys are unable to retain water. This should not be confused with diabetes mellitus (see below) which is caused by insufficient amounts of insulin. (Diabetes means 'overflow'; insipidus means 'tasteless'; mellitus means 'honey'.)

Thyroid disorders

Hyperthyroidism

This is sometimes called thyrotoxicosis. It is caused by an excessive production of thyroxin and may be accompanied by an enlarged thyroid gland or goitre. The condition causes weight loss, anxiety, palpitations, heat intolerance and sweating. It is more common in females than males.

Hypothyroidism

This is sometimes called myxoedema. It is caused by underproduction of thyroxin. Sufferers will complain of weight gain, feeling cold, and skin changes such as dryness and coarseness. The hair becomes dry, brittle and unmanageable; sufferers are prone to alopecia (hair loss). The facial features will swell and look puffy. It is five times more frequent in females than males and is one of the most common endocrine disorders.

Proving the point

List the sexual characteristics associated with the male and female gender.

Simple goitre or thyroid enlargement
Eating too much or too little iodine in the diet can cause the thyroid gland to become enlarged and swollen. It is more common in developing countries where access to health care may be difficult.

Disorders of the adrenal medulla
Stress-related disorders
Stress stimulates the production of the 'fight or flight' hormone, adrenaline. Adrenaline causes a rise in blood sugar levels, blood pressure, pulse and metabolism. It also decreases the immune response so that the body is more susceptible to infectious illnesses. The hormones produced in times of stress are vital to life, but if the stress is unrelenting there will be unpleasant consequences. There are a number of stress-related disorders such as hypertension (abnormally high blood pressure), duodenal ulcers, migraines and irritable bowel syndrome. Relaxing therapies can help clients combat tensions.

Disorders of the adrenal cortex
Cushing's syndrome
This is caused by excessive production of glucocorticoids. Its many symptoms include enlarged abdomen, wasting of the limbs, facial hair, thinning of the skin and hair, and a swollen or 'moon face'.

Addison's disease
This is caused by a lack of glucocorticoids. Its symptoms include low blood pressure, muscular weakness and excessive skin pigmentation, especially in sun-exposed areas.

Adreno genital virilism
Otherwise known as adrenogenital syndrome, this is a disorder of the adrenal cortex which results in over-production of androgens. In women it results in virilism or masculinisation. Women may grow a beard and other body hair. The clitoris may become enlarged and the breasts may shrink. Menstruation usually stops.

Disorders of the pancreas
Diabetes mellitus
Some people are unable to control the level of their blood glucose because they suffer from the condition diabetes mellitus. There are two kinds of diabetes mellitus:
- Type 1 diabetes appears early in life. Type 1 diabetics do not produce enough insulin, so blood glucose cannot be stored in the cells as glycogen. If untreated, this condition is fatal, so Type 1 diabetics have to inject

themselves with insulin several times a day.
- Type 2 diabetes tends to occur in older people, so is often referred to as maturity-onset diabetes. It results from either a reduced efficiency at producing insulin or a reduced sensitivity of the target cells to the hormone. Type 2 diabetes is generally associated with a poor diet high in carbohydrate and leading to obesity. It can be controlled by a combination of exercise and diet although insulin injections may also be necessary.

Symptoms of diabetes include:
- increased thirst
- increased urination
- slow wound healing
- loss of skin sensitivity
- feeling generally unwell.

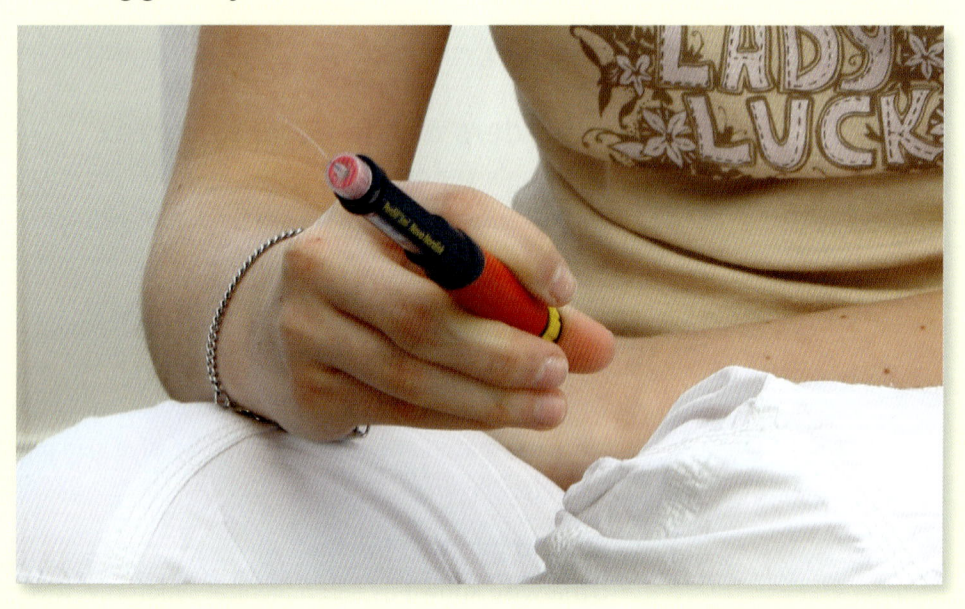

▲ Type 1 diabetics have to inject themselves with insulin several times a day.

Link to practice

When treating diabetic clients, you should consider the following:
- Diabetics may experience a sudden fall in blood sugar (hypoglycaemic attack) so should not be treated without prior medical consent.
- Diabetics often experience a lack of sensation in the hands and feet, so manicures, pedicures or any treatments involving extremes of heat or cold are usually contra-indicated or require GP approval.
- Since minor wounds can be very slow to heal, any minor cut is potentially very serious as there is the added risk of infection and/or ulceration.
- Therapists must never give dietary advice to a diabetic client – only a medically qualified dietician can do this.

Fascinating fact

Men can father children very late in life – Pablo Picasso and Charlie Chaplin are famous examples of men who had children in their eighties.

The effects of ageing on the endocrine system

As the body ages, there is a loss of bone mass and muscle tissue, leading to 'frailty'. These changes can be linked to the endocrine system, in particular the reduction of growth hormone (GH). Some older people experience slow thyroid function, since the rate of metabolism slows slightly with age; thus older people are more prone to weight gain (sometimes called 'middle-age spread'). Maturity onset (Type 2) diabetes is common in elderly people, especially those who have had poor diets or are obese.

The production of sex hormones slows down from middle age onwards in both sexes but the effects of this are more dramatic in women. Although the production of the male hormone testosterone decreases later in life, elderly men can still produce active sperm in normal numbers. (Link to The Reproductive System, page 191)

The menopause

This is when menstruation ceases completely, but there are several years leading up to it when the functions of the ovaries slow down. The fall in oestrogen levels can cause many physiological changes, including:
- hot flushes
- palpitations
- irritability
- fatigue
- anxiety
- loss of concentration
- excessive hair growth (hirsuitism)
- bone weakening (osteoporosis).

Hormone replacement therapy (HRT) given to menopausal women has been shown to help women through this often distressing time.

Case study
Level 3/Holistic

Lois is 35 years old and is currently on maternity leave after giving birth to her first child some five months ago. She is not a regular client but has been treated to a pamper day by her mother, who is worried that her once bright and vivacious daughter has changed since the birth of her child and is in need of cheering up. Lois complains of feeling cold all the time, has no energy and is not motivated to leave the house and participate in any hobbies, despite offers of free babysitting. Her features have become thickened and her hair is coarse. Identify the problem, its cause and a solution/remedy.

Case study
Level 2

Rani is a 50 year old diabetic who has been coming to the salon regularly for facials. She has treated herself to a pair of strappy sandals and wants a pedicure treatment before she wears them. Identify the problem, its cause and a solution/remedy.

SECTION 2

Case study
Level 3/Holistic

Laura is in her late-forties and has come to the salon having won a pamper day in the local primary school raffle where she works as the head teacher. In addition to working full-time Laura is the single mother of two teenage children. Her working life is extremely busy and involves a lot of late nights and occasions when she has to take work home. Laura has dry skin with some congestion in the T-zone. She complains of insomnia, headaches and a tendency to lose her temper with her colleagues and children. Last week she found herself in tears for no reason. Identify the problem, its cause and a solution/remedy.

Knowledge check

1. Define 'hormone'.
2. Distinguish between an endocrine and exocrine gland.
3. Name the part of the brain that controls the pituitary gland.
4. Some of the hormones from the anterior lobe of the pituitary contain the suffix - *trophic*. What does this suffix mean?
5. Name the two divisions of the pituitary gland.
6. Explain why the pituitary gland is called the master gland?
7. What is the term used to describe the way in which the endocrine system is regulated?
8. Name the mineral essential for the production of thyroxin.
9. Describe three symptoms of an overactive thyroid gland.
10. Name the thyroid disorder most likely to result in dry, thin hair.
11. Name the two divisions of the adrenal gland and describe the effects of the hormones from each.
12. Describe three disorders of the adrenal cortex.
13. Name the specialised cells of the pancreas that secrete insulin.
14. State the function of insulin.
15. State the function of glucagon.
16. Name two male and two female secondary sexual characteristics.
17. Which trophic hormones regulate the hormones from the ovaries?
18. Name and describe two stress-related disorders.
19. Describe the difference between diabetes insipidus and diabetes mellitus.
20. Make a chart to highlight the key differences between the nervous and endocrine systems.

SECTION 2

CHAPTER 10 The Digestive System

The human body requires energy for it to complete all its complex functions, rather like a car needs petrol and oil to run efficiently. A car will convert petrol into energy, which it can use to make the engine run and produce movement, and it will produce waste that leaves via the exhaust pipe. The human body is more complicated than a car but works according to the same principle – the food that goes in has to be converted into useable units that allow the body to function effectively.

This chapter deals with the metabolism and utilisation of food, the processes which make food digestable, and what happens once food has been digested.

You will learn

In this chapter you will learn about:
- the organs and structures of **digestion**
- the process of digestion from **ingestion** to **elimination**
- the **metabolism** of food including absorption and utilisation of nutrients
- the functions of **enzymes**
- the storage and breakdown of **adipose** tissue
- the absorption and elimination of water.

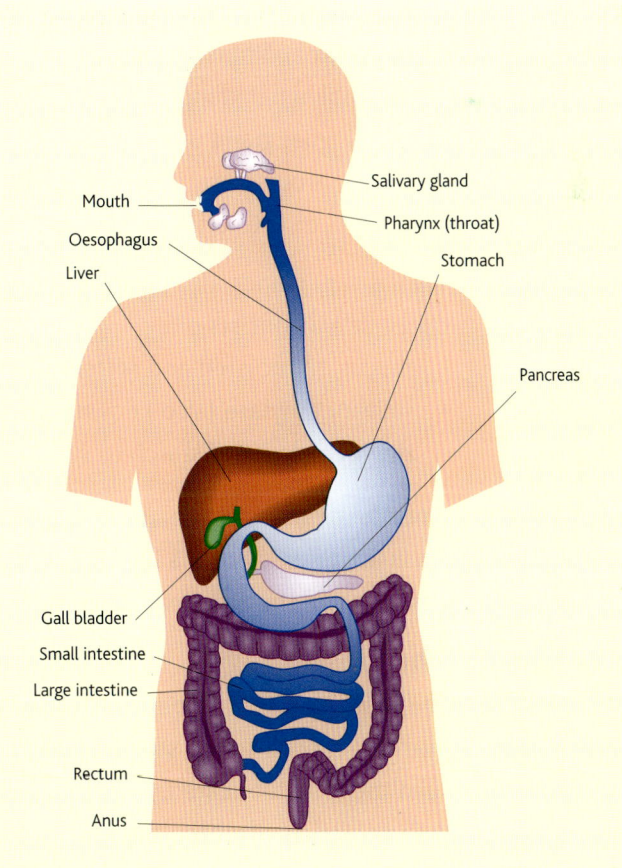

▲ The digestive system

PAGE 149

The organs, structures and process of digestion

The mouth
The process of digestion begins in the mouth. The front teeth bite off pieces of food and the back teeth (the molars) grind the food, breaking down fibres and reducing it further in order for it to be swallowed easily. Inside the mouth are **salivary glands** which secrete saliva containing digestive enzymes. These start to break down simple carbohydrates, such as those found in bread. Saliva mixes with the food to make swallowing easier.

Taste
Whilst food is held in the mouth, molecules of food connect with over 10,000 taste buds on the tongue and send messages to the brain. From these, you will decide whether the food you are eating is sweet, sour, salty, bitter or umami – and ultimately whether it is palatable.

The salivary glands
The salivary glands are formed of **epithelial cells** which produce either mucous (slimy) or serous (watery and protinaceous) secretions. (Link to Cells and Tissues, page 20) They are also known as the accessory glands and there are three major pairs:
- the parotid glands: the largest, found below and in front of the ear
- the submandibular glands: found under the jaw
- the sublingual glands: situated under the tongue.

The sublingual gland produces mucous secretions, whereas the parotid gland produces serous secretions. The submandibular gland contains a mixture of both types of cells and produces a mixture of the two liquids.

The salivary glands also produce saliva, which empties into the mouth via ducts. Saliva consists of:
- mucus, to moisten and soften food
- salivary amylase (also known as ptyalin), which is an enzyme that begins the breakdown of starch to sugar.

Once food has been chewed sufficiently, the mouth and tongue form it into a ball-shape, known as a bolus. This is then swallowed and passes into the **oesophagus**, the tube leading to the stomach.

The oesophagus
The oesophagus is a tube approximately 25 cm (10 inches) long, which runs from the mouth to the stomach. It is soft and muscular and secretes mucus to keep the food lubricated. It expands open as the bolus of food passes through, then constricts after the food has passed. This movement helps to push the food onwards to the stomach.

Fascinating fact

Many people do not take the time to chew their food properly. The old fashioned advice was to chew food a hundred times before swallowing, which is a bit excessive. However, the body cannot successfully digest food which has not been chewed properly; this can lead to indigestion and other more serious problems.

Fascinating fact

Foods that taste 'umami' are certain **amino acids**, like monosodium glutamate. Umami is a relatively new taste – it was first identified in 1909.

Proving the point

Although taste buds can detect differences in food, the sense of smell can reveal more. For example, your taste buds can tell you that you are eating sweet ice-cream, but you need a sense of smell to know what flavour of ice-cream you are eating. Try eating a crisp while holding your nose. Can you tell what flavour it is? Let go and taste the difference!

CHAPTER **10** The Digestive System

Proving the point
Try eating a cracker biscuit quickly. What happens? What does this show you about the function of chewing and saliva?

Fascinating fact
If you are upside down and swallow some food, it is still able to make its way to the stomach. This is due to the muscular walls of the oesophagus constricting and pushing the food onwards.

Fascinating fact
Heartburn has nothing to do with the heart. The painful sensation occurs when acid in the stomach juice goes the wrong way through the cardiac sphincter, causing a burning sensation in the oesophagus. Because the cardiac sphincter is at the same level as the heart, it feels as though the heart is burning.

Link to learning
To understand how the folds of the stomach allow it to expand, imagine a very creased piece of material – if you iron it smooth, it will increase in size.

At the end of the oesophagus, where the tube joins with the stomach, there is a **sphincter** which allows the passage of food in one direction only – into the stomach. Because of its proximity to the heart, it is called the cardiac sphincter, but it is also known as the lower oesophageal sphincter.

The stomach

The stomach is an organ which is shaped like a pear; it is often described as J-shaped. It is approximately 30 cm (12 inches) in length and 15 cm (6 inches) wide at the widest part. It has muscular and elastic walls which are able to expand and constrict.

The structure of the stomach walls is fairly complex, consisting of various layers of membranes and three layers of muscle tissue.

- The muscular layers are circular, longitudinal and diagonal. These layers of muscle produce a churning effect, which stirs the food and mixes it with the digestive juices. This begins the process of digestion for all other nutrients.
- The inner lining of the stomach is composed of specialised epithelial cells. These secrete various substances which form **gastric juice** (see below). The lining is also structured to allow the stomach to expand and contract. It consists of folds which are known as rugae (pronounced roo-gee) when the stomach is empty, but can stretch and unfold to accommodate approximately 1 litre (2 pints) of food and drink.

▲ The oesophagus runs from the mouth to the stomach.

▲ The stomach, showing the structure of the walls and lining

PAGE 151

Fascinating fact
Gastric juice and the salivary glands are stimulated at the smell and thought of food. This is known as the cephalic phase (cephalic means relating to the brain) because food does not have to be present to start these secretions.

Fascinating fact
The process of digestion slows down when the body is carrying out physical activity and when it is completely at rest. Therefore it is not a good idea to eat just before exercising and just before going to bed. (Link to Muscles and the Muscular System, page 73)

Fascinating fact
Because alcohol is absorbed in the stomach, it enters the bloodstream quite soon after consumption. If the stomach is empty, the alcohol is absorbed far more rapidly and enters the blood in a matter of minutes. This will have the effect of making you feel drunk. If the stomach is full, i.e. you have eaten beforehand, the alcohol is absorbed more slowly over a longer period of time. This is why it is always advisable to eat before you drink or only drink alcohol with food.

Functions of the stomach

The stomach has four main functions, as shown below.

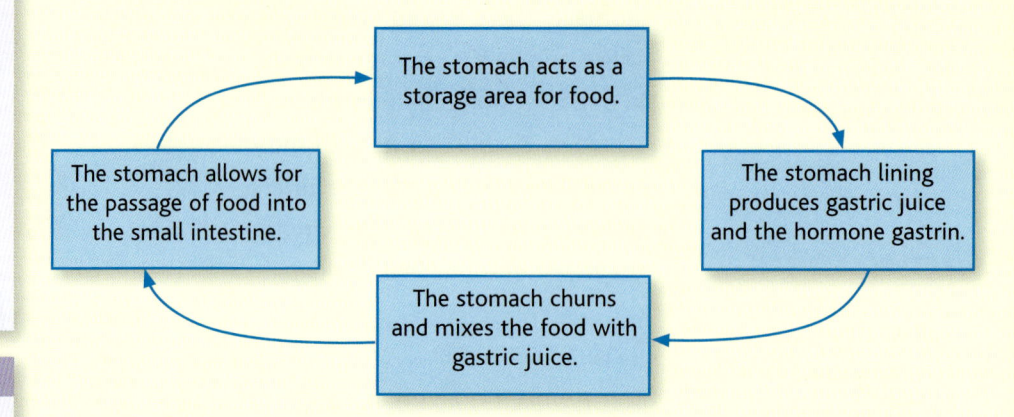

- The stomach acts as a storage area for food.
- The stomach lining produces gastric juice and the hormone gastrin.
- The stomach churns and mixes the food with gastric juice.
- The stomach allows for the passage of food into the small intestine.

- **Storage**: Food enters the stomach mainly undigested. For the digestion processes to begin the contents have to be acidic and the food has to be transformed into a liquid state. Depending upon the type and how much food you have eaten, it can take anywhere from 30 minutes to several hours for the enzymes to break down the food. For example, fat and protein take longer to digest than fruits.

- **Gastric juice** is secreted by specialised epithelial cells in the inner lining of the stomach. It is composed of:
  - *Hydrochloric acid* (HCl): this is produced to kill any bacteria which may have been ingested and to break down the fibrous tissue in meat.
  - *Pepsin*: an enzyme which digests protein. It is produced by the stomach in an inactive form but is activated by the presence of food and in acidic conditions, i.e. when hydrochloric acid is produced.
  - *Intrinsic factor*: a protein which is necessary for the absorption of vitamin B12 when it enters the small intestine.
  - *Water*: this helps to liquefy the food.
  - *Mucus*: this acts as a barrier to protect the stomach wall against the action of hydrochloric acid. It also protects against mechanical injury to the stomach wall by lubricating the food.

  When the food has completely mixed with gastric juice and has liquefied, it is known as **chyme**. Gastrin, a hormone which is produced when food is in the stomach, regulates the amount of acid produced.

- **Absorption**: a limited amount of absorption occurs through the stomach wall. Substances which are absorbed through the stomach lining include:
  - water
  - alcohol
  - sugars
  - minerals (water soluble, i.e. salt)
  - vitamins (water soluble, i.e. vitamin C and B-vitamins)
  - drugs, i.e. aspirin.

CHAPTER 10 The Digestive System

> **Case study**
> **Holistic**
> During a reflexology treatment, areas of imbalance show up on a client's stomach area. When asked about her eating habits, the client reveals that although she normally eats healthily, she often goes for long periods with no food. During the treatment, the client was feeling particularly hungry. Explain what is happening physiologically when this client goes for long periods without eating. Give suggestions as to why this is not good for the health of the digestive system.

The pyloric sphincter

At the far end of the stomach, there is another sphincter muscle called the pyloric sphincter or pylorus. This leads to the first part of the small intestine – the **duodenum**. The pylorus only opens when the food inside the stomach is sufficiently acidic. When the correct acid level is reached, the sphincter opens to allow a small amount of food through into the duodenum. The food remaining in the stomach moves forward, but because it is not as acidic, the pyloric sphincter closes again. In this way, the amount of food passing through into the duodenum is regulated.

> **Link to learning**
> Use the phrase 'Some People Can't Play' to remember the main functions of the stomach:
> **S**ome – Stores food until acidic
> **P**eople – Produces gastric juice and gastrin
> **C**an't – Churns food with gastric juice
> **P**lay – Passes food into small intestine.

The small intestine

The small intestine is divided into three parts: the duodenum, the **ileum** and the **jejunum**. The job of the small intestine is to continue digestion of food and allow for absorption of digested nutrients. For this reason it is the longest part of the digestive tract – about 3 metres (10 feet). The reason it is known as the small intestine is because its diameter is smaller than that of the large intestine – the small intestine is about 2.5 cm (1 inch) in diameter, whereas the large intestine is about 6 cm (2¼ inches) in diameter.

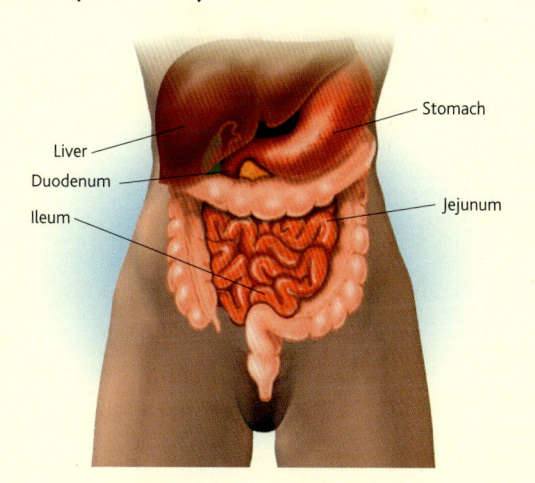

▶ The small intestine consists of the duodenum, ileum and jejunum

Absorption of nutrients inside the small intestine

The small intestine is structured so that the inside surface area is maximised. Finger-like projections, known as villi, increase the surface area. The epithelial cells lining the villi also have tiny finger-like projections, known as micro-villi, which further increase the overall surface area of the large intestine.

PAGE 153

SECTION 2

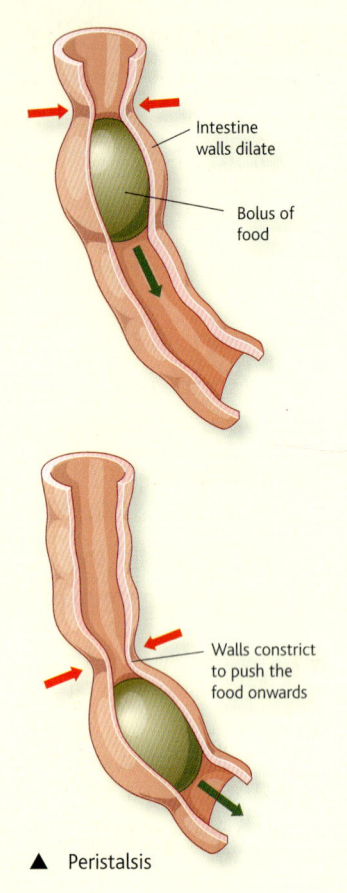

The villi contain a rich blood supply which, once the digested food has absorbed through the villi wall, take the nutrients away to the liver via the hepatic portal vein. (Link to The Blood Circulatory System, page 85) Food or chyme (as it is correctly known) is pushed through the small intestine by **peristalsis**, a wave-like movement brought about by the **involuntary muscle** tissue in the walls of the intestines.

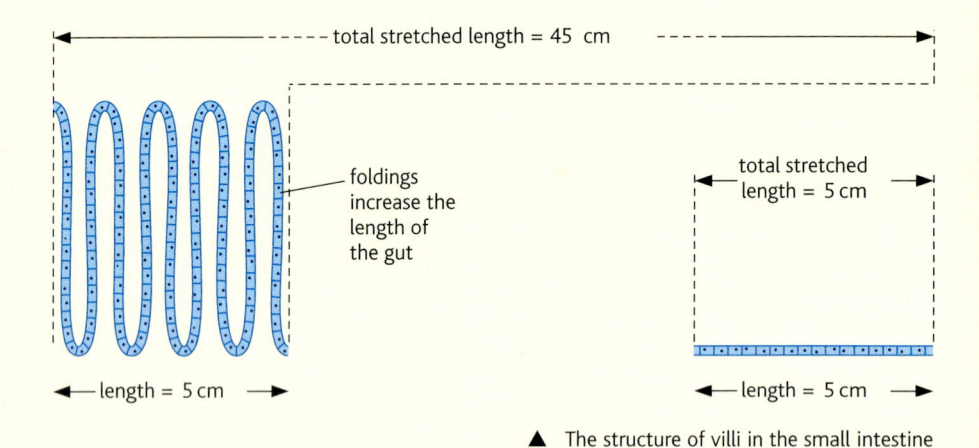

▲ Peristalsis

▲ The structure of villi in the small intestine

Most of the digestive processes which take place in the small intestine do so because of the enzymes in pancreatic juice (see below). However, the small intestine produces intestinal juice. These transform complex carbohydrates into simple sugars.

The duodenum

The duodenum is approximately 25 cm (10 inches) long. In the duodenum:
- Juice from the pancreas arrives via a duct. Pancreatic juice contains enzymes which continue the breakdown of protein.
- **Bile** from the gall bladder arrives via the bile duct. Bile emulsifies fat.

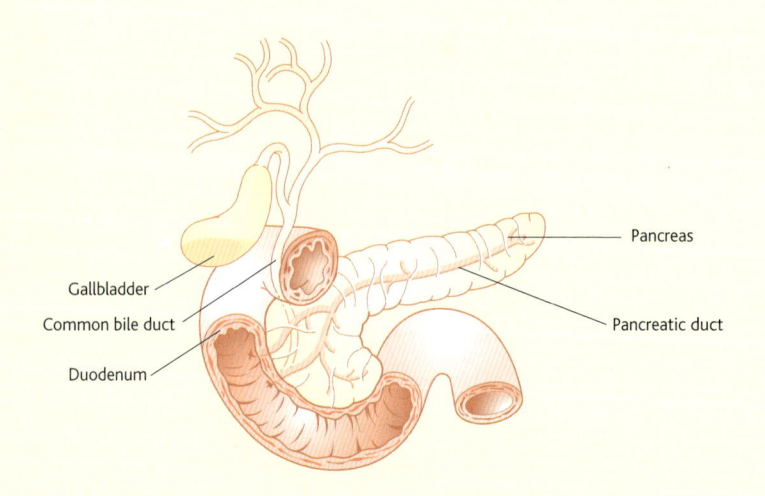

▲ The pancreas, gall bladder, duodenum and liver

During emulsification, fat droplets are suspended in a solution. Bile acids cause the fat globules to break down into smaller droplets, which greatly increases the surface area and allows the enzymes access to the fat droplets.

The duodenum walls contain glands which secrete a substance (carbonate) which protects the walls from the acidic food (the pH in the duodenum is between 6.0 and 6.5, so is slightly acidic). The internal walls are similar in structure to the stomach.

The jejunum

This section of the small intestine is about 2 metres (6.5 feet) in length. It has virtually the same internal structure as the ileum. The pH in the jejunum is almost neutral (pH 7.0). The pH is significant because certain enzymes which act on certain food types need varying alkaline conditions, and the contents gradually neutralise the further they pass through.

The ileum

The ileum is about 3 metres (10 feet) in length. Most absorption of food takes place here because the ileum has an excellent blood supply. The ileum contains lymphoid tissue called Peyer's patches, which produces lymphocytes that destroy micro-organisms that have entered the body through the mouth. The pH in the ileum is usually between pH 7.0 and 8.0 (neutral or slightly alkaline). The ileum joins the large intestine via the ileo-caecal valve.

The ileo-caecal valve

The ileo-caecal valve lies at the very end of the ileum and connects it to the first part of the large intestine, the caecum. The ileo-caecal valve has two main functions:

- it prevents the backflow of contents from the large intestine to the small intestine
- it prevents the contents of the ileum from passing into the large intestine prematurely.

Gastrin, the **hormone** produced when food is in the stomach, regulates the amount of acid produced. When chyme mixed with gastrin approaches the ileo-caecal valve, the gastrin causes the valve to relax and this lets the chyme through. If there is no chyme present, the valve remains shut.

The appendix

This is a worm-like structure at the start of the large intestine. Although not a great deal is known about its function, it is thought that it has a role in developing immunity since it is rich in lymphoid tissue. If the entrance to the appendix becomes blocked, it can become inflamed and appendicitis occurs, requiring surgical removal of the appendix.

The large intestine

The large intestine, or colon, is a tube of circular muscle about 1 metre (3.3 feet) in length and 6 cm (2¼ inches) in diameter. The function of the large intestine is to absorb water and eliminate waste (**faeces**). Hardly any absorption of food takes place here.

The material which passes into the large intestine is water and undigested matter. Water is absorbed from this undigested material and passes back into the blood. Any undigested food matter is used by the intestinal bacteria to make vitamin K and B-vitamins, and these are absorbed in very small amounts. Gas is also formed here.

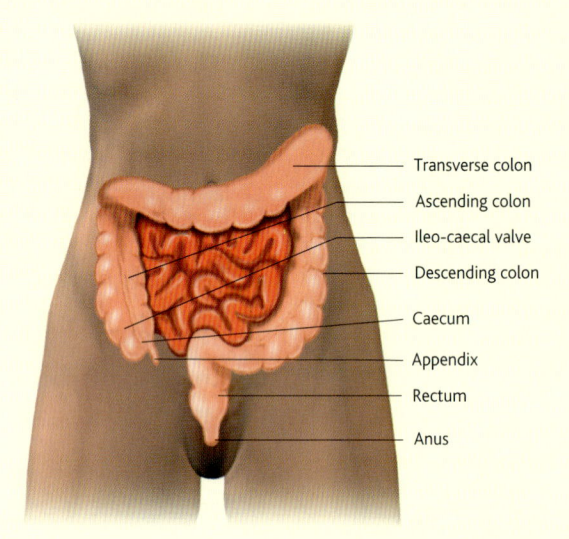

▲ The large intestine.

- Transverse colon
- Ascending colon
- Ileo-caecal valve
- Descending colon
- Caecum
- Appendix
- Rectum
- Anus

It is important for the body that sufficient amounts of indigestible material are consumed in food – this is commonly refered to as fibre. Fibre adds bulk to the faeces and propels it forwards through the colon. If insufficient amounts of fibre are ingested, the faecal matter is not propelled through the colon and constipation occurs.

Faeces

Faeces is the waste matter of digestion. (Link to The Excretory and Urinary System, page 177) It is composed of:
- about 70 per cent water
- undigested food
- undigestible material (fibre)
- intestinal debris – this includes worn out cells from the walls of the intestine (which are constantly replaced) and intestinal bacteria.

The semi-solid faeces are passed into the rectum by peristalsis and expelled by the anus.

The process of digestion and the passage of food from ingestion to elimination can last from 1 to 3 days. This passage is dependent upon many different factors, including the type of food ingested, the emtional state of the person, certain antibiotics and the presence of disease and micro-organisms.

Fascinating fact

It used to be that the appendix was removed as a matter of course if other abdominal surgery was being carried out, in order to prevent possible problems later in life. Now the appendix is spared so that it can be used in reconstructive surgery of the bladder or ureter.

Fascinating fact

If, for some reason, water in the large intestine is not returned to the blood, dehydration would occur, e.g. with diarrhoea or food poisoning.

Link to practice

Constipation can be assisted by massage to the abdomen. The movements performed should be reinforced stroking and gentle kneading. Movements are always performed in the direction that food travels – up the ascending colon, along the transverse colon, down the descending colon. Kneading should not be performed over the sigmoid flexure.

The pancreas

This **gland** is situated behind the duodenum (see page 154). It is both an **endocrine** and an **exocrine** gland.

As an endocrine gland it secretes the hormones **insulin** and **glucagon**, which regulate the amount of sugar circulating in the blood. (Link to The Endocrine System, page 135)

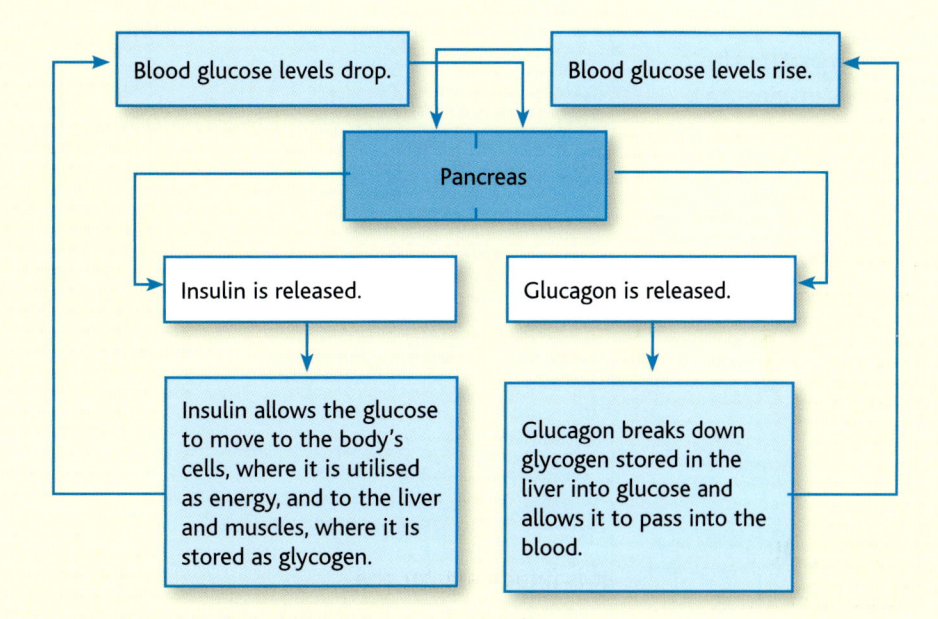

Fascinating fact
When red blood cells die, the pigments in **haemoglobin** break down to form a substance called bilirubin. The liver removes the bilirubin from the blood and it becomes part of bile. It is the bilirubin which makes the faeces brown in colour.

```
Blood glucose levels drop. → Pancreas ← Blood glucose levels rise.
Pancreas → Insulin is released. → Insulin allows the glucose to move to the body's cells, where it is utilised as energy, and to the liver and muscles, where it is stored as glycogen.
Pancreas → Glucagon is released. → Glucagon breaks down glycogen stored in the liver into glucose and allows it to pass into the blood.
```

Fascinating fact
The word 'pancreas' is a Greek word; it is formed from *pan* meaning 'all' and *kreas* meaning 'meat'. This could be because the pancreas of certain animals was considered a delicacy in Ancient Greece.

As an exocrine gland, the pancreas produces pancreatic juice which contains important enzymes for the digestive process. Pancreatic juice is a clear alkaline fluid which helps to neutralise the acid of the stomach. Pancreatic juice enters the duodenum via the pancreatic duct. It contains the following enzymes:

Enzyme	Enzyme
Trypsin	Converts proteins to amino acids
Lipase	Converts fats to fatty acids and glycerol
Amylase	Digests starch
Chymotrypsin	Converts proteins to peptides and amino acids

The liver

The liver is the largest gland in the body and the largest organ after the skin. It weighs about 1.3 kg (3 lbs) and is situated under the diaphragm, to the right of the stomach (see diagram page 149). It is made up of many lobules.

The liver has a very rich blood supply which it receives through two vessels:
- the hepatic artery carries **oxygenated** blood to supply the liver
- the hepatic portal vein carries blood that has come from the intestines and which is rich in nutrients. (Link to The Blood Circulatory System, page 85)

Link to learning

Deamination is the process by which amino acids are broken down and converted to energy and ammonia. Ammonia is toxic to the body so it is converted to uric acid and urea, which can be safely excreted by the body in urine. (Link to The Excretory and Urinary Systems, page 174)

The functions of the liver

The liver is an amazing organ because it has numerous functions. The most important of these functions can be categorised into three main areas: production, metabolism and storage.

Production	Bile	Emulsifies fats Produced continuously by the liver; stored in the gall bladder until needed
	Heparin	Prevents blood clotting inside blood vessels
	Energy	Used by the body for various activities
	Heat	Carried around body to maintain temperature
	Uric acid and **urea**	A by-product of protein breakdown
Metabolism	Fats	Desaturated (conversion of fats from saturated to unsaturated) and oxidised so they can be used and stored by the body
	Proteins	Some harmful amino acids are **deaminated** (see box right) and converted to usable carbohydrate or urea (a waste product)
	Carbohydrate	Excess is converted to fat for storage
	Drugs and poisons	Destroyed or neutralised to become harmless
Storage	Vitamins A and D and B-vitamins	Stored in the liver until needed
	Iron	Produced as a result of the breaking down of worn-out red blood cells; stored until needed for new red blood cells
	Glycogen	Formed from glucose; can be transformed back into glucose depending upon needs of the body; regulated by the hormones insulin and glucagon

The gall bladder

The gall bladder is a small muscular sac situated on the inner surface of the liver. It is basically a storage sac for bile produced by the liver. (For a diagram of the gall bladder, see page 154.)

When chyme enters the duodenum, it triggers the contraction of the gall bladder. This releases bile into the common bile duct and takes it to the duodenum. Bile contains:

- water
- bile pigments
- bile salts
- waste matter (which is excreted eventually with the faeces)
- alkali salts (which emulsify fats and neutralise the acidic chyme).

CHAPTER 10 The Digestive System

> **Link to learning**
>
> The liver is the main heat-producing organ of the body. It provides the body with the heat necessary to maintain body temperature, although the skin regulates body temperature and the blood circulatory system transports the heat. This is a good example of how the body systems work as a whole!

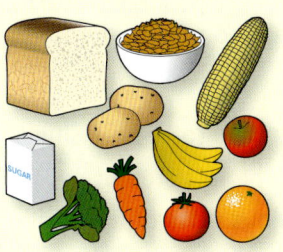

▲ Carbohydrates include bread, potatoes, rice and pasta

> **Proving the point**
>
> Research the foods which contain the essential amino acids. Try to work out what foods a vegetarian or vegan would need to eat to ensure a full intake of essential amino acids.

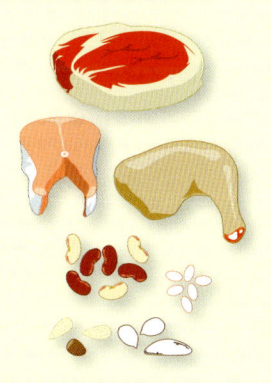

▲ Sources of protein include meat, fish, nuts, seeds and pulses

The digestion, absorption and utilisation of nutrients

Digestion occurs through two processes:
- Mechanical digestion takes place in the mouth, using the teeth to mechanically grind food, and in the stomach where the food is churned.
- Chemical digestion takes place throughout the digestive tract and requires enzymes to chemically break down food so that it may be absorbed.

In order to appreciate how food is digested, it is necessary to look at the specific food groups.

Carbohydrates

Carbohydrates provide the body with energy. They can be simple, for example, sugar, which are used almost instantly by the body, or they can be more complex, such as bread and cereals, which are used more slowly. Carbohydrates should make up 50–60 per cent of a person's daily intake of calories. Excess carbohydrates are converted to fat and stored in the body. Typical foods which fall into this category are bread, pasta, potatoes, rice, and fruit and vegetables.

Carbohydrates consist of three main groups:
- Sugars – obtained from fruit, honey, sugar, malt and milk. The sugars are known as glucose, fructose, sucrose, maltose and lactose respectively.
- Starch – obtained from plants such as potatoes and rice. In their uncooked state they are indigestible.
- Fibre (also known as non-starch polysaccharides or NSP) – obtained from cereals, fruit and vegetables.

Carbohydrate breakdown begins in the mouth (starch), but most digestion takes place in the duodenum, and absorption occurs mainly in the ileum.

Proteins

Protein is needed by the body to repair and maintain body tissue. It can also be used as an energy source. Protein is obtained from animal and vegetable sources, including eggs, cheese, meat, fish, peas, beans and lentils (pulses) and certain vegetables. During digestion, proteins are broken down into peptides and amino acids. It is these units which are used by the body for maintenance, building and repair of body tissues, and as a source of energy. Protein digestion begins in the stomach, continues in the duodenum and is completed in the ileum.

Amino acids are organic compounds which when combined together form proteins. It has been determined that humans need around 20 amino acids. Some are obtained from the food we eat, meat, fish, cheese, eggs, some

> **Proving the point**
>
> Take a lump of butter or margarine or a spoonful of oil. Rub it well into your hands then try to rinse your hands under cold water. What happens? Now add some handwash or washing-up liquid and rub this in well, then rinse under warm water. What is the difference? The second method shows you how fats emulsify in the body.

vegetables and grains. These are known as essential amino acids. Non-essential amino acids are made by the body from a combination of the essential amino acids.

Fats

Fats serve three main functions:
- They provide a rich energy source for the body; they are needed for general body activities and for heat, and are stored as an energy reserve.
- Fat is needed for the absorption and utilisation of other nutrients, for example, certain vitamins.
- Fat provides a cushioning tissue under the skin. (Link to The Skin, Hair and Nails, page 32)

Fats are obtained from animal sources (butter, meat and fish) and vegetable sources (oils, nuts and some fruits i.e. avocados). Animal sources are generally saturated fats; vegetable sources are unsaturated. Having too much saturated fat in the diet is harmful and can lead to heart disease.

Fats are broken down into fatty acids and glycerol. They have to be emulsified and liquefied for the body to be able to absorb them. If the fats are not needed straight away, they are taken to the **adipose** cells in various parts of the body and stored.

Fat digestion begins to a very small degree in the stomach, and bile emulsifies fat in the duodenum. Most fats are absorbed through the walls of the small intestine into special lymphatic capillaries called lacteals. Here, the fat mixes with lymph creating a milky substance called chyme. This is carried through the lymphatic system and enters the blood near the heart. (Links to The Blood Circulatory System, page 87 and The Lymphatic System, page 103) The utilisation of fat occurs as soon as it has been digested and absorbed into the bloodstream. Any excess is stored in the body in adipose cells.

Enzymes

Each food group requires a set of enzymes to break it down. Enzymes are catalysts which assist with the process of digestion in that they create change and speed up biological processes. They do this in numerous processes throughout the body. Around 1,500 have been identified.

> **Fascinating fact**
>
> Protein is classified according to how many amino acids it contains. If it contains all the amino acids the body needs (essential amino acids) it is known as having a high biological value; protein which does not contain all the amino acids is said to have a low biological value. Generally, all meat products have a high biological value. Essential amino acids are harder to obtain from vegetables, therefore vegetarians (those who do not eat meat) and vegans (those who do not use any animal products) must eat a greater range of foods to gain the essential amino acids the body needs.

CHAPTER 10 The Digestive System

Proving the point

If the amount of calories you consume exceeds the amount you use up, the remainder is stored as a reserve of fat. If you use more calories than you consume, the body draws on these reserves of stored fat.

Although exact needs will differ, the average estimated energy requirement for an adult female (aged 19–50 years) is 1,940 calories (Kcal) and for adult males (aged 19–50 years) 2,550 calories (Kcal). Using the calorie listings on food packets in your home and a calorie counter (these are available online), work out roughly how many calories you and members of your family consume daily. Does this exceed the recommended daily requirement or is there a deficit?

Fascinating fact

Some enzymes are used in 'Biological' washing powders, to break down protein and starch stains on clothes.

Nutrient	Class of food	Enzyme	End product
Carbohydrates	Starch	Salivary amylase	Maltose
	Maltose	Maltase	Glucose
	Sucrose	Sucrase	Glucose and fructose
	Lactose	Lactase	Glucose and galactose
Fats	Fats and oils	Lipase	Fatty acids and glycerol
Proteins	Peptides	Pepsin	Peptides
		Erepsin	Amino acids
		Trypsin and chymotrypsin	Peptides and amino acids
	Milk	Rennin (in babies)	Rennin (in babies)

Vitamins and minerals

Vitamins are needed for the body to carry out numerous functions. They have no use as body builders or sources of fuel but are essential as regulators of tissue activity. They are obtained from a wide variety of foods but mainly fruit, vegetables and grains. They are divided into two groups:
- water-soluble (B-vitamins and vitamin C)
- fat-soluble (vitamins A, D and K).

The different vitamins and their function in the body are described below.

Name	Function	Food source	Deficiency
Vitamin A (retinol)	Vision; maintenance of epithelial tissue	Liver; dairy foods; green vegetables	Night blindness; dry skin
Vitamin B1 (thiamine)	Facilitates release of energy from food	Meat; vegetables; wholemeal bread	Nervous disorder: beri-beri
Vitamin B2 (riboflavine)	Facilitates release of energy from food	Milk	Rare
Vitamin B3 (nicotinic acid)	Facilitates release of energy from food	Meat; potatoes; wholemeal bread	Skin disease; pellagra
Vitamin B12	Synthesis of nuclear matter in cells	Liver; yeast extract	Anaemia
Vitamin C (ascorbic acid)	Maintains connective tissue	Citrus fruit; vegetables	Bleeding gums, scurvy
Vitamin D (calciferol)	Facilitates exchange of blood and phosphorous between blood and bones	Egg yolk; margarine; exposure to sunlight	Rickets
Vitamin E	Maintains cell membranes	Plant oils	Rare
Vitamin K	Blood clotting	Dark green leafy vegetables	Rare

Minerals all have different jobs in the body. Although only tiny amounts of each mineral are required, they are essential to health. The body also needs other substances known as trace elements. These include copper, iodine and fluoride.

SECTION 2

> **Fascinating fact**
>
> Some unlikely sources of water include:
> - cabbage = 92 per cent water
> - milk = 87 per cent water
> - lean meat = 75 per cent water.

Name	Function	Food source	Deficiency
Sodium	Transmission of nervous impulses; kidney function; tissue fluids	Salt; bread; cereals	Calcium loss in urine; raised blood pressure
Calcium	Growth and repair of bones and teeth; blood clotting; muscle contraction	Milk; cheese; bread	Osteoporosis; kidney stones; increased blood pressure
Phosphorous	Healthy bones and teeth; production of DNA and RNA; muscle contraction	Milk; cereals; bread	Loss of bone tissue (particularly post-menopause)
Potassium	Transmission of nervous impulses; cell metabolism	Fruit and fruit juices; vegetables; milk; meat	Increased blood pressure; reduced heartbeat
Chloride	Tissue fluid and gastric secretions	Salt	Rare
Iron	Production of haemoglobin	Liver; watercress	Anaemia
Iodine	Production of thyroxin	Seafood; salt	Goitre

Vitamins and minerals are absorbed through the walls of the small intestine. Water-soluble vitamins pass directly into the blood; fat-soluble vitamins are absorbed with fat. Some B-vitamins and vitamin K are produced in the colon and absorbed through the wall of the large intestine.

Water

Water is necessary for the body to carry out all its processes. It is absorbed in the large intestine.

> **Case study**
>
> **Level 3**
>
> Keira has booked in for a massage. During the consultation she says that she has been having trouble with stomach aches and diarrhoea lately, so does not want massage over the stomach area. What further questions might you ask Keira and why?

Diseases and disorders of the digestive system

Bowel cancer

Also known as colorectal cancer, this can occur anywhere in the colon or rectum. The lining of the inside of the colon is constantly being shed and replaced. If the cells do not form correctly, tiny lumps or polyps occur, which may develop into a tumour. If the tumour is malignant and the cancer is not treated, it can spread to other parts of the body, commonly the liver.

Factors which affect the likelihood of developing bowel cancer are:

- age (most sufferers are aged 50 years and over)
- a previous history of polyps or cancer in the bowel

> **Fascinating fact**
>
> The largest user of essential oils is the food industry.
> - It has long been known that the herbs aniseed and fennel have an effect on the appetite. Roman soldiers used to chew fennel to stave off hunger, and aniseed is used to flavour many drinks which are taken as an aperitif (before eating to stimulate digestion) in countries such as France and Greece.
> - The herb peppermint is used extensively as a stomach calmer; it is added to indigestion remedies and other medicines.

- a previous history of other bowel diseases
- Crohn's disease (see below)
- irritable bowel syndrome (IBS) (see below)
- ulcerative colitis (see below)
- a diet which is high in red meat and fat and low in vegetables and fibre
- being overweight
- smoking
- drinking alcohol to excess
- family history of bowel cancer.

Treatment for bowel cancer includes surgery to remove the tumour, radiotherapy and chemotherapy. Treatment and survival rates for bowel cancer have improved dramatically in the last 20 years.

Constipation
This is when the faeces remain in the bowel longer than required. Elimination becomes increasingly difficult as more water is absorbed through the colon wall making the stools even firmer and harder to eliminate.

Colitis
Inflammation of the colon.

Crohn's disease
This is **chronic** (long-term) inflammation of the digestive tract, usually the ileum. There is no known cause. It produces symptoms such as cramps, pain, diarrhoea and raised temperature. Bouts may occur once or twice only or may recur throughout life.

Cirrhosis
Deterioration of the liver due to internal scarring which reduces the functioning of the liver. The commonest cause is alcoholism.

Diarrhoea
Watery and very loose stools. Many different factors can cause diarrhoea, for example, low fibre diets, certain drugs, stress, food poisoning and gastroenteritis (see below). If diarrhoea persists for longer than 48 hours, medical advice should be sought.

Flatulence
Gas in the gut may be caused by a number of factors but is usually due to the type of food ingested. High fibre foods tend to create more gas, as do foods high in complex carbohydrates, i.e. beans and potatoes.

Gall stones
These are hard lumps caused by a build-up of solid particles in the gall bladder. The exact cause is unknown, but sufferers also have high cholesterol levels in

> **Fascinating fact**
>
> Vitamin K plays an important part in blood clotting. A very small number of newborn babies (about 1 in 10,000) suffer from vitamin K deficiency, which can result in internal bleeding and is a potentially fatal condition. To protect against this, all newborn babies are offered vitamin K injections in the first few days after birth.

the blood and one of the jobs of the liver is to remove this cholesterol. Gall stones generally require surgery to remove, although some drugs containing bile acid may be given to attempt to dissolve small stones; newer experimental techniques involve injecting the gall bladder directly with drugs.

Gastritis

Inflammation of the lining of the stomach, often caused by viral infections or a side-effect of medication (e.g. aspirin). More commonly it results from over-indulgence of food, alcohol or smoking.

Gastroenteritis

Inflammation of the digestive tract caused by:
- a virus which may be passed to others (may be termed gastric flu)
- eating contaminated food (food poisoning)
- an alteration in the intestinal bacteria, i.e. eating a dramatically different diet when abroad.

Halitosis

Bad breath. May be caused by poor digestion.

Hepatitis

Inflammation of the liver. There are different types of Hepatitis; the most common ones are viruses named Hepatitis A, B and C. Hepatitis A can be caught by anyone. Good personal hygiene and proper sanitation can help prevent it. Vaccines are available. Hepatitis B and C are transmitted mainly through infected blood and can be life-threatening. A vaccine is available for Hepatitis B.

Heartburn

Reflux of stomach acid into the oesophagus, causing pain and a burning sensation.

Hiatus hernia

To reach the stomach, the oesophagus passes through a space in the diaphragm known as the oesophageal hiatus. If there is a weakness at this spot in the diaphragm muscle, the abdominal organs protrude through and appear as a rounded lump. This is known as a hiatus hernia and can be repaired by surgery.

Irritable bowel syndrome (IBS)

IBS is irregular peristaltic movements in the bowel which interferes with the normal progress of matter through the bowel. This causes bouts of diarrhoea and constipation, pain, discomfort and bloating. There are thought to be several causes but the exact cause is not known. Emotional stress is a contributing factor.

Indigestion
Also called dyspepsia, indigestion is a series of symptoms, which may differ from person to person. Symptoms commonly include: heartburn, belching, bloating, abdominal distension, pain in the chest region and acid reflux into the mouth. It may be caused after eating a specific type of food; if anxious; during pregnancy; eating too quickly, or after eating a very rich meal.

Jaundice
This is a symptom of a disease which may be affecting the liver, pancreas or gall bladder. The skin and whites of the eyes turn yellow due to a build-up of bilirubin, a by-product of the breakdown of worn-out red blood cells. (The liver normally processes bilirubin and sends it to the gall bladder in bile; see also page 154.)

Malnutrition
This generally means a diet insufficient in nutrients; however, it can also be applied to a diet which contains an incorrect amount of nutrients.

Nausea
A feeling of sickness. Can be a physiological reaction brought about to induce vomiting to expel stomach contents, or psychological.

Pancreatitis
Inflammation of the pancreas. It may be acute (short term) or chronic (long term). Sufferers tend to have gallstones as well and are heavy drinkers. Causes intense pain, vomiting and retching. Indigestion usually occurs during bouts.

Ulcer
A 'raw' spot in the lining of either the stomach or duodenum. May be caused by a variety of factors, including excessive drinking and smoking, taking frequent painkillers, rushed and irregular eating habits. Stress is also a contributing factor.

Ulcerative colitis
Ulcerative colitis is an inflammatory bowel disease. It can cause frequent bouts of diarrhoea that may contain blood and mucus, and abdominal pain. The cause is not fully understood but it tends to run in families.

Vomiting
Muscular contractions of the diaphragm which cause the stomach contents to be expelled. This is usually an involuntary response which occurs when the stomach contains something which would be harmful to the body if retained.

The effects of ageing on the digestive system

As people age, they tend to slow down and do less exercise; this can lead to a decreased need for energy in the form of food taken in. If this happens, a person may eat less and in doing so, will reduce the amount of nutrients going into the body, potentially leading to malnutrition. When the body is in a state of malnutrition, it is harder for the body to resist infection and fight disease. Taste can diminish with age, which has a negative effect on appetite, also possibly leading to malnutrition.

Ageing can cause changes which do not have a wholly negative effect on the functioning of the digestive system. The oesophagus muscles weaken but this does not seem to affect the passage of food. The stomach empties more slowly, but again, this does not seem to have any obvious effects. The enzyme which digests milk (lactase) may be inhibited, which can cause lactose intolerance in some people, and this may produce symptoms such as flatulence or diarrhoea. Movement through the large intestine may be slower, producing constipation.

Knowledge check

1. State the function of the mouth and salivary glands in the digestive process.
2. Name the organs and glands involved in digestion.
3. Describe what is meant by digestion.
4. List the functions of the stomach.
5. State the constituents of pancreatic juice.
6. What is bile and where is it stored?
7. Where do pancreatic juice and bile enter the digestive tract?
8. List the main functions of the liver.
9. Name the two blood vessels supplying the liver and give an explanation for why the liver is supplied with two vessels.
10. State the parts and functions of the small intestine.
11. Give a brief overview of the structure of the small intestine.
12. What is a lacteal?
13. List the functions of the large intestine.
14. Name the nutrients required by the body.
15. State the main functions of each nutrient.
16. List the enzymes required to break down protein, fats and carbohydrates.
17. What is the difference between mechanical and chemical digestion?
18. State the function of insulin.
19. Explain what happens to excess fat and carbohydrates in the body.
20. What is the function of fibre in the diet?

SECTION 2

CHAPTER 11 The Excretory and Urinary System

> **Link to learning**
>
> The excretory system refers to the kidneys, skin, bladder, ureter and large intestine.

The **excretory** system is not really a system as such. It is a term used to collectively describe other systems or parts of systems which share a common excretory function. These systems are:
- the **urinary** system
- the digestive system (Link to The Digestive System, page 149)
- the skin. (Link to The Skin, Hair and Nails, page 31)

The term **excretion** describes the process of elimination from the body and is used to describe the physiological processes which remove waste. The most obvious examples of excretion from the body are the elimination of **urine** from the urinary system and the elimination of **faeces** from the digestive system. Sweating is a process of excretion which involves the removal of waste from the sweat glands in the skin. **Exhalation** is a type of excretion as it involves elimination of the waste products of **respiration** from the mouth or nose. (Link to The Respiratory System, page 111)

> **Link to practice**
>
> Treatments such as reflexology, aromatherapy and Swedish body massage can result in excessive urination due to stimulation of the urinary system.

Excretion is an important physiological function because without it the body would become poisoned by the waste products of other physiological functions such as digestion and breathing. The body performs a careful balancing act which makes sure that the 'good' things like nutrients, oxygen, water and minerals are retained, and the 'bad' things such as undigested food, carbon dioxide, excess salts and excess water are expelled. These are examples of **homeostasis**. Disorders of those systems involved in excretion can lead to disharmony in the body, which has a negative effect on normal body functioning and can lead to disease.

> **You will learn**
>
> In this chapter you will learn about:
> - regulation of body fluids
> - regulation of salts
> - maintenance of **pH**
> - the structure and function of the urinary system
> - the location, structure and function of the kidneys
> - urine production and excretion
> - the location, structure and function of the large intestine
> - the composition and elimination of **faeces**
> - the absorption and elimination of water in the digestive system
> - the structure and function of sweat glands
> - diseases and disorders of the excretory system
> - the effects of ageing on the excretory system.

Homeostatic mechanisms

The role of the excretory systems is to help the body to maintain the best internal environment for healthy, normal functioning. This balance is known as homeostasis and is maintained by the excretory systems through the regulation of body fluids, the regulation of salts and the maintenance of pH levels.

Regulation of body fluids

About 60 per cent of a person's body weight is made up of water, which is distributed around the body in fairly constant amounts.

- 70 per cent of the body's total water content is inside cells and is called intracellular fluid.
- The remaining 30 per cent is not in cells and is called extracellular fluid. This water makes up the body fluids such as blood, **lymph** and **sebum**.

These volumes of water are separated by thin, **permeable** cell walls or capillary walls and water is constantly passing from one area to another. Despite this, the volume of water in different areas of the body remains pretty constant throughout life. (Link to Cells and Tissues, page 14)

A person will eat and drink different kinds of things in varying amounts from day to day and carry out different levels of physical activity that cause the body to sweat in varying amounts. Despite these variations, there is the same amount of water in the body at any given time. This is another remarkable example of homeostasis, and a number of the body's systems work together to ensure this balance is maintained.

In order to maintain optimum water levels, water taken into the body must be in equal amounts to the water eliminated. On average, adults in the West consume about 2.5 litres (4.5 pints) of water each day – around 1.5 litres (2.6 pints) of this comes in the form of drinks and about 1 litre (1.8 pints) is in the form of food. Water is excreted from different systems of the body in different amounts. Each day, on average:

- about 400–500 ml of water is excreted by the lungs as water vapour (Link to The Respiratory System, page 117)

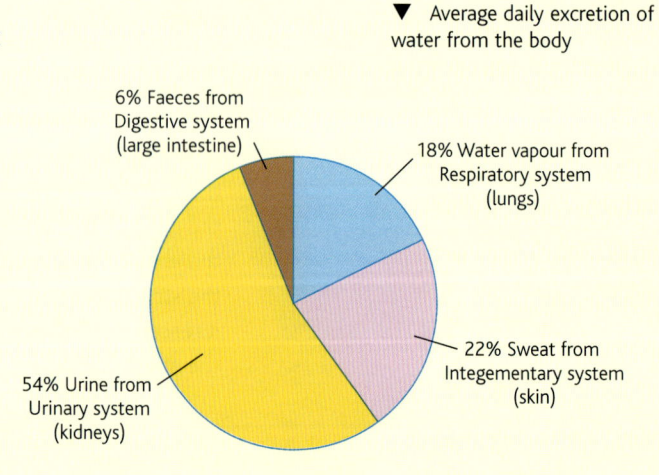

▼ Average daily excretion of water from the body

- 6% Faeces from Digestive system (large intestine)
- 18% Water vapour from Respiratory system (lungs)
- 22% Sweat from Integumentary system (skin)
- 54% Urine from Urinary system (kidneys)

Link to learning

The prefix *intra* – means 'within' (a structure) while the prefix *inter* – means 'between' (structures.) For example, an international football match is a competition between nations.

Link to learning

As water in the body passes from one area to another its composition changes so that tissue fluid can become **lymph**, and lymph fluid can become blood, and blood can become urine. This is a bit like the process of recycling an aluminium can, which might become part of a car or a cooker or even another aluminium can!

Fascinating fact

When it is cold during the winter months, you might notice that you urinate more frequently. This is because you lose less water through sweat. During the warmer summer months, on the other hand, you urinate less because you sweat more.

- about 500–600 ml of water is excreted by the skin as sweat (Link to The Skin, Hair and Nails, page 37)
- about 1,000–1,500 ml is excreted by the kidneys as urine
- about 100–150 ml is excreted in the faeces. (Link to The Digestive System, page 156)

Of course, the amount of water consumed and excreted does vary between and within individuals and these figures, therefore, represent average amounts. The important thing to remember is that the body is able to regulate fluids so that a constant balance is maintained (homeostasis). Certain conditions might cause a person to consume more fluids, such as hot weather or excessive thirst caused by illness or physical activity. Also, in such conditions the body is likely to excrete greater amounts of fluid in sweat. As more water is lost through sweat, the body regulates this by lowering the amount of water excreted through urine. Thus, via the unconscious processes of sweating more, urinating less and feeling thirsty, as well as the conscious process of drinking more fluids, the body works to regulate its water balance.

Regulation of salts in body fluids

It is vital that volumes of water in the body remain constant in order that cells and tissues can function effectively. However, this is only half of the story. As well as being present in the right amounts, bodily fluids must be of the correct composition if the body is going to be able to function properly. Water in the body contains minute dissolved particles of mineral salts which are obtained from food. These tiny particles or **ions** carry an electrical charge and are called **electrolytes**.

> **Link to practice**
> There are two types of electrolytes:
> - those which have a positive (+) charge are called **cations**
> - those which have a negative (-) charge are called **anions**.

As positively charged and negatively charged ions balance each other out, the number of anions and cations in body fluids must be regulated in order that the composition of body fluids remains evenly balanced. A healthy balanced diet should contain all the essential minerals the body needs; as they are needed in such small amounts, a deficiency is rare. (Link to The Digestive System, page 161) Because of this, minerals are sometimes called *micronutrients*. Some of the essential minerals are listed in the table below. Of these:
- some carry a positive charge, such as calcium, magnesium, sodium and potassium
- some carry a negative charge, such as chloride and phosphates.

The body maintains the right balance of electrolytes by absorbing what is required and excreting what isn't. This passes from the body in urine.

Mineral salt (ion)	Body fluid	Electrolyte
Sodium	Plasma and interstitial fluid	(+) anion
Potassium	Intracellular fluid	(+) anion
Chloride	Plasma and interstitial fluid	(-) cation
Calcium	Traces	(+) anion
Magnesium	Traces	(+) anion
Phosphate	Intracellular fluid	(-) cation

> **Fascinating fact**
> Kidney stones are an example of crystallised mineral salts. Normal urine composition allows for excess salts to be excreted from the body; if this balance is not maintained, crystals form which can block the passage of urine and cause considerable discomfort.

> **Fascinating fact**
> Overly acidic pH levels in the body can lead to infection. One sign of this is cloudy urine.

> **Link to learning**
> *Renal* is used as a prefix or suffix to denote something to do with the kidneys, e.g. renal medulla, renal disease, renal failure, adrenal glands.

Maintenance of pH

As well as maintaining levels of water and electrolytes, the body must maintain the **pH** of body fluids so that the various cell activities can take place effectively. All body fluids are slightly alkaline with an average pH of 7.4 (although levels vary slightly in different types of fluid). Venous blood is slightly less alkaline than arteriole blood because of the presence of waste products such as carbon dioxide and other acids which are produced in the tissues. Interstitial and intracellular fluid (in cells and tissues) is slightly more alkaline than pH 7.4.

In order that the correct pH balance is maintained, alkalis and proteins neutralise the acids which are produced during chemical reactions in the tissues, and acids such as carbonates and chloride neutralise alkalis. This balancing of pH levels is yet another example of homeostasis.

If the body fluids become less alkaline, a condition called **acidosis** can occur and this can lead to coma and death. If the body fluids become more alkaline than normal, it can lead to a condition called **alkalosis**. This can be caused by loss of acid from excessive vomiting, by retention of an alkali such as potassium as a result of kidney failure, or by taking in high levels of alkaline salts such as sodium bicarbonate.

The urinary system

The urinary system is concerned with maintaining fluid balance in the body. Put very simply, it consists of internal 'pipework' which allows for the storage and transport of fluid, rather like the pipe work in your house. In a house, there is a central water tank for the storage of cold water, and maybe a boiler or immersion heater for the storage of hot water. These are linked by a network of pipes which supply sinks, dishwashers, washing machines, baths, showers and toilets with running water. There is also a second network of pipes which transports waste water away from these structures via plugholes and drains to an external sewerage system. The structure of the water system in your body is very similar to that which takes place in your house in that there are inlets and outlets and places of storage, all connected by a series of tubes.

CHAPTER 11 The Excretory and Urinary System

The urinary system consists of a number of organs which store fluid. These are a pair of kidneys and the bladder. The kidneys are linked to the bladder by a pair of muscular tubes called the ureters, and the bladder is linked to the external genitalia by a single tube called the urethra. The kidneys filter one bodily fluid, blood, and produce a second fluid, urine.

Urine is transported from the kidneys along the ureters by a series of contractions called **peristalsis**. This is a series of squeezing movements the same as those which move food along the digestive tract. (Link to The Digestive System, page 154) From the ureters, urine arrives at the bladder where it is stored until excretion takes place. When the levels of urine in the bladder reach a certain point, this is felt as the need to release urine. When passing urine from the body, it leaves the bladder via a tube called the urethra.

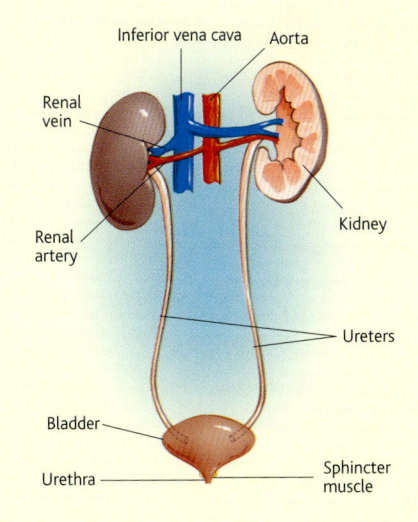

▲ The structure of the urinary system

The urinary structures play a key role in removing excess fluid from the body and also in removing toxic waste materials in the form of urine.

The kidneys

> **Link to practice**
>
> Body massage techniques, such as tapotement, should be adapted directly over the kidneys to avoid damage or bruising to these vulnerable structures.

The kidneys are located in the lumbar curve of the lower back between the 12th thoracic vertebra and the 3rd lumbar vertebra, one on either side of the vertebral column. (Link to The Skeletal System, page 48) The kidneys are positioned to the posterior part of the abdomen and are more vulnerable than other internal organs as they are not enclosed by skeletal structures such as the pelvis or the thorax.

The kidneys are bean-shaped organs and are relatively large, measuring about 11 cm long, 6 cm wide and 3 cm thick. Each kidney is surrounded by a capsule of fibrous tissue and is embedded in a bed of fat.

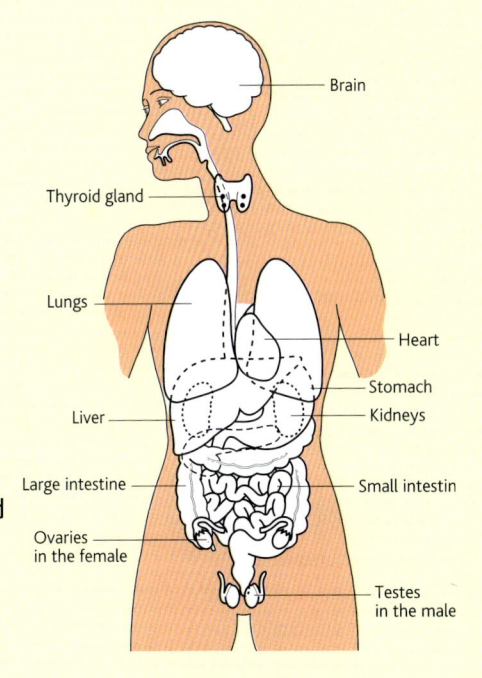

▲ The kidneys in relation to the other main organs of the body

PAGE 171

SECTION 2

> **Link to practice**
>
> Dark circles under the eyes may be an indicator of poor kidney function. Foods which enhance kidney function are root vegetables such as onions, beetroot and celery, fruits such as blueberries, blackberries and cranberries, and fish such as trout and salmon.

A cross-section diagram of a kidney illustrates two distinct parts. The darker outer part of the kidney is the renal cortex, and the paler inner section is the renal **medulla**.

The key functions of the kidneys are to receive and filter blood in order to produce and secrete urine. They receive approximately 1 litre (2 pints) of blood each minute from the renal artery.

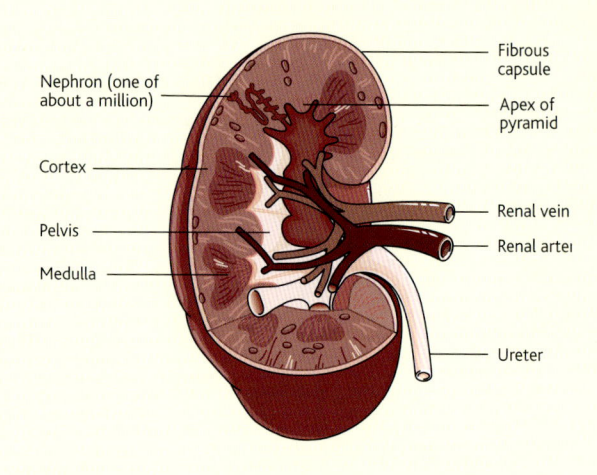

▲ Cross-section diagram of a kidney

This blood is filtered into useful substances which can be reused and waste substances for excretion.

Nephrons

There are over one million tiny, twisted tubes in each kidney called **nephrons** – the cross-section diagram of a kidney above shows one of these structures drawn in. A more detailed drawing of a nephron is given below.

> **Link to learning**
>
> The terms medulla and cortex are used to describe the inside and outside of structures such as the kidneys, the hair and the adrenal glands.

The kidneys are unique in that they are the only organs which transport blood through two sets of capillaries. This is in order to carry out the filtration processes necessary to remove excess water and waste products from the blood and produce urine.

It is the structure of each nephron which enables this process to take place.

> **Link to learning**
>
> The terms afferent and efferent are used to mean travelling towards a structure and travelling away from a structure (such as afferent and efferent nerves in the CNS).

> **Fascinating fact**
>
> If the tubules in each kidney were unravelled they would stretch more than 40 miles (65 kilometres) in length.

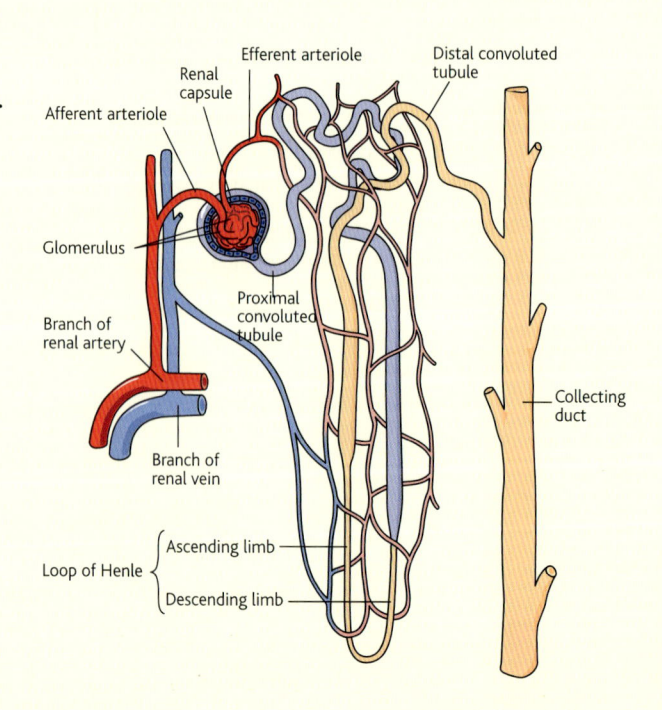

▶ A nephron and its blood supply

CHAPTER 11 The Excretory and Urinary System

> **Link to learning**
> By filtering, reabsorbing and secreting, nephrons help to maintain homeostasis of the blood's volume and composition.

The structure of a nephron

At one end of each nephron is a cup called the glomerular capsule (also known as the renal capsule or Bowman's capsule). This structure holds a bundle of capillaries leading from the renal artery which are collectively called the **glomerulus**.

- The arteriole which brings blood to the glomerulus is called the **afferent** arteriole or vessel.
- The arteriole which takes blood away from the glomerulus is the slightly smaller **efferent** arteriole or vessel.

> **Link to learning**
> The walls of the glomerulus are like a sieve with very fine holes. Tiny particles like water can be filtered through, but larger particles like blood cells and protein cannot.

The nephron twists down into the renal medulla and back up into the renal cortex. It ends with a straight tubule in the renal medulla. The efferent vessel then divides to form a second set of capillaries where blood is collected by small venules that empty into the renal vein.

Urine production and excretion

Blood is the body's system of transport and is filtered by the kidneys to produce urine. Components of blood which are filtered by the kidneys are the products of digestion:

- glucose from the digestion of carbohydrates
- amino acids from the digestion of protein
- fatty acid from the digestion of lipids (fats)
- vitamin and mineral salts
- water. (Link to The Digestive System, page 162)

> **Fascinating fact**
> In the presence of kidney disease, vital substances such as blood cells and proteins are also filtered and are found in the glomerular filtrate.

Urine production
Filtration under pressure

The walls of the glomerulus are semi-permeable, meaning that they allow certain substances to be filtered through them into the Bowman's capsule but not others. The reason for this **diffusion** from one structure to another is that blood in the glomerulus is under pressure (since the renal artery branches off the aorta and enters the

▼ Diffusion from the glomerulus to Bowman's capsule – the filtering system of the kidney

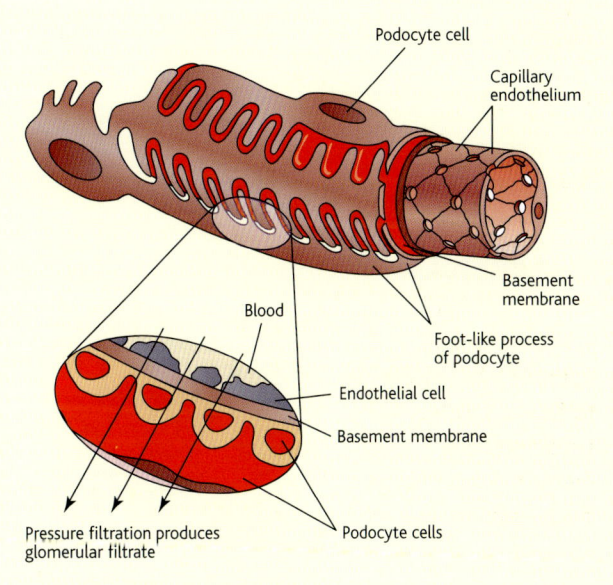

Podocyte cell
Capillary endothelium
Basement membrane
Foot-like process of podocyte
Blood
Endothelial cell
Basement membrane
Pressure filtration produces glomerular filtrate
Podocyte cells

PAGE 173

> **Fascinating fact**
> Pregnancy tests are carried out by measuring the levels of particular hormones present in urine.

much narrower efferent arteriole). (Link to The Blood Circulatory System, page 85) Because of the high pressure of the blood, water and other small particles are forced through the walls of the glomerulus into the Bowman's capsule but larger blood cells and proteins remain in the blood. This is the process called **filtration** under pressure.

The fluid in the Bowman's capsule is called **glomerular filtrate** and has a similar composition to plasma, the liquid part of blood. It contains water, **glucose**, **amino acids**, salts, fatty acids and **urea**.

Selective reabsorption

The glomerular filtrate now passes from the Bowman's capsule into the renal tubule and collecting duct. Here, blood in the capillaries around the renal tubule absorbs some of the substances from the glomerular filtrate. Only those substances which are needed by the body are absorbed. This is the process called **selective reabsorption**.

- All of the glucose in the glomerular filtrate is reabsorbed and so is most of the water and salts.
- The fluid which remains contains no glucose but does contain urea and salts. This fluid is called urine.

Active secretion

Finally, substances from the blood in the second capillary network that are not needed by the body are secreted into the renal tubule and collecting duct for excretion. These substances include:

- waste products
- excess secretions of hormones
- medication such as antibiotics
- excess ions (to maintain the electrolyte balance of the body).

These substances are passed into the urine.

> **Fascinating fact**
> Healthy, fresh urine is cleaner than your mouth or your hands – Ancient civilizations have used urine as soap and mouthwash!

> **Fascinating fact**
> The acidity of urine varies according to the levels of salts, which help to maintain the pH of blood at about 7.4.

> **Fascinating fact**
> The colour of urine can vary according to diet. Beetroot can cause urine to be red in colour while excess vitamin C in the diet will result in urine that is a bright orange colour.

▼ The three stages of the production of urine.

1. Blood from renal artery enters glomerulus
2. Ultra filtration takes place in the glomerulus
3. Filtrate enters Bowman's Capsule
4. Some substances are reabsorbed back into the blood
4. Some substances are reabsorbed back into the blood
5. Urine to pelvis of kidney
6. Blood to renal vein

First coiled region of tubule
Second coiled region of tubule
Blood capillaries
Loop of Henle
Collecting duct

Blood composition g per 100cm³
Water	91
Urea	0.03
Salts	0.4
Glucose	0.1
Proteins	8

Filtrate composition g per 100cm³
Water	99
Urea	0.03
Salts	0.7
Glucose	0.1
Proteins	0

Urine composition g per 100cm³
Water	96
Urea	3
Salts	1.2
Glucose	0
Proteins	0

▲ Filtration under pressure   ▲ Selective reabsorption   ▲ Active secretion

Urine storage and release

Urine is an acidic fluid consisting of:

- 96 per cent water
- 2 per cent urea
- 2 per cent uric acid and salts.

However, this composition can be affected by the kinds of food and drink consumed as well as by certain illnesses.

Urine is stored in a muscular reservoir called the bladder. The size, shape and position of the bladder can vary slightly according to how much or how little urine it holds. The lower part remains fixed, about 3–4 cm behind the pubis symphysis, but as the bladder fills up, it moves upwards and forwards into the abdominal cavity.

The bladder can hold over 500 ml (1 pint) of fluid, but this would cause great discomfort and usually the desire to empty the bladder is felt when it contains about 250–300 ml (½ pint) of urine. The average quantity of urine excreted in a 24-hour period is about 1.5 litres (3 pints) in order to maintain fluid balance in the body.

Urine passes from the bladder through a sphincter muscle into a tube called the urethra. This sphincter muscle is under conscious control. In females, the urethra is about 4 cm in length, which is the distance from the bladder to the external genitalia. In males, however, the urethra is considerably longer (approximately 20 cm) as it extends from the bladder and along the length of the penis. In males, the urethra is a passage for sperm as well as urine and so this structure plays a role in the reproductive as well as the urinary system. (Link to The Reproductive System, page 183)

Summary of the structure and function of the urinary system

	Structure	Function
Kidneys	Two bean-shaped organs located in the lower, posterior abdomen	Secretion and excretion of urine
Ureters	Pair of long, thick-walled tubes, one leading from each kidney	Transport urine from the kidneys to bladder
Bladder	Organ in lower pelvis with a fixed opening behind pubis symphysis	Reservoir for storage of urine with a maximum capacity of 500 ml (1 pint)
Urethra	Single tube extending from the bladder which is 20 cm long in males and 4 cm long in females	Elimination of urine from the body. In males the urethra also functions as part of the reproductive system

---

Fascinating fact

Try to find out the names of some medical conditions which can be detected by the composition of urine.

Fascinating fact

A client in the later stages of pregnancy may need to pass urine more frequently as the growing baby pushes down on the bladder, decreasing its volume.

Fascinating fact

Poor bladder function can lead to symptoms including poor bladder control, frequent or infrequent urination, and headache. A common symptom of diabetes is frequent and excessive urination.

Link to learning

There are several examples of homeostasis in the urinary system. These include regulation of fluids, regulation of salts and regulation of pH.

SECTION 2

Link to practice

It is not the holistic or beauty therapist's job to diagnose conditions or prescribe specific treatment. Referrals should be made to a qualified herbalist, naturopath or dietician.

The large intestine

The large intestine, or colon, is a muscular tube about 1.5 metres (4.9 feet) long. This is the final part of the digestive tract which leads from the **small intestine** to the anus. (Link to The Digestive System, page 136)

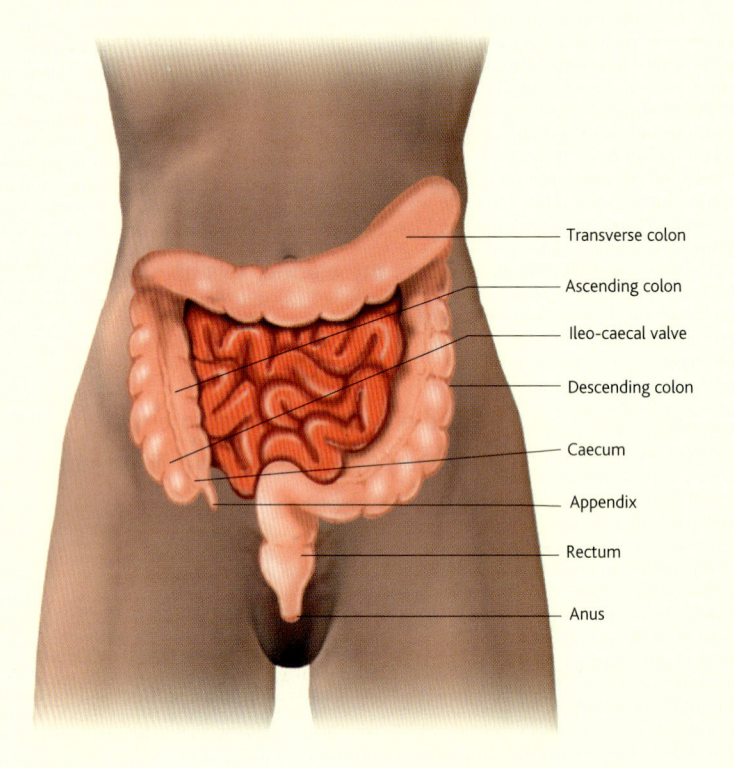

- Transverse colon
- Ascending colon
- Ileo-caecal valve
- Descending colon
- Caecum
- Appendix
- Rectum
- Anus

◀ The large intestine

Link to practice

Colonic irrigation or hydrotherapy is a procedure which flushes the colon with warm water to remove stagnant faeces, undigested food and toxins such as medication. Benefits can include relief from digestive disorders such as those listed above, increased physical and mental energy, improved circulation and improvement in the condition of the skin. Colonic irrigation should always be performed by a qualified practitioner following a thorough consultation.

Link to practice

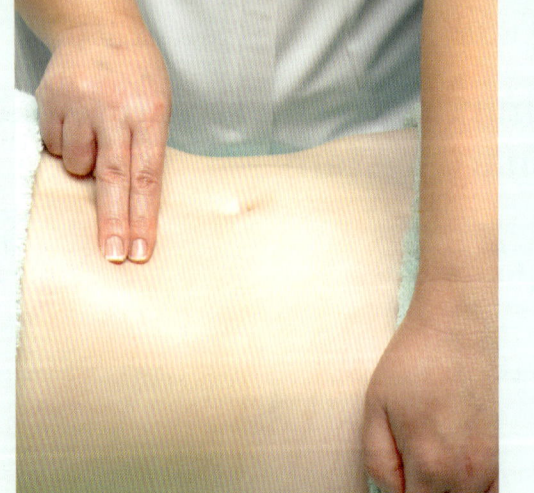

Massage of the abdomen must always follow the direction of the large intestine:
- up the right in line with the ascending colon
- then across from right to left in line with the transverse colon
- then down the left in line with the descending colon
- before coming back in towards the sigmoid colon
- and going down again in line with the rectum.

Fascinating fact

The brown colour of faeces comes from the decomposition of old red blood cells which mixes with the other waste components.

PAGE 176

> **Fascinating fact**
>
> The **appendix** is a small structure attached to the caecum which has no function in modern humans due to evolutionary changes to diet. The appendix of humanity's ancient ancestors was much bigger as it was responsible for the digestion of foliage. Animals which eat foliage (foliovores) have a much larger appendix than humans.

The composition and elimination of faeces and water

By the time 'food' enters the large intestine, it contains very little nutrients as most of these have been absorbed into the bloodstream. (Link to The Digestive System, page 149) The material entering the large intestine contains water, salt, indigestible cellulose and bacteria. Most of the water and salts that remain are absorbed by the walls of the large intestine and in their absence, much of the bacteria cannot survive. This leaves only cellulose and dead bacteria, which combine with a little water to form a paste called faeces. Faeces, therefore, has a solid part which is about 50 per cent dead bacteria and 50 per cent cellulose, and a liquid part which is water.

Peristalsis occurs about 3–4 times a day in the large intestine and it is these contractions which move faeces from the colon to the rectum. As the rectum fills with faeces, it becomes distended. This triggers a reflex contraction of the sphincter muscle which expels faeces along the anal canal. At this point, the urge to excrete faeces is felt in a process called **defecation**. If defecation is delayed, more water is absorbed from the faeces, which reduces the sensation of fullness but can, in time, lead to constipation.

Common excretory problems associated with defecation

Problem	Possible cause	Possible solution
Small, hard pellets	Congestion in the liver	Milk thistle supplement
Light coloured or yellowy	Undigested fats	Increase intake of essential fatty acids from fish and seeds
Presence of food	Undigested food	Chew your food properly
Bad odour which takes a while to disperse	Sluggish digestion; high acid	Take digestive enzymes as a supplement
Bloating or wind	Poor digestion	Cut out junk food; cut down on wheat and dairy foods; eat slowly and without drinks

The structure and function of sweat glands

Sweat glands, or **sudoriferous glands**, are structures of the **dermis** of the skin. (Link to The Skin, Hair and Nails, page 37) There are two types of sweat gland:
- The larger **apocrine** sweat glands are attached to hair follicles in the groin, the axilla and the nipples. These glands are stimulated during times of stress, anxiety or excitement.
- The smaller **eccrine** sweat glands are located all over the body, but there

are more of them in certain areas such as the palms of the hands and soles of the feet. The main function of eccrine sweat glands is to maintain body temperature (homeostatic function).

Sweat glands also have an excretory function as sweat comprises water, salts and other waste products – the same as urine. Alcohol, food and medication can also be excreted in sweat. The average amount of sweat which is excreted in a 24-hour period is 500–600 ml (approximately 1 pint), although this will vary depending on the amount of urine excreted. If less fluid is excreted in urine, more fluid will be excreted in sweat and vice versa. This is in order to maintain fluid balance in the body (homeostasis)

> **Case study**
>
> **Level 3/Holistic**
> Marinda is a new client who has booked a course of body massage treatments. You have treated her twice but are dreading her next visit as she suffers from excess, unpleasant smelling perspiration. Identify the problems, its possible cause, what further information is required and the treatment advised.

> **Link to practice**
> Disorders of the excretory system can cause discomfort in the abdomen and lower back, in which case they would contra-indicate treatment.

> **Fascinating fact**
> Normal perspiration does not smell, although spicy foods and alcohol can sometimes be detected.

Diseases and disorders of the excretory system

The urinary system
Cancer of the kidney
Hypernephroma is the name given to a cancerous tumour of the kidney. This is most commonly found in males over the age of 50 years. Symptoms include pain in the pelvic area and the passage of blood.

Kidney disease
Typical characteristics of kidney disease include lower back pain and coloured discharge or blood in the urine.

Kidney stones
Kidney stones or renal calculus are salt crystals which, if small enough, are passed in urine or, if larger, may become lodged in the urinary tract and require surgical intervention. Typical symptoms of kidney stones include difficulty urinating, blood in the urine and abdominal pain.

Nephritis
Nephritis is inflammation of the kidneys which results in retention of excess water and salts. Symptoms typically include high blood pressure, passage of blood in urine, pain in the pelvic area and swollen ankles.

Urinary tract infection
An infection or inflammation of the urinary tract is usually characterised by

CHAPTER 11 The Excretory and Urinary System

> **Fascinating fact**
> The body contains enough bacteria to fill a tin of beans; most of this lives in the digestive tract. Some of the bacteria in the colon are 'good' bacteria, and these can be replaced or topped up with supplements such as acidophilus or probiotic drinks, which help maintain healthy digestion.

> **Fascinating fact**
> Eating corn, which is not wholly digestible, is a good way to find out how efficiently your digestive system is working. A healthy body will digest corn in about six hours. If it takes much longer than this to appear in your faeces, it can be an indicator of poor digestion.

> **Fascinating fact**
> Function of the colon can be adversely affected by stress, smoking, medication and poor diet. These factors can cause the body to fail to excrete its waste products and instead hold onto them (constipation).

a constant desire to pass urine, the passage of blood in the urine or another unusual discharge, abdominal pain and an intense burning sensation on passing urine.
- Urethritis is the name given to inflammation of the urethra.
- Cystitis is the name given to inflammation of the bladder.

Both these disorders are caused by a bacterial infection and are more common in females due to the relative shortness of the urethra compared to males.

The skin

Hyperhidrosis
An over-secretion of sweat. This condition usually affects particular areas of the body such as the hands, feet and/or underarms (axilla).

Anhidrosis
A partial or complete lack of perspiration.

Bromhidrosis
Unpleasant smelling perspiration. This can be the result of an infection, poor hygiene or wearing close-fitting clothing made of artificial fabric.

Miliaria rubra
Excess perspiration can cause the sweat ducts to become blocked, which can lead to a condition called miliaria rubra. This disorder is characterised by small raised itchy spots and is often referred to as heat rash, sweat rash or prickly heat.

The effects of ageing on the excretory system

As with all the body's systems, age-associated changes may be apparent in the organs of excretion.
- Some clients may experience excessive sweating (hyperhidrosis), which is a common symptom of the **menopause**, while more mature clients might not sweat at all as the function of the sudoriferous glands slows down with age.
- Mature clients may experience bladder weakness and feel the desire to pass urine more frequently as the bladder sphincter becomes less taut.

Clients should be advised to maintain a balanced diet to ensure the health of the digestive system and regular bowel movements.

Fascinating fact

A lack of perspiration may be a symptom of a thyroid disorder. (Link to The Endocrine System, page 144)

Fascinating fact

The 'good' bacteria in natural yoghurt can help alleviate the itching associated with prickly heat. But don't eat it! Smooth the yoghurt on your skin for a natural remedy.

Knowledge check

1. Name three methods of excretion from the body.
2. Define the term homeostasis.
3. Explain how water balance is maintained in the body.
4. Name three mineral salts found in body fluids.
5. Explain how the balance of mineral salts is maintained in the body.
6. Name and describe the main components of the kidney.
7. Describe the stages of urine production.
8. List the components of urine.
9. Name three disorders of the urinary system.
10. Name and locate the structures of the large intestine.
11. Describe the stages of faeces production.
12. List the components of faeces.
13. Explain the importance of the sequence of an abdominal massage.
14. Describe three disorders of the large intestine.
15. Explain the difference between apocrine and eccrine sweat glands.
16. Explain how sweat glands assist in the removal of waste from the body.
17. Give two examples of peristalsis in the body.
18. Describe three disorders of the sweat glands.
19. Describe the effects of ageing on the organs of excretion.
20. List the advice for maintaining a healthy excretory system.

SECTION 2

Chapter 12 The Reproductive System

Link to practice

The reproductive system is extremely relevant to the therapist because many treatments can be affected by changes in hormonal levels in women. For example, clients may be more sensitive to the painful effects of electrolysis treatment during **menstruation**. As a therapist, you may notice changes in clients' skin depending on the stage of the **menstrual cycle**; for example, acne is often more marked when the client is premenstrual.

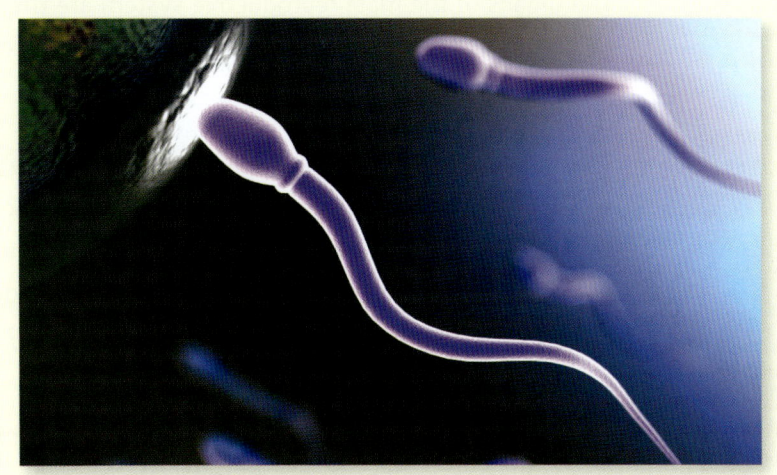

◀ A female ovum (egg) and male sperm come together to begin a new human life

Reproduction is the amazing process which ensures that the thread of life is sustained. When the largest human **cell**, the female **ovum**, or egg, is combined with the male **sperm**, they form a single cell called a **zygote**. This cell divides and grows so that life can begin.

Mammals need a male and a female partner in order to reproduce, as each sex cell, known as a **gamete**, contains only half the required number of **genes**. (Link to Cells and Tissues, page 11) The organs of male and female reproduction have become highly **specialised** for this purpose. These reproductive organs, or **gonads**, become active at **puberty** and remain so until the **menopause** for women and the end of life for men. The male **testes** produce the sperm and the female **ovaries** produce ova. In women the reproductive organs are protected by the pelvic girdle. In men the testes are situated on the outside of the body because the sperm are more suited to a temperature lower than body temperature.

The gonads are also glands that produce **hormones** which control the production of sperm and ova. (Link to The Endocrine System, page 142)

You will learn

In this chapter you will learn about:
- the structure and function of the male reproductive system
- the structure and function of the female reproductive system
- the menstrual cycle
- fertilisation, pregnancy and birth
- the process of **meiosis**
- the menopause
- the structure and function of the female breast
- diseases and disorders of the reproductive system
- the effects of ageing on the reproductive system.

PAGE 181

SECTION 2

> **Proving the point**
>
> The hormone **testosterone** is responsible for the development of the male secondary sexual characteristics that emerge at puberty. (Link to The Endocrine System, page 140) Make a list of these characteristics.

> **Link to learning**
>
> The penis and the scrotum are referred to as the male genitalia.

The male reproductive system

The organs of the male reproductive system are the testes, their ducts, the penis and a number of glands that secrete substances that form semen.

The testes

The testes are about 5 cm (2 inches) in length and about 2.5 cm (1 inch) across, and are suspended between the thighs in a sac of skin called the **scrotum**. They develop in the abdominal cavity and move down into the scrotum before birth. The position of the testes, on the outside of the body, ensures that the sperm are kept at an optimum temperature of 35°C (95°F), which is slightly below body temperature (36.7°C or 98.1°F).

- The testes are made up of tiny tubules called seminiferous tubules which produce sperm. Sperm are stored in the epididymis until they are mature and can swim.
- As the mature sperm leave the epididymis they enter the vas deferens. The vas deferens is housed in the spermatic cord. It curves behind the urinary bladder and is joined by the duct from the seminal vesicle.
- The seminal vesicle produces a fluid called **semen** which nourishes and transports the sperm.
- At the base of the bladder is the **prostate gland**. This produces an alkaline secretion which helps to neutralise the acidity of the female vagina during sexual intercourse.

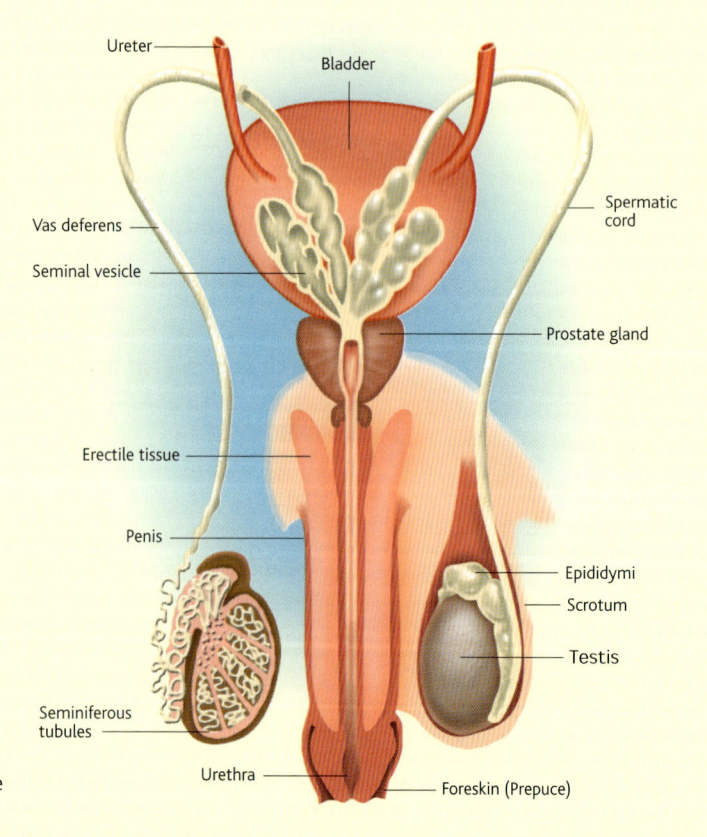

▶ The male reproductive system

PAGE 182

CHAPTER 12 The Reproductive System

> **Fascinating fact**
>
> The average volume of semen produced at ejaculation is 2 to 5 ml; this will contain between 40 and 100 million sperm (about 20 million sperm per ml). Only one sperm is needed to fertilise an egg!

The penis

The penis has a dual function:
- it carries urine from the bladder to the outside (Link to The Excretory and Urinary Systems, page 175)
- it transports sperm and semen into the female vagina.

The penis is a soft, spongy organ that contains spaces that fill with blood when stimulated so that it can become erect. During sexual intercourse it ejaculates sperm into the female vagina.

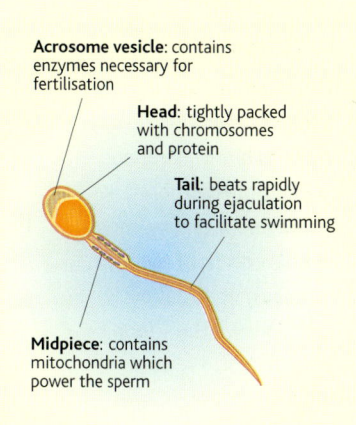

Acrosome vesicle: contains enzymes necessary for fertilisation

Head: tightly packed with chromosomes and protein

Tail: beats rapidly during ejaculation to facilitate swimming

Midpiece: contains mitochondria which power the sperm

▲ The structure of a single sperm

The female reproductive system

The female reproductive organs are the ovaries, the fallopian tubes, the uterus, the vagina and the vulva. They are all contained within the pelvic cavity except the vulva.

> **Fascinating fact**
>
> The word ovaries means 'egg receptacle'.

> **Fascinating fact**
>
> Describe the effects of oestrogen on the body. (Link to The Endocrine System, page 143)

> **Fascinating fact**
>
> A woman's first menstruation is known as the 'menarche'.

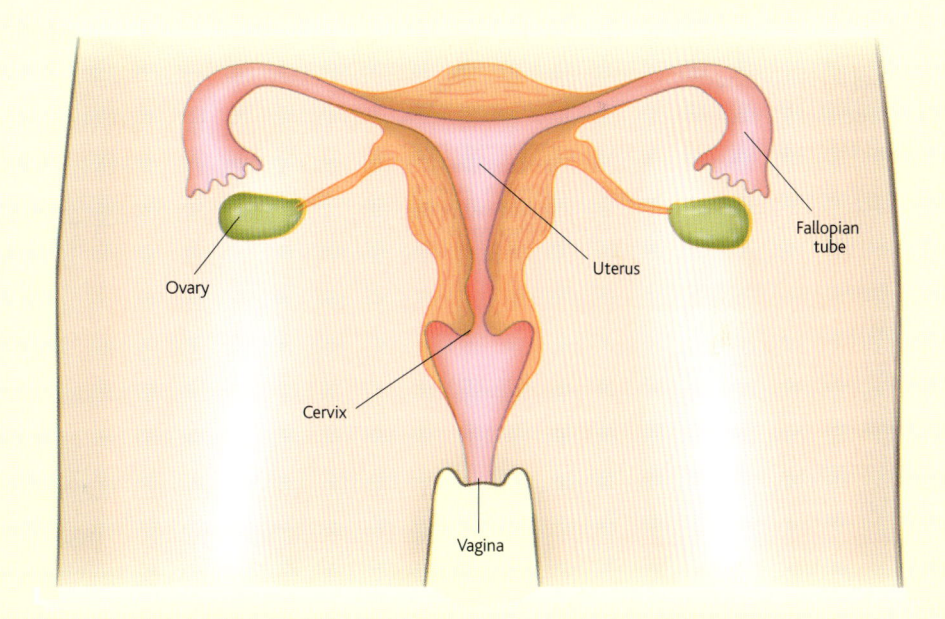

Ovary — Uterus — Fallopian tube — Cervix — Vagina

▲ The female reproductive system

The ovaries

The ovaries, situated in the pelvic cavity on either side of the **uterus**, are the size and shape of an almond, measuring about 4 cm (1.6 inches) in length and 2 cm (0.8 inches) across. They are held in place by a broad **ligament** called the ovarian ligament. The two major roles of the ovary are:
- to produce a mature egg for **ovulation** each month
- to secrete the reproductive hormones **oestrogen** and progesterone.

PAGE 183

SECTION 2

Fascinating fact
The word 'menstruation' is taken from the 28-day cycle of the waxing and waning of the moon. However, in reality, most women do not have a regular menstrual cycle that follows the moon's cycle.

Fascinating fact
It has been observed that groups of women living together, such as best friends, sisters, mothers and daughters, and lesbian couples, often menstruate at the same times. This is known as 'menstrual synchronicity', and it has also been observed in rats, mice and lemurs.

Proving the point
Make a list of all the possible symptoms of pre-menstrual tension (PMT). What are the hormonal changes that take place that might explain these symptoms?

Fascinating fact
Women have always attempted to prevent pregnancy. Roman women used sponges soaked in vinegar and hollowed-out lemons inserted over the cervix as contraceptives.

Producing a mature ovum for fertilisation

The ovaries contain ova (eggs) in an unripened state, known as **follicles**. Each follicle has the ability to mature into a ripened egg, to be released from the ovary for fertilisation. A woman is born with all the follicles she will ever produce in a lifetime. Once she reaches **puberty**, generally between the ages of 12 and 14 years, a woman will have up to one million follicles. During a woman's fertile years (typically between 12 and 45 years of age), only about 400–500 of these follicles will ripen and produce eggs for fertilisation. These eggs are released as part of a regular monthly cycle known as the menstrual cycle (see page 185).

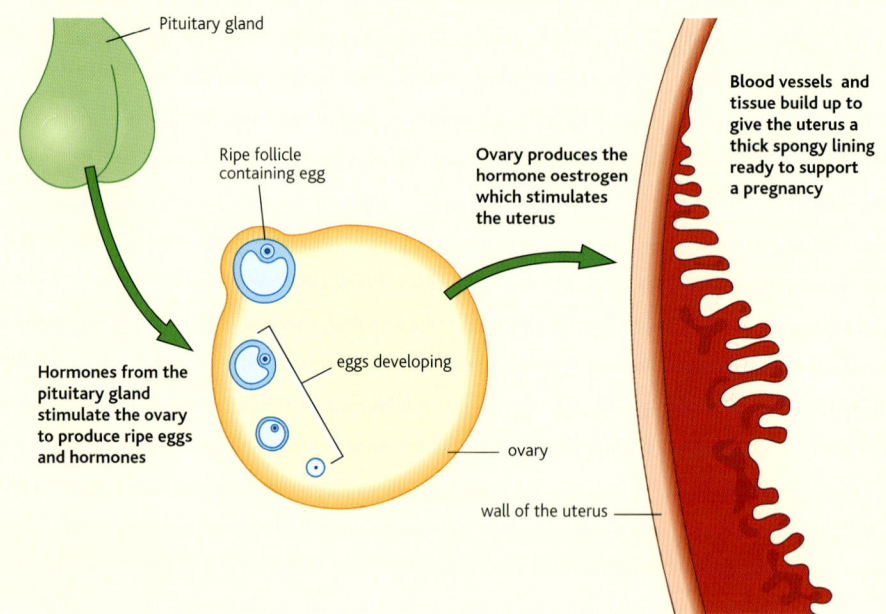

▲ The maturation of a female ovum, from follicle to ovulation

When the ovum has ripened (matured), the follicle ruptures, releasing it from the ovary – this is called ovulation and it occurs once roughly every 28 days. The ovum travels to the **fallopian tube** in preparation for fertilisation.

The secretion of reproductive hormones

- In the ovary, the hormone **oestrogen** is released into the bloodstream. (Link to The Endocrine System, page 142) Oestrogen is a powerful hormone that regulates the secondary sexual characteristics and prepares the body for pregnancy every month.
- The rupture of the follicle at ovulation leaves behind a patch of scar tissue called the **corpus luteum**; this secretes the hormone progesterone. Progesterone further prepares the body for pregnancy by thickening the wall of the uterus and developing the breast tissue.

The fallopian tubes

The fallopian tubes are about 10 cm (4 inches) in length. After ovulation, they carry the mature ovum from the ovary towards the uterus. The end of the fallopian tube is fimbriated or fringed to enable it to collect the ovum after ovulation. It takes about five days for the ovum to reach the uterus from the ovary but this will vary between individuals. The egg can only be fertilised within 24 hours of ovulation so, if sexual intercourse has taken place, fertilisation will occur in the fallopian tube.

The uterus

The uterus, or womb, is a muscular chamber which resembles an upside-down pear and is about 7.5 cm (3 inches) long. It is the site of menstruation, pregnancy and labour. The womb lining of the uterus is a specialised tissue called **endometrium**; this layer is shed during menstruation.

The base of the uterus is narrow and is known as the neck of the uterus or **cervix**, which forms a barrier between the uterus and the vagina. The cervix contains a tiny mucus-filled opening, usually only the diameter of a pinprick. This opening dilates to approximately 10 cm (4 inches) during labour, allowing the baby's head to pass into the vagina or birth canal.

The vagina

The vagina is a muscular tube approximately 7.5 cm (3 inches) long. It connects the uterus with the outside world, receives the penis during intercourse and is used as the birth canal. The walls of the vagina are muscular, and are formed in folds to permit enlargement during childbirth. Tiny glands called Bartholin's glands secrete mucus to lubricate the vagina during intercourse and childbirth.

The vulva and perineum

The **vulva** (meaning 'to wrap around') is the external part of the female reproductive system. It includes two pairs of lips, or **labia**, and the **clitoris**, a small organ of great sensitivity. The entire pelvic floor is called the **perineum**, a diamond-shaped area between the thighs and buttock in males and females.

The menstrual cycle

The menstrual cycle is a series of events that takes place in women approximately every 28 days from puberty to the menopause. It is regulated by the **pituitary** hormones Follicle stimulating hormone (FSH) and Lutenising hormone (LH).

The following chart gives a breakdown of the processes involved in a typical 28-day menstrual cycle, although the length of a menstrual cycle can vary

---

Link to practice

Common disorders of the menstrual cycle include:
- *Dysmenorrhoea* – pain associated with menstruation.
- *Amenorrhoea* – absence of menstruation; pregnancy is the most common cause but it can also be caused by anorexia, over-rigorous athletic training or stress.
- *Pre-menstrual tension* (PMT) – characterised by mood swings, irritability, clumsiness and emotional distress in the post-ovulatory phase of the menstrual cycle. Doctors now recognise PMT as a medical condition with psychological and physical symptoms that are so severe they may even disrupt the lives of some women.

Link to practice

Many women experience an outbreak of acne when they are premenstrual. This is a result of an increase in sebum production, which is linked to raised levels of progesterone during the second half of the menstrual cycle.

Fascinating fact

The word *mens* means 'monthly' and *pause* means 'to stop'.

SECTION 2

Proving the point
Make a list of any inherited characteristics you have acquired from a member of your family.

Fascinating fact
Gender in humans is determined by the male sperm. The mother's sex chromosome in the ovum is always female (shaped like an 'X') but the father's sex chromosome in the sperm can be either female (shaped like an 'X') or male (shaped like a 'Y'). During fertilisation, the sperm and egg will fuse to form either a female ('XX') or male ('XY') sex chromosome, and this determines the baby's gender.

Link to practice
Some treatments are contra-indicated by pregnancy. Contra-indicated treatments are usually those that are stimulating to the body or those that may cause a change in blood pressure. The most vulnerable time for treatment is in the first trimester (the first 13 weeks of pregnancy).

Proving the point
List all the treatments contra-indicated by pregnancy.

considerably from individual to individual.

Days 1–5	The endometrium breaks down; menstruation takes place.
Days 6–13	Follicle stimulating hormone (FSH) levels rise The ripening follicle secretes oestrogen The ovum develops The endometrium begins to build up
Day 13	Levels of Lutenising hormone (LH) rise
Day 14	Ovulation occurs, leaving corpus luteum in the ovarian follicle
Days 15–28	The corpus luteum secretes progesterone The endometrium is prepared to receive the fertilised ovum The breasts are prepared for milk production If fertilisation has not occurred, the levels of oestrogen and progesterone fall and the endometruim degenerates; this results in tearing causing bleeding (menstruation)

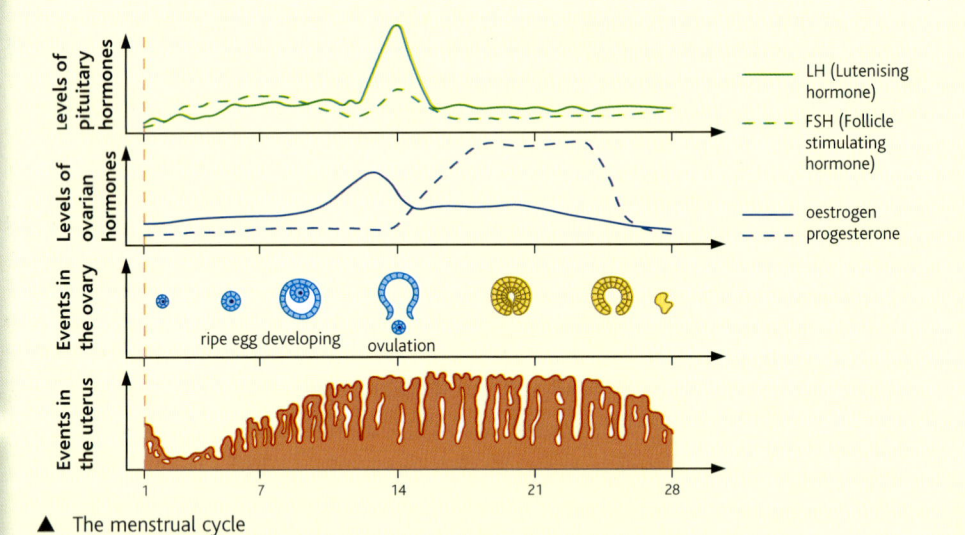

▲ The menstrual cycle

Fertilisation, pregnancy and birth
Pregnancy begins when the ovum is fertilised by a sperm in a process called meiosis, which usually takes place in the fallopian tube.

Meiosis
The human gametes – the sperm and ovum – each contain only 23 **chromosomes** (every other human cell contains 23 pairs of chromosomes). During fertilisation, the male and female gametes merge to form a single cell called a **zygote**. The zygote contains the full set of 46 human chromosomes – 23 chromosomes from the father (the sperm) and 23 chromosomes from the mother (the ovum). This makes a unique individual formed from the pairing of the 23 chromosomes from each parent. The chromosomes carry **genetic** information that can be passed on from both parents. Characteristics such as eye colour, height and some illnesses are passed onto the new baby in the **genes**.

CHAPTER 12 The Reproductive System

> **Link to learning**
>
> **The contraceptive pill**
> The 'pill' became widely used in the 1960s. The most common contraceptive pill contains a combination of oestrogen and progesterone and is called the combined pill. The pill works by maintaining higher than normal levels of oestrogen, preventing ovulation; the effect of progesterone is to make the mucus around the cervix hostile to sperm. The effects of the combined pill on the skin and hair are similar to those seen in pregnancy. Although the pill is an effective contraceptive, it does not offer any protection against sexually transmitted diseases, which are on the increase again.

The zygote starts to divide rapidly by a process of cell division known as **mitosis**. The first few days of life are spent travelling down the fallopian tube towards the uterus. Once the fertilised egg arrives at the womb, typically after about 5 days, it is called an **embryo**. The embryo implants in the rich womb lining (endometrium), a process which takes roughly a week, and then a **placenta** starts to form. The embryo is connected to the placenta by the **umbilical cord**. Nourishment and oxygen pass from the mother's blood to the baby's blood via the placenta, although their blood does not mix and they have separate blood streams. From this point on, the new baby develops very quickly. After eight weeks the baby is called a foetus. Development in the womb typically lasts for 38 weeks from conception (40 weeks from the last menstrual period).

> **Development in the womb**
> - **Weeks 4–6**: The embryo is the size of a poppy seed; its heart is a single tube with a few uncoordinated beats; its bones begin to form.
> - **Week 8**: The embryo has become a foetus. It is about 2.5 cm (1 inch) long and makes slight movements. The face is developing and the mouth starts to open.
> - **Week 12** (3 months): The foetus is just over 5 cm (2 inches) long. Its vocal organs and sexual organs have formed. It is starting to suck and use the muscles it will later use in breathing.
> - **Week 20** ($4\frac{1}{2}$ months): The foetus is about 25 cm (10 inches) long. The baby kicks, twists, jumps and somersaults. Its eyebrows and eyelashes start to form.
> - **Week 28**: The baby is about 38 cm (14 inches) long and weighs just less than 1 kg (about 2lb). Its heartbeat speeds up when it hears its mother's voice. It could survive with medical assistance if born.
> - **Week 40** (9 months): The baby is ready to be born. It weighs about 4 kg (8 lb) and is about 55 cm (20 inches long).

> **Proving the point**
> Name the pituitary hormone responsible for milk production. (Link to The Endocrine System, page 136)

During pregnancy, the placenta produces the hormones oestrogen and progesterone. These support the pregnancy and prepare the breasts for **lactation** or breastfeeding.

Pregnancy ends when labour begins. There are three distinct stages to childbirth: the first stage when contractions are felt; the delivery of the baby; and the expulsion of the placenta.

> **Fascinating fact**
> The first stage of childbirth can last many hours. It was originally called labour because it is hard work!

After the birth, the hormones that maintained pregnancy gradually return to their original levels, and prolactin, the hormone that maintains lactation, now takes over. Lactation will continue as long as the baby is suckled at the breast – this can last for several years but many mothers will stop breastfeeding once their baby is fully weaned (eating solid foods).

> **Link to practice**
>
> **Hormonal changes during pregnancy**
> The hormones oestrogen and progesterone are secreted by the placenta during pregnancy. These hormones maintain the pregnancy and prepare the breasts for breastfeeding but they can have unexpected effects on the body. These include:
> - *Linea nigra*: a brown line seen on the abdomen, extending from the naval to the pubis.
> - *Chloasma* or the mask of pregnancy: an increase in pigmentation around the eyes and cheekbones.
> - *Stretch marks,* or striae, on the abdomen and breasts as they enlarge.
> - Fine, downy hair may appear on the cheeks and upper lip.
> - Hair loss (alopecia).

The menopause

The end of a woman's reproductive life is called the menopause or 'change of life'. It usually occurs between the ages of 45 and 55 years, but some women may experience the menopause much earlier or later. At this time menstruation becomes more infrequent and finally stops altogether. The ovaries are reduced to scar tissue and stop producing oestrogen. The reproductive organs begin to shrink and pregnancy becomes impossible.

The physical effects of the menopause are unpleasant and are usually characterised by hot flushes, hair loss, depression and weight gain. Even more worrying is the effect of the low levels of oestrogen on the bones: women show a rapid loss in bone density in the ten years following the menopause. The bones can become thin and porous giving rise to a condition called osteoporosis (this literally translates as 'porous bone'), causing bones to break easily. (Link to The Skeletal System, page 58) Hormone Replacement Therapy (HRT) is used to prevent osteoporosis, but a diet rich in calcium as well as regular exercise throughout life may help.

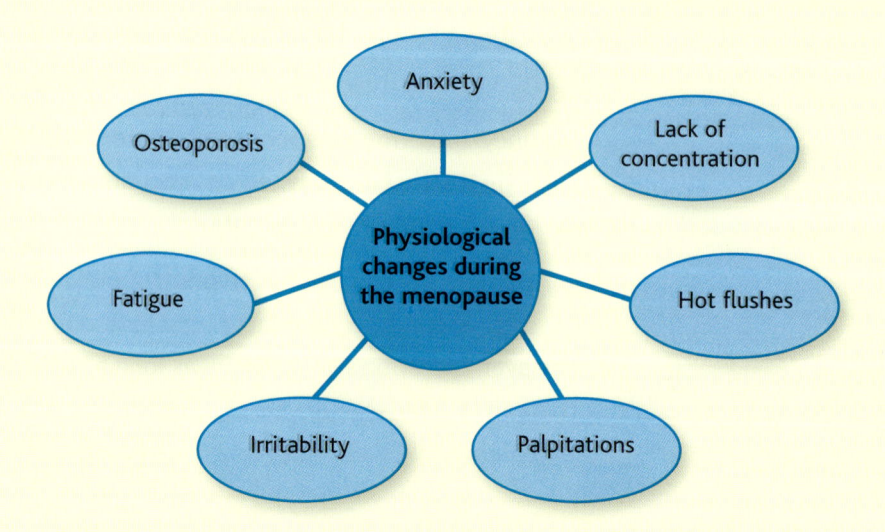

Physiological changes during the menopause:
- Anxiety
- Lack of concentration
- Hot flushes
- Palpitations
- Irritability
- Fatigue
- Osteoporosis

> **Link to practice**
>
> **Hirsutism**
> Post-menopausal women often develop male pattern hair growth. This is caused by the reduced levels of oestrogen and the dominance of testosterone from the **adrenal cortex**. (Link to The Endocrine System, page 140) Hirsutism can be treated by a combination of medical therapy and electrolysis; it also responds well to laser treatment. Many women find this condition very embarrassing and should be treated tactfully when they present for treatment.

Case study

Level 2 and 3/Holistic
Ann is a 54-year-old woman who is going through the menopause. She has had an unpleasant time coping with hot flushes and night sweats. These have left her with permanently reddened cheeks, which become more noticeable after drinking red wine or eating spicy food. Identify the problem, its possible cause and suggest a suitable remedy.

Case study

Level 3
Johanna is 54-years-old and has almost passed through her menopause. She has developed a strong hair growth on her upper lip and a number of strong coarse hairs on her chin. She has had Type 1 diabetes since she was 18 years old. Previous epilation treatments at another salon have left clearly visible scarring. Identify the problem, its possible cause and suggest a suitable remedy.

The structure and function of the female breast

The breasts, or **mammary glands**, are the female accessory reproductive organs. Their function is to produce milk for the baby, and the process of milk production is called lactation. The breasts develop at puberty when fat is deposited between the lobes, but do not become fully functional until the end of pregnancy.

Fascinating fact

Women are advised to check their breasts for lumps every month just after a period (since breasts can often contain normal lumps before a period). Any unusual findings should be reported to a doctor. Because the lymph drainage is into the axilla (underarm) area, this area should be checked too.

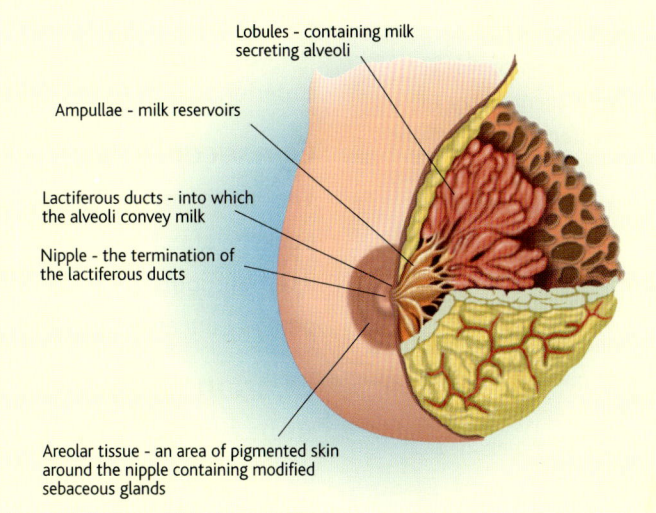

▶ The structure of the mammary glands

Labels:
- Lobules – containing milk secreting alveoli
- Ampullae – milk reservoirs
- Lactiferous ducts – into which the alveoli convey milk
- Nipple – the termination of the lactiferous ducts
- Areolar tissue – an area of pigmented skin around the nipple containing modified sebaceous glands

> **Link to practice**
>
> Very occasionally a therapist performing an underarm wax on a female client may notice a lump under the client's skin. Without alarming the client, the therapist should advise the client to make an appointment with her doctor.

The breast contains a number of lobes supported by **adipose** tissue. Milk is formed in the lobes and carried to the nipple by a lactiferous sinus. Around the nipple is a pigmented area called the areola. This consists of areolar tissue which turns from pink to brown during pregnancy.

Blood supply is from the mammary artery, and venous return is via the mammary vein. The breast has a plentiful supply of **lymphatic vessels** which drain any excess tissue fluid or infections into the **axillary nodes**.

The breast is supported internally by delicate ligaments known as Cooper's ligaments. These run between the skin and the deep tissue to support the milk lobes. The size of the breast is determined by the amount of adipose tissue present. The breast is supported by the pectoralis major. (Link to Muscles and the Muscular System, page 70)

Diseases and disorders of the reproductive system

Breast cancer

The majority of breast lumps are discovered by women themselves and are **benign** (non-cancerous), but successful treatment for breast cancer is often dependent on early detection. Breast cancer affects one woman in twelve but is rarely seen in women under 30 years of age or men. Women over 50 years are regularly screened for breast cancer using a technique called mammography.

Endometriosis

Occasionally the lining of the uterus or endometrium can develop outside the uterus; in such cases, it can be found in the pelvic cavity, the abdomen and, occasionally, in the thorax. Endometriosis usually occurs in women between the ages of 25 and 40 years who have not had children. Sufferers usually experience very painful periods and can become infertile.

Gynaecomastia

This is the development of breast tissue in the male. It is very common at puberty, affecting one or both breasts in 50 per cent of boys. It usually resolves itself without any treatment but can be very embarrassing for the young person concerned.

Ovarian cysts

Single cysts can develop on the ovaries: these are simply fluid-filled sacs which do not usually have any systemic effects on the body but can grow very large, causing swelling of the abdomen and discomfort.

> **Link to practice**
>
> **The pelvic floor and female incontinence**
>
> After the menopause (and childbirth), some women notice stress incontinence. This means that they leak small amounts of urine every time the bladder experiences any pressure. This may happen during coughing, laughing, sneezing or during exercise. Naturally this is uncomfortable and embarrassing. Exercises to strengthen the pelvic floor can help to reduce this type of stress incontinence. Advise your client to try to tighten her pelvic floor at least three times a day. She should try to imagine that she is stopping a flow of urine and to slowly tighten and release the muscles involved. If the problem is severe, advise your client to seek medical advice.

Polycystic ovarian syndrome

Otherwise known as Stein Levental Syndrome, this condition is characterised by multiple cysts which form on the ovaries and is relatively common in young women. Polycentric (*poly* means 'many') ovaries will secrete **androgens** or male sex hormones which slowly produce an effect on the body. It gives rise to a number of symptoms including:

- irregular or absent periods
- hirsutism
- weight gain
- infertility.

Because the development of these symptoms is gradual, the client may not realise that there is anything wrong and may see an electrolygist before seeking medical advice. Such clients must always be referred to a doctor.

Prostate cancer

Prostate cancer is the most common cancer in men; each year over 26,000 men are diagnosed with it in the UK; an even greater number of men will be diagnosed with an enlarged prostate gland (this presses on the neck of the bladder making the bladder feel full). The prostate makes a fluid that forms part of the semen to nourish and protect the sperm on their journey towards the vagina. In prostate cancer the cells begin to divide abnormally; unless treated, the cancer will spread to other parts of the body. The cause of prostate cancer is not fully understood but it is thought that diet and lifestyle may put some men at a higher risk. If treated early, the chances of recovery are good and men are advised to visit 'well man' clinics for screening.

The effects of ageing on the reproductive system

The activities of the female reproductive system have a limited time span as they are restricted by the onset of the menopause. Fertility declines with age as women enter their thirties and ovulation becomes less regular. The fallopian tubes become weaker making them less able to support a fertilised ovum. Much later, the female organs can become weak and prolapse (sinking) of the uterus is a common complaint amongst elderly women.

Men are at their most fertile in their mid-twenties; however, there are numerous examples of elderly men fathering children (such as Rod Stewart). Men do not experience a 'change of life', however, the reduction of testosterone results in a decline in muscle strength and decreased sexual desire, although this does not usually affect the production of viable sperm. Age can affect the prostate gland which becomes enlarged, pressing on the bladder causing frequency of urination; this is usually treated by an operation.

SECTION 2

Case study
Level 3

Sunita is a 29-year-old woman who has requested electrolysis. Her face and shoulders are covered by dark terminal hair. She is slightly overweight, carrying a lot of adipose tissue on the abdomen. She has no children and complains of painful periods. Identify the problem, its possible cause and suggest a suitable remedy.

Case study
Level 3

Hilary is 35 years old and has come for a body massage. During the course of the consultation she expresses concern about her breasts – she says that they do not feel as firm as they used to be. She has always had large breasts and felt they were her best feature; she does not want to have an operation. Identify the problem, its possible cause and suggest a suitable remedy.

Knowledge check

1. When do the gonads become active?
2. Name the male gonads.
3. Name the male sex hormone.
4. List the order in which sperm travel to reach the outside.
5. Which glands, apart from the testes, produce secretions to aid the sperm?
6. Explain how the position of the testes assists the process of reproduction.
7. Name the pituitary hormone that regulates male and female reproduction.
8. Describe how the ovaries are held in position.
9. Explain the function of the ovaries.
10. Define ovulation.
11. Name the two hormones produced by the ovaries.
12. Briefly describe the menstrual cycle.
13. At what point in the menstrual cycle are the levels of hormones at their lowest?
14. Define meiosis.
15. Name the structure formed by the union of the sperm and the ovum.
16. What is a gene?
17. Name the pigmented area around the nipple.
18. Explain lactation.
19. How many lymph nodes are in the breast?
20. Explain how the contraceptive pill works.

GLOSSARY

absorption (of food) when digested nutrients pass through the walls of the digestive tract into blood circulatory (and lymphatic) vessels

acid mantle a combination of sweat and sebum that provides a protective layer for the skin

acidity a relatively high level of hydrogen ions concentration in a solution. Acidity is measured on the pH scale and an acidic reading is below 7

acidosis condition where pH of body fluids is less alkaline than normal

actin protein in muscle

acute short-term

adenosine triphosphate (ATP) form of energy produced in muscles

adipose a type of connective tissue, commonly called fat

adrenaline hormone released in large amounts by the adrenal gland in times of stress

afferent nerve or vessel that carries an impulse or substance towards another part of the body

alkalinity a relatively low concentration of hydrogen ions. Alkalinity is measured on the pH scale and an alkaline reading is above 7

alkalosis condition where pH of body fluids is more alkaline than normal

alveoli small sacs or pouches found at the end of the bronchiole

amino acids building blocks of protein

anabolism when units are used by the cell to build, repair and produce energy so that the cell can sustain its life cycle.

anagen the growing time of the hair growth cycle

androgen male sex hormone

anion negatively-charged ion or mineral salt

antagonists pair of muscles which have opposite actions

antibody a type of protein which attaches to substances that do not belong in the body, such as toxins or disease-causing bacteria; they are produced by lymphocytes

antigen any substance that causes immune system to produce antibodies against it

antioxidant chemical that reduces the rate of particular oxidation reactions

apocrine sweat glands found in the underarm (axilla) and pubic regions

aponeurosis flattened sheet of tendon

appendicular skeleton appendages of the skeleton including upper and lower limbs

arousal state of flux in response to an emotional stimulus

arterial relating to the arteries

arteriole smaller vessel which branches off from an artery and connects to a capillary

artery the largest of the blood vessels carrying blood away from the heart; they contain muscular walls to withstand high blood pressure

assimilation the conversion of nutrients into living tissue; constructive metabolism

atrium one of the chambers of the heart that receives blood directly from a vein (plural: atria)

atrophy reduce in size and therefore strength, or to become weaker

automatic occurring without conscious thought

autonomic nervous system (ANS) part of the PNS which controls automatic activity

axial skeleton core structures of the skeleton including skull, thorax and vertebral column

axon long fibres of a neurone which transmit impulses away from the cell body

basal layer stratum germinitavum; the deepest layer of the epidermis

bile digestive juice secreted by the liver and stored in the gall bladder; aids in the digestion of fats

blood the thick red liquid in the vessels; it is classed as a connective tissue

blood circulatory system system of the body responsible for internal transport of oxygen, nutrients and waste; composed of the heart, blood vessels, lymphatic vessels, lymph and the blood

blood glucose main sugar found in the blood and the body's main source of energy

blood pressure measurement of the force applied to the walls of the arteries as the heart pumps blood through the body

body systems a group of organs that work together

buffer system substances which prevent sharp changes in the concentration of hydrogen ions. They include bicarbonates, phosphates and proteins such as haemoglobin

calcification process of bone formation involving the deposition of calcium

cancellous tissue lighter, less compact bone tissue

capillary smallest of all the blood vessels; their walls are just one-cell thick to allow substances to pass through

carbon dioxide gas which is a waste product of metabolism, excreted through the lungs during breathing

cardiac relating to the heart

cardiac cycle route the blood takes through the heart to the lungs and back to the heart to be pumped around the body

cardiac muscle muscle tissue surrounding the heart

cartilage firm, tough connective tissue which consists of a tough matrix, yet is also flexible. There are two basic types: hyaline and fibro-cartilage

cartilaginous joints where two bones are connected by a pad of fibrocartilage, e.g. between the bones of the spinal column

catabolism when useful products, such as nutrients, are broken down into useable units in a cell

cation positively-charged ion or mineral salt

cell smallest living unit in the human body and the basic building block of the human body

cell membrane encloses the cell and allows substances to pass in and out of it

cellulite appearance of fat cells (adipose tissue) beneath the skin's surface

GLOSSARY

central nervous system (CNS) has overall control of the nervous system and consists of the brain and spinal cord

cerebral hemispheres left and right portions of the cerebrum or forebrain

cerebrum also known as the forebrain; largest part of the brain which is responsible for co-ordinating movement

cholesterol fatty substance found in tissue and fat

chromosome rod-like structure found in all living cells, containing the chemical patterns which control what an animal or plant is like

chronic long-term

chyme food that has completely mixed with gastric juice and has liquefied

cilia hair-like projections on the surface of columnar cells

clear layer stratum lucidum; the layer of the epidermis found on the soles of the feet and the palms of the hands

cognitive connected with thinking or conscious mental processes

collagen rubbery connective tissue found in the dermis

compact tissue hard, dense bone tissue

congenital a disease or condition that exists at or from birth

connective tissue tissue that connects, supports, binds, or separates other tissues or organs

constriction blood vessels narrowing to restrict blood flow to an area in a capillary

contraction movement produced when muscle is excited by a stimulus

coronary relating to the circulation to the heart

corpus luteum gland that forms on the surface of the ovary at the site of ovulation and produces progesterone during the second half of the menstrual cycle

cortex pigmented part of the hair

cortisol hormone released at times of stress; known as the 'stress hormone'

cuticle flat scale-like cells that form the outer surface of the hair (for nails, see eponychium)

cytoplasm gel-like substance which fills the cell from the membrane to the nucleus

defecation act of passing faeces

degenerative cause of progressive deterioration

dementia medical condition that affects especially old people, causing gradual worsening of the memory and other mental abilities, and leading to confused behaviour

dendrite short projection of a neurone which transmit impulses towards the cell body

deoxygenated blood blood that is low in oxygen concentration

dermis the true skin; composed of areolar connective tissue supported by collagen and elastin; contains blood vessels, nerve endings, sweat glands, hair, hair follicles and sebaceous glands

desquamation natural shedding of the cells of the stratum corneum

diaphysis shaft of a long bone

diastolic pressure blood pressure when the heart relaxes and the heart cavities fill with blood; blood pressure is then at its lowest

differentiation way in which different cells are specialised to carry out a specific function in the body

diffusion movement of particles from a high solution on one side of a thin membrane to a low solution on the other side

digestion breaking down of nutrients into a useable form

digestive system organs that take in food and turn it into products that the body can use to stay healthy. Waste products that body cannot use leave the body through bowel movements

dilation blood vessels widening to allow greater amounts of blood to flow through a capillary

diuretic substance that promotes fluid loss by increasing urine volume

DNA deoxyribonucleic acid; provides the genetic blueprint for the physical characteristics of all living organisms.

duodenum first part of the small intestine

eccrine sweat glands located all over the body

efferent nerve or vessel that carries an impulse or substance away from another part of the body

elastin connective tissue found in the epidermis which gives the dermis its elastic quality

electrolyte charged ion or mineral salt

electromagnetic spectrum ordered array of wavelengths including cosmic rays, visible light and radio waves

elimination excretion of waste products from the digestive system

embryo developing baby in the first eight weeks of pregnancy

emulsify mixing of two liquids which do not readily make a smooth mixture, e.g. water and oil

endocrine gland organs of the body which produce and release hormones into the blood to be carried around the body

endocrine system system of ductless glands that regulate bodily functions via hormones secreted into the bloodstream including the hypothalamus, pituitary gland, thyroid, adrenal glands, and gonads

endometrium lining of the uterus

endorphin hormone which acts on the nervous system and reduces feelings of pain

enzyme any of a group of chemical substances which are produced by living cells and which cause particular chemical reactions to happen while not being changed themselves

epidermis the outer layer of the skin

epiphysis ends of a long bone

epithelial tissue (or epithelium); lines and protects areas and organs of the body, such as the skin

eponychium cuticle of the nail, overlying the nail body

erythema reddening of the skin caused by dilation of the blood vessels

erythrocyte red blood cell

excretion removal of waste products from metabolism as water, urine or carbon dioxide

exhalation also known as expiration

exocrine gland externally secreting gland, such as a salivary gland or sweat gland that releases its secretions directly or

GLOSSARY

through a duct

faeces the solid waste excreted from the body through the bowels

fibril filament of muscle protein

fibrous joint located where two bones dovetail together, e.g. between the bones of the skull

filtration under pressure first stage of urine production which involves filtration of fluid in the nephron of the kidneys

foetus developing baby after the first eight weeks of pregnancy

follicle tubular sheath below the surface of the skin that contains the mechanism that creates the hair

gamete reproductive cell; sperm or ova

gaseous exchange movement of oxygen and carbon dioxide between the blood and the air in the lungs

gastric relating to the stomach

gene part of the DNA in a cell which controls physical development and behaviour

genetic inherited characteristics relating to genes

gland organ of the body which secretes liquid chemicals that have various purposes

glomerulus bundle of capillaries in the kidneys

glucose simple sugar produced from digested carbohydrates

glucagon hormone produced by the pancreas that increases the level of glucose (sugar) in the blood

glycogen form that glucose is stored in muscle

gonad sex glands; ovaries or testes

granular layer stratum granulosum; the waterproof layer of the epidermis

haemoglobin iron-containing pigment in erythrocytes

heart the muscular organ composed of cardiac muscle tissue that is responsible for pumping blood around the body

hirsutism male-pattern hair growth; usually androgen-related in women

homeostatic mechanism the process and activity that helps to maintain homeostasis

homeostasis describes the state of being the same

hormone chemical produced by an endocrine gland

horny layer stratum corneum; the outer layer of the epidermis consisting of flattened, scale-like cells

human anatomy study of organs and organ systems of the human body

human physiology study of the mechanical, physical, and biochemical functions of humans, human tissues or organs

hydrostatic pressure pressure of the fluid (blood) travelling in the capillaries

hypertonic excess tension

ileum mid-section of the small intestine

immune system complex system that is reponsible for protecting against infections and foreign substances

immunity resistance to disease

ingestion taking in of substances, usually food, in to the digestive system

inhalation also known as inspiration; breathing air, smoke, or gas into the lungs

insertion point where muscle attaches to bone

insulin hormone in the body which controls the amount of sugar in the blood

integumentary system body system comprising the skin, hair and nails

interstitial fluid fluid filling the minute spaces between cells of the body; also known as tissue fluid

involuntary muscle (see smooth muscle)

ion atoms or groups of atoms with an electrical charge resulting from the loss or gain of one or more electrons

irritability ability of cells to respond to an external stimulus, whether physical, chemical or thermal

jejunum the final section of the small intestine

joint place where two or more bones meet

keratin waterproof protein found in the granular layer of the epidermis

keratinisation hardening of epithelium; occurs in skin, hair and nails, and provides a tough, impermeable barrier

lactation production of milk from the breasts

lactic acid waste product formed due to lack of oxygen in muscles

lanugo soft, downy hair present in foetal life and usually shed just before or just after birth

leucocyte white blood cells that engulf and digest bacteria and fungi; an important part of the body's defence system

ligament band of strong fibrous, connective tissue

lumbar inward curve of the lower back

lumen diameter of the inside of blood vessels

lymph colourless liquid which takes useful substance around the body, and takes waste matter away from body tissue in order to prevent infection

lymphatic system circulatory network of vessels carrying lymph, and the lymphoid organs such as the lymph nodes, spleen, and thymus, that produce and store infection-fighting cells

lymphatic tissue tissue making up the lymphatic system

lymphocytes type of white blood cell of which there are three types; they are concerned with defending the body from viruses and other types of infections

lymph capillary minute vessels of the lymphatic system

lymph duct one of the lymphatic or absorbent vessels, which carry lymph and discharge it into the veins

lymph node bean-shaped structure scattered along vessels of the lymphatic system. These nodes act as filters, collecting bacteria or cancer cells that may travel through the lymphatic system

lymph vessel network of vessels that circulate lymph and branch into all the tissues of the body

malnutrition poor nourishment of the body

mammary pertaining to the breast

matrix non-living material found between cells

medulla inner region

meiosis cell division in gametes

melanin pigment or colour found in the basal layer of the epidermis

melanocyte specialised cell in the skin which absorbs UV rays

GLOSSARY

from the sun

melatonin hormone produced by the pineal gland that regulates the sleep/wake cycle

menopause the end of a women's reproductive life

menstrual cycle monthly cycle of hormonal changes

menstruation monthly shedding of the endometrium from the uterus; results in blood flow from the vagina

metabolism process by which cells utilise energy from food and produce waste products

mitosis process by which cells are constantly growing and dividing; simple cell division

motor nerves (see efferent nerves)

muscle fatigue when muscle feels tired and sore due to a build up of lactic acid

muscle tone state of partial contraction which muscles are in under normal, resting circumstances

myelin sheath protective sheath which surrounds a bundle of neurons

myology the study of muscles

myosin protein in muscle

negative feedback process which acts to counter the potentially disruptive effects of external inputs; it can act as a stabilizing mechanism

nephron minute twisted tubule in kidneys

nerve plexus network of nerves which supplies a particular area of the body

nervous system system of cells, tissues and organs that regulate the body's responses to internal and external stimuli

neuroglia connective tissue which supports neurones by insulating and protecting them

neurological relating to nerves

neurone basic tissue of the nervous system; very specialised nerve cells which transmit messages

neurotransmitters naturally occurring chemicals in the brain which transmit messages from one nerve cell to another

nucleus membrane-bound structure that contains the cell's genetic information and controls the cell's growth and reproduction

oedema excess fluid surrounding the tissue

oestrogen the female sex hormone from the ovaries that regulates female secondary sexual characteristics

olfactory relating to the sense of smell

oncology the branch of medicine concerned with tumours

organ part of the body which perfoms a particular job

origin point where muscle attaches to bone

osmoregulation regulation of the quantity of water and minerals in the body, which occurs in the kidneys

osmosis passage of dissolved substances through a membrane

ossification process of bone formation

osteoblast cell which produces new bone tissue

osteoclast cell which destroys old bone tissue

osteocyte mature bone cell

osteoporosis disorder of bones common in post-menopausal women

ovary egg producing gland

ovulation release of the ovum from the ovary

ovum female reproductive cell

oxygen colourless gas that forms a large part of the air on earth and which is needed by people, animals and plants to live

papilla small projection or elevation

parasympathetic nervous system part of the ANS which responds to pleasant emotions

pathogen any invading micro-organism, virus, bacterium or fungus

peripheral nervous system (PNS) all parts of the nervous system other than the brain and spinal cord

peristalsis wave-like movement by involuntary muscles in the digestive system, which moves food materials onwards

permeable able to pass through

peronychium part of the cuticle at the side of the nail

pH percentage of hydrogen. The pH scale ranges from 0 (strongly acidic) to 14.0 (strongly alkaline), with 7.0 as neutral (neither acidic or alkaline)

phagocyte cell that ingests and destroys foreign matter

placenta structure used to supply the developing baby with nourishment and oxygen and remove waste products

plasma yellowish fluid that is the liquid part of blood

platelets cell-like particles that stick together to help form blood clots

prickle cell layer stratum spinosum; layer of the epidermis in which the basal cells begin to change their shape, developing spindles or prickles

prostate gland at the base of the bladder

puberty physical process of changing from a child into an adult

pulmonary circulation circulation to the lungs

pulse regular beating of the heart

red blood cell (see erythrocyte)

reflex action movement which occurs in response to a stimulus without conscious control

releasing hormones hormone produced by the hypothalamus that influences another gland

respiration release of heat energy from oxygen and glucose

respiratory system organs that are involved in breathing including the nose, throat, larynx, trachea, bronchi, and lungs

reproductive system specific organs that regulate all sexual functioning

RNA ribonucleic acid; a chemical cousin of DNA, RNA is responsible for translating the genetic code of DNA into proteins

salivary gland gland which secretes saliva containing digestive enzymes

sebaceous gland gland in the skin that secretes sebum

sebum grease or oil that prevents the skin and hair from cracking

secondary sexual characteristics traits that distinguish the two sexes but that are not directly part of the reproductive system

secrete production and release of a liquid

selective reabsorption final stage of urine production which

GLOSSARY

involves the reabsorption of glucose, water and salts required by the body

semen secretion from the seminal vesicles that nourishes the sperm

semi-permeable some but not all substances are able to pass through

sensory nerves (see afferent)

septum wall in the heart dividing it in two

skeletal muscle also known as voluntary muscle and striated (striped) muscle which is under conscious control

sliding filament theory fibrils of actin and myosin slide past each other during muscle contraction

smooth muscle also known as involuntary muscle; muscle tissue which is not under conscious control

somatic nervous system part of the PNS which controls voluntary movement

specialised adapted to carry out a particular function in the body

sperm male reproductive cell

sphincter circular muscle which allows the passage of food in one direction only

sprain injury caused by over-exertion of a muscle or joint

stem cell cell that, by sucessive division, can give rise to different types of specialised cells

steroid hormone produced by the adrenal cortex and sex glands (ovaries and testes)

striated muscle (see skeletal muscle)

subcutaneous layer underneath the initial layer of skin

sudiferous gland sweat gland; found all over the skin, their main function is to cool the body by producing sweat

sympathetic nervous system branch of the ANS which responds to strong emotions

synapse minute space between neurones where communication of information occurs; also known as reflex arc

synovial joint type of freely moveable joint

synthesis to assemble a substance from other substances

systemic circulation circulation to the systems of the body (i.e. not the pulmonary)

systolic pressure blood pressure when the heart contracts and blood is pumped out from the heart; blood pressure is then at its highest

target cells any cell that has a specific receptor for antigen or antibody or hormone

telogen resting part of the hair growth cycle

tendon bands of connective tissue which attach muscle to bone

terminal coarse hair; it can occur anywhere on the body but is more common on the head, eyebrows, pubic area, legs and underarms

testes male sex glands; they secrete testosterone and manufacture sperm

testosterone the male sex hormone

thyroxin hormone from the thyroid gland that regulates metabolism

tissue formed when cells of the same type combine with other cells

tissue fluid (see interstitial fluid)

tonicity the state of contraction of a muscle at rest, e.g. muscles with high tonicity are those which have a supportive function in posture

trophic hormones also known as stimulating hormones; they are sent to other glands to increase their output

tumour when cells divide and do not reproduce exactly, the abnormal cells then group together to form a tumour. A tumour can be benign (usually harmless) or malignant (cancer-causing)

ultraviolet radiation (UV) radiation lying in the ultraviolet range with wave lengths shorter than light but longer than x rays

urea soluble crystalline body which is the chief constituent of urine

urinary system Group of organs and their interconnections that permits excess, filtered fluids to exit the body

urine liquid waste produced by the kidney

uterus womb

valve device which opens and closes to conrol the flow of blood in the heart and the veins

vasoconstriction process by which, if the body temperature starts to fall, the body retains heat by closing down (constricting) blood vessels in the skin

vasodilation process by which, if the body temperature starts to rise, blood vessels in the skin become wider (dilate)

vein blood vessel that carries blood towards the heart

vellus short, downy, non-pigmented (colourless) hair found all over the body

venous relating to the veins

venous return return of blood to heart; affected by pressure gradient across circulation, respiratory pump and muscle pump

ventricle muscular chambers of the heart that are responsible for pumping blood from the heart into the arteries

venule small blood vessel that carries blood from a capillary to a vein

voluntary actions which are under conscious control

voluntary muscle (see skeletal muscle)

vulva external female genitalia

wavelength the distance between two waves of energy

white blood cells (see leucocytes)

zygote formed during fertilisation, when the ovum and sperm fuse; the start of a new human life

INDEX

A

abduction 8, 54
absorption 33, 152, 153, 159
acidity 15
acidosis 27, 80, 170
acne 43
actin 65
active secretion 174
adduction 8, 54
adenoids 108
adenosine triphosphate (ATP) 72
adipose tissue 18, 21, 22, 32, 190
adrenal glands 129, 139–140, 143, 145
adrenaline 90, 129, 139–140, 143, 145
aerobic exercise 139
ageing 29, 31
    circulatory system 97
    digestive system 166
    endocrine system 147
    excretory system 179
    lymphatic system 110
    muscular system 75–76
    nervous system 133–134
    reproductive system 191–192
    respiratory system 119
    skeletal system 59–60
    skin 31, 45–46
AIDS 109
alcohol 90, 93, 139, 152, 163
alkalinity 15
alkalosis 27, 80, 170
allergic reactions 38
alopecia 44, 144, 188
alveoli 114
Alzheimer's disease 132
amenorrhoea 185
amino acids 150, 159–160, 174
ammonia 158
amylase 150, 157
anabolism 14
anaemia 82, 94
anagen 41
androgens 142, 145, 190
aneurysms 94
angina 94, 96

anhidrosis 38, 179
antibodies 82, 83, 100, 104
anti-coagulants 94–95, 98
anti-diuretic hormone 78, 137, 143
anti-oxidants 45
anus 156
apocrine glands 37, 177
aponeuroses 56, 65
appendicular skeleton 48, 49
appendix 155, 156, 176
areolar connective tissue 22, 32
arrector pili 41
arrhythmia 96
arteries 38, 84–85
arterioles 85
arteriosclerosis 95
arthritis 27, 58
ascorbic acid 46, 51, 95, 161
aspirin 98, 164
asthma 118
autonomic nervous system 24, 121, 129–131
axial skeleton 48
axillary nodes 190
axons 122

B

bacteria 79, 179
Bartholin's glands 185
basal cell carcinoma 43
basal layer 35
basophils 82
bile 154, 158
bilirubin 157
blackheads 38
bladder 156, 171, 174, 175
bloating 177
blood 18, 21, 23, 50, 77, 78, 168
blood glucose 94, 141, 143, 145
blood pressure 90–93, 96, 106
blood shunting 93
blood vessels 84–87, 91, 92
body fluids 168–169
body temperature 14, 15, 31, 64
boils 43
bolus 150

bone mass 147
bones 18, 21, 23, 51–59
Botox™ 24
bow legs 69
brain 122, 123–125
breasts 70, 189–190
breathing 111, 115, 116
bromhidrosis 38, 179
bronchi 113
bruising 9, 95
bursitis 59

C

caecum 155
calcitonin 138
calcium 50–51, 59, 162, 170
calories 160
cancer 108, 112, 119, 162, 191
capillaries 86, 87, 114
carbohydrates 158, 159, 161
carbon dioxide 111
cardiovascular system 6, 19, 25, 62, 88, 91
cartilage 18, 21, 23, 51, 56
catabolism 14
catogen 41
cell debris 102
cell membrane 11
cells 2, 4, 11
    disorders 27–28
    epithelial 150
    homeostasis 14–16
    metabolism 13–14
    properties 13
    structure 11–12
cellulite 28, 32
central nervous system (CNS) 121, 123–126
cerebral palsy 75, 132
cerebrospinal fluid 123
cerebrum 124
cervix 185
chilblains 95
chloasma 43, 188
chloride 162, 170
chromosomes 186

chyle   100
chyme   152, 160
chymotrypsin   157
cilia   113
circulatory system   11, 77–98
   ageing   97
   blood   18, 21, 23, 50, 77, 78, 168
   diseases   94–97
   heart   88–89
   pulse   85, 89–90
circumduction   8, 55
cirrhosis   163
cisterna chyli   103
clitoris   185
cold sores   44
colitis   163
collagen   22, 32, 37, 65
connective tissue   11, 18, 21–23, 26, 121
constipation   45, 156, 163, 179
contra-action   10
contraception   184, 187
contra-indication   10, 186
Cooper's ligaments   190
corpus luteum   184
cortex   172
cranial nerves   127
Crohn's disease   162, 163
Cushing's syndrome   143, 145
cutaneous membranes   26
cuticle   40
cystitis   179
cytoplasm   11

D

dandruff   44
deep vein thrombosis (DVT)   119
defecation   177
dehydration   124, 156
dementia   132, 133
dendrites   122
dermatitis   34, 42
dermis   32, 37–39
desquamation   36
diabetes   97, 98, 143–147, 175
diaphragm   113

diaphysis   52
diarrhoea   156, 163
diastolic pressure   90
digestion   152, 159
digestive system   6, 11, 149–166
   ageing   166
   diseases   162–165, 179
   efficiency   179
   organs   150–158
dihydroxyacetoine   36
dislocation   59
diuretics   137
DNA   12
ducts   17
duodenal ulcers   145
duodenum   153, 154
dysmenorrhoea   143, 185

E

eccrine glands   37, 177
eczema   42
effector nerve   127
efferent nerve   123
effleurage   74
elastin   22, 32, 65
electrolysis   140
electrolytes   169
elevation   8
embryo   187
emphysema   118–119
emulsification   154–155, 160
endocrine system   6, 17, 107, 135–148
endometrium   185, 190
endorphins   136
enzymes   150, 154, 157, 160
eosinophils   82
epidermis   31, 32, 34–35
epididymis   182
epidurals   127
epilepsy   132
epiphyses   52
epithelial cells   17, 20–21, 26, 31, 150
eponychium   42
erythema   39, 77
excretion   7, 14, 34, 102, 167–170, 178–179

exhalation   116, 167
exocrine glands   17, 136
extracellular fluid   168
eyes   1, 172

F

faeces   156, 167, 168, 176, 177
fallopian tube   184, 185
fat   22, 39, 104, 154, 158, 160, 161
fatty acids   160
fertilisation   186
fibre   156, 159
fibroblasts   22
fibrous joints   53
fibrous tissue   22
flatulence   163
folliculitis   43
fracture   57
fructose   159
furuncle   43

G

gall bladder   154, 158
gall stones   163–164
gametes   181
gaseous exchange   87, 114, 115
gastric juice   151, 152
gastrin   152, 155
gastroenteritis   164
gender   186
genes   181, 186
glands   17, 109, 135
glomerulus   173
glucagon   94, 141, 143, 157
glucocorticoids   140, 145
glucose   72, 159, 174
glycogen   94, 141, 158
goitre   144, 145
Golgi body   13
gonadotrophins   142
gonads   181
granular layer   35
granulocytes   80, 81–82
growth hormone   136, 142, 147
gynaecomastia   190

INDEX

H

haemoglobin 81, 157
haemophilia 95
hair 39, 40–41, 44
halitosis 164
hangnail 44
head lice 44
health 9, 90
heart 19, 25, 62, 88–89, 91, 96
heartburn 151, 164
heat 33, 38, 79, 93, 158
heparin 158
hepatic portal vein 153
hepatitis 164
herpes 44
hiatus hernia 164
high blood pressure 90
hirsutism 44, 140, 143, 144, 147, 189
histamine 38, 82
HIV 109
Hodgkin's disease 108
homeostasis 14–16, 111, 135, 138, 167, 168–170
hormone replacement therapy (HRT) 147
hormones 14, 38, 135–148, 174, 181, 188
horny layer 36
hydrochloric acid 152
hydrotherapy 176
hyperhidrosis 38, 179
hypernephroma 178
hypertension 96, 145
hyperthyroidism 143, 144
hypoglycaemia 146
hypotension 96
hypothalamus 78, 137
hypothermia 15
hypothyroidism 143

I

IBS 145, 163, 164
ileo-caecal valve 155
ileum 153, 155
immunity 11, 79, 83, 99, 107, 109
impetigo 44
indications 10–11
indigestion 150, 163, 165
inflammation 13

inhalation 116
insulin 14, 94, 141, 143, 146, 157
integumentary system 6, 31
intercostals 116
interstitial fluid 106
intracellular fluid 168
intrinsic factor 152
involuntary muscle 24, 62, 154
iodine 138, 139, 145, 162
ions 169
irritable bowel syndrome 145, 163, 164

J

jaundice 165
jejunum 153, 155
joints 8–9, 53–56, 58–59, 60

K

keratin 21, 34, 35, 41
kidneys 15, 78, 143, 170, 171, 175, 178

L

labia 185
lactation 187, 189
lacteals 104
lactic acid 72
lactose 159
large intestine 156, 176–177
larynx 112, 113, 118
leucocytes 79, 81, 100
leukaemia 96, 109
ligaments 21, 56
linea nigra 188
lipase 157
liver 153, 157–158, 159
lungs 88, 113–114, 115, 119
luteinising hormone 136, 185
lymph 99, 168
lymphatic system 28, 99–110
lymph nodes 101–102, 107
lymphocytes 80, 82, 100, 104
lymphoma 109
lymph vessels 101, 190

M

macrophages 83, 85, 102, 108
malaria 107
malnutrition 165
mammary glands 70, 189–190

massage 33, 34, 39
    abdomen 176
    aromatherapy 103
    cancer 108
    circulatory system 77, 81, 87
    constipation 156
    gyratory 74
    Indian head 84, 107
    kidneys 171
    lymphatic system 99, 103, 104, 106
    muscle performance 73
    muscular disorders 75
    oncology 108
    shoulder muscles 66
medulla 172
melanin 35
melanocytes 34, 35
melanoma 43
melatonin 139, 140, 143
membranes 19, 25
meninges 26, 123
meningitis 28, 132
menopause 147, 179, 188
menstrual cycle 185–186
menstruation 140, 143, 181
metabolism 13, 87, 111, 135, 138
migraines 145
milia 43
miliaria rubra 38, 179
minerals 50–51, 161
mitochondria 13
mitosis 35, 187
moles 42
monocytes 80, 83
motor nerves 123, 126
motor neurone disease 75, 132
mucous membranes 26
mucus 112, 113, 150, 152
multiple sclerosis (MS) 75, 133
mumps 133
muscle tissue 19, 24–25, 62, 147
muscular system 61–76
    abdomen 70
    ageing 75–76
    arms 68
    back 71
    chest 70

INDEX

disorders 74, 75
   facial muscles 66
   legs 69
   shoulders 67
myelin sheath 122
myosin 65, 72
myxoedema 143

N

naevus 42
nails 41–42, 44–45
negative feedback 94, 138
nephritis 178
nephrons 172–173
nervous system 6, 11, 19, 27, 39, 121–134
neuroglia 27
neurones 19, 27, 122–123
neurotransmitters 75
neutrophils 82
nicotinic acid 161
non-Hodgkin's lymphoma 109
nucleolus 12
nucleus 11–12, 122
nutrients 159–162, 169

O

obesity 96, 146, 147
oedema 28, 105, 109, 110
oesophagus 150
oestrogen 135, 140, 142, 144, 183, 184
olfactory system 128
organelles 12
osmoregulation 14
osmosis 87
ossification 51
osteoarthritis 27
osteoblasts 51
osteoclasts 51
osteocytes 51–52
osteoporosis 51, 58, 147, 188
ovarian cysts 190
ovaries 142, 143, 144, 183
ovulation 183, 184
ovum 181
oxygen 111
oxytocin 137, 143

P

pancreas 94, 108, 140–146, 154, 157
pancreatitis 165
papilla 37, 40
parathyroid glands 138–139, 140, 143
Parkinson's disease 75, 125, 133
pelvic floor 190
penis 175, 183
pepsin 152
peptides 159
perichondrium 26
perineum 185
periosteum 26
peripheral nervous system (PNS) 121, 126–127
peristalsis 25, 130, 153, 171, 177
peronychium 42
Peyer's patches 101, 155
pH 15, 80, 170
pharyngeal tonsils 108
pharynx 113
phosphorus 162
physiology 2
pineal gland 139, 143
pituitary gland 135–137, 142–143, 144
placenta 187
plasma 23, 78, 80, 106, 135
platelets 79, 84
pleura 114, 119
pneumonia 119
polycystic ovarian syndrome 190
potassium 162, 170
prefixes 4, 168, 170
pregnancy 105, 143, 174, 186
pre-menstrual tension 135, 184, 185
prickle cell layer 35
prickly heat 180
progesterone 142, 183
prolactin 136
prolapse 191
pronation 8, 55
prostaglandins 143
prostate gland 182, 191
proteins 158, 159–160, 161
psoriasis 36, 43
ptyalin 150, 157
puberty 139, 181, 184

pulmonary artery 115
pulmonary circulation 88
pulmonary embolism 119
pulmonary vein 115
pulse 85, 89–90
pyloric sphincter 153

R

rectum 156
red blood cells 80, 81
reflex action 130–131
reflex arc 123
reflexology 84, 116, 138, 153
repetitive strain injury 59, 65
reproductive system 6, 181–192
respiration 6, 16, 102, 167
respiratory system 6, 11, 111–120
retinol 46, 51, 158, 161
rheumatism 58
rheumatoid arthritis 27
ribosomes 12
rickets 36
ringworm 44, 45
RNA 12

S

salivary glands 150
scabies 44
sciatica 59, 74, 75, 126, 133
sebaceous cysts 43
sebaceous glands 32, 37–38
seborrhoea 39
sebum 34, 38, 168
secretion 34
selective reabsorption 174
semen 182, 183
seminiferous tubules 182
senile dementia 133
sensory system 6, 32–33, 121, 123, 127–128, 146
septicaemia 97, 109
serous membranes 26
sex hormones 140, 147
sexual intercourse 182
shingles 44
shivering 64
shock 97
sickle cell anaemia 94

PAGE 201

INDEX

simple epithelium   17, 20
skeletal system   6, 47–60
skin   26, 31–39
    ageing   31, 45–46
    dermis   37
    diet   45
    diseases   42–44
    functions   32–33
    split capillaries   86
    structure   32, 34–35
    subcutaneous layer   39
small intestine   153–155
smoking   88, 90, 98, 112, 113, 117–118
smooth muscle   19, 24–25
sodium   162, 170
solar plexus   126
somatic nervous system   126
sperm   181, 183
sphincters   151
spider veins   86
spinal cord   125
spleen   106, 107–108
spondylosis   58
sprains   59, 74
Stein Levental syndrome   190
stem cells   80, 81
steroids   142, 143
stomach   151–153
strata   21
stratified epithelium   17, 20
stress   90, 93, 140, 145
stretch marks   188
striated muscle   24
sucrose   159
sudoriferous glands   *see* sweat glands
suffixes   4
sugar   159
sun protection factor   (SPF) 35
supination   8, 55
surface area   113, 153
sweat   33, 34, 168
sweat glands   37, 177–178
synapse   123
synovial joints   54
synovial membranes   26
systemic circulation   88
systolic pressure   90

T

tapotement   171
target cells   135
taste   150
teeth   150
telogen   41
tendonitis   59, 65
tendons   18, 21, 56, 63, 65
testes   142, 143, 181, 182
testosterone   140, 142, 143, 144, 182
tetany   143
thalamus   127
thiamine   161
thrombosis   97
thymus gland   108, 139, 143, 147
thyroid gland   17, 138, 143, 144–145, 180
thyroid stimulating hormone (TSH)   136
tinea   44
tissues   4, 11, 16–27
    disorders   27–28
    epithelial   17, 20–21, 31
    fibrous   22
    lymphatic   101
T-lymphocytes   108, 139
tonicity   64
tonsillitis   110
tonsils   101, 107, 108
total blood volume   91, 92
trachea   113
treatments
    see also massage
    body wraps   105
    colonic irrigation   176
    electrical muscle stimulation   66, 126
    electrolysis   140
    galvanic   33
    heat   93
    petrissage   74
    reflexology   84, 116, 138, 153
    vacuum suction   105
trypsin   157
tuberculosis (TB)   119
tumours   28

U

ulcer   165
ulcerative colitis   165
ultraviolet (UV) rays   34, 35
umami taste   150
umbilical cord   187
urea   102, 158, 174
ureters   156, 175
urethra   171, 175
urethritis   179
uric acid   158
urinary system   11, 170–176, 178–179
urine   168, 173–174, 175
uterus   183, 185, 191

V

vaccinations   83
vagina   182, 185
varicose veins   97
vas deferens   182
vasoconstriction   33
vasodilation   33, 92
vasopressin   78, 137, 143
veins   38, 86
vellus   41
venous return   64, 87
venules   86
verruca   44
villi   153
vitamins   46, 51, 94, 95, 152, 158, 161, 163
vitiligo   42
vocal cords   112
voice box   *see* larynx
voluntary muscle   24, 62–64, 65
vomiting   165
vulva   185

W

warfarin   98
warts   44
water   29, 78–79, 152, 156, 162, 168–169
white blood cells   79, 81, 100
wind   156, 163, 177
windpipe   *see* trachea

Y

yoga   140

Z

zinc   95
zygotes   181, 186